Unanswered Questions in Periodontology

Editor

FRANK A. SCANNAPIECO

DENTAL CLINICS OF NORTH AMERICA

www.dental.theclinics.com

October 2015 • Volume 59 • Number 4

ELSEVIER

1600 John F. Kennedy Boulevard • Suite 1800 • Philadelphia, Pennsylvania, 19103-2899

http://www.dental.theclinics.com

DENTAL CLINICS OF NORTH AMERICA Volume 59, Number 4
October 2015 ISSN 0011-8532, ISBN: 978-0-323-40080-0

Editor: John Vassallo; j.vassallo@elsevier.com
Developmental Editor: Kristen Helm

Dental Clinics of North America (ISSN 0011-8532) is published quarterly by Elsevier Inc., 360 Park Avenue South, New York, NY 10010-1710. Months of issue are January, April, July, and October. Business and Editorial Offices: 1600 John F. Kennedy Boulevard, Suite 1800, Philadelphia, PA 19103-2899. Periodicals postage paid at New York, NY and additional mailing offices. Subscription prices are $280.00 per year (domestic individuals), $485.00 per year (domestic institutions), $135.00 per year (domestic students/residents), $340.00 per year (Canadian individuals), $628.00 per year (Canadian institutions), $410.00 per year (international individuals), $628.00 per year (international institutions), and $200.00 per year (international and Canadian students/residents). International air speed delivery is included in all *Clinics* subscription prices. All prices are subject to change without notice. **POSTMASTER:** Send address changes to *Dental Clinics of North America*, Elsevier Health Sciences Division, Subscription Customer Service, 3251 Riverport Lane, Maryland Heights, MO 63043. **Customer Service (orders, claims, online, change of address): Elsevier Health Sciences Division, Subscription Customer Service, 3251 Riverport Lane, Maryland Heights, MO 63043. Tel: 1-800-654-2452 (U.S. and Canada). Fax: 314-447-8029. E-mail: journalscustomer service-usa@elsevier.com (for print support); journalsonlinesupport-usa@elsevier.com (for online support).**

Reprints. For copies of 100 or more, of articles in this publication, please contact the Commercial Reprints Department, Elsevier Inc., 360 Park Avenue South, New York, NY 10010-1710. Tel.: 212-633-3874; Fax: 212-633-3820; E-mail: reprints@elsevier.com.

The *Dental Clinics of North America* is covered in *MEDLINE/PubMed (Index Medicus), Current Contents/Clinical Medicine, ISI/BIOMED* and *Clinahl.*

Contributors

EDITOR

FRANK A. SCANNAPIECO, DMD, PhD
Professor and Chair, Department of Oral Biology, School of Dental Medicine, University at Buffalo, The State University of New York, Buffalo, New York

AUTHORS

AKIRA AOKI, DDS, PhD
Junior Associate Professor, Department of Periodontology, Graduate School of Medical and Dental Sciences, Tokyo Medical and Dental University (TMDU), Tokyo, Japan

WENCHE S. BORGNAKKE, DDS, MPH, PhD
Department of Periodontics and Oral Medicine, University of Michigan School of Dentistry, Ann Arbor, Michigan

HSUN-LIANG CHAN, DDS, MS
Clinical Assistant Professor, Department of Periodontics and Oral Medicine, University of Michigan School of Dentistry, Ann Arbor, Michigan

YONG-HEE PATRICIA CHUN, DDS, MS, PhD
Assistant Professor, Departments of Periodontics and Cellular and Structural Biology, University of Texas Health Science Center at San Antonio, San Antonio, Texas

SEBASTIAN G. CIANCIO, DDS
Department of Periodontics and Endodontics, University at Buffalo, The State University of New York, Buffalo, New York

RALUCA COSGAREA, DDS, Dr med dent
Assistant Professor, Department of Periodontology, Philipps University Marburg, Marburg, Germany; Department of Prosthodontics, Iuliu Hatieganu University, Cluj-Napoca, Romania

JIA-HUI FU, BDS, MS
Assistant Professor, Discipline of Periodontics, Faculty of Dentistry, National University of Singapore, Singapore, Singapore

ERNEST HAUSMANN, DMD, PhD
Professor Emeritus, Department of Oral Biology, School of Dental Medicine, University at Buffalo, The State University of New York, Buffalo, New York

KENNETH R. HOFFMANN, PhD
Professor, Department of Neurosurgery, School of Medicine and Biomedical Science, University at Buffalo, The State University of New York, Buffalo, New York

ALAN D. HUTSON, PhD
Professor, Department of Biostatistics, University at Buffalo, The State University of New York, Buffalo, New York

SØREN JEPSEN, DDS, MSc, PhD
Department of Periodontology, Operative and Preventive Dentistry,
Center of Dento-Maxillo-Facial Medicine, Faculty of Medicine, University of Bonn,
Bonn, Germany

AMY C. KILLEEN, DDS, MS
Assistant Professor, Department of Surgical Specialties, University of Nebraska Medical
Center College of Dentistry, Lincoln, Nebraska

PIN-CHUANG LAI, DDS
Divisions of Periodontology and Biosciences, College of Dentistry, The Ohio State
University, Columbus, Ohio

MARJA L. LAINE, DDS, PhD
Department of Periodontology, Academic Centre for Dentistry Amsterdam (ACTA),
University of Amsterdam, VU University Amsterdam, Amsterdam, The Netherlands

BRUNO G. LOOS, DDS, MSc, PhD
Professor and Chairman, Department of Periodontology, Academic Centre for Dentistry
Amsterdam (ACTA), University of Amsterdam, VU University Amsterdam, Amsterdam,
The Netherlands

MARK MACEACHERN, MLIS
Informationist, Taubman Health Sciences Library, University of Michigan, Ann Arbor,
Michigan

RICHARD J. MIRON, DDS, MS, PhD
Head of Laboratory of Oral Cell Biology, Department of Periodontology, School of Dental
Medicine, University of Bern, Bern, Switzerland

THOMAS W. OATES, DMD, PhD
Professor and Vice Chair, Department of Periodontics, University of Texas Health Science
Center at San Antonio, San Antonio, Texas

GEORGIOS PAPANTONOPOULOS, DDS, MSc
Department of Mathematics, Center for Research and Applications of Nonlinear Systems,
University of Patras, Patras, Greece

RICHARD A. REINHARDT, DDS, PhD
BJ & Ann Moran Professor, Department of Surgical Specialties, University of Nebraska
Medical Center College of Dentistry, Lincoln, Nebraska

GEORGE ROMANOS, DDS, PhD, Prof Dr med dent
Professor, Department of Periodontology, School of Dental Medicine, Stony Brook
University, Stony Brook, New York

FRANK A. SCANNAPIECO, DMD, PhD
Professor and Chair, Department of Oral Biology, School of Dental Medicine, University at
Buffalo, The State University of New York, Buffalo, New York

FRANK SCHWARZ, Prof Dr med dent
Professor, Department of Oral Surgery, Heinrich Heine University, Düsseldorf, Germany

ANTON SCULEAN, DMD, Dr med dent, MS, PhD
Professor and Chairman, Department of Periodontology, School of Dental Medicine,
University of Bern, Bern, Switzerland

DAGMAR E. SLOT, MSc, PhD
Department of Periodontology, Academic Centre for Dentistry Amsterdam (ACTA), University of Amsterdam, VU University Amsterdam, Amsterdam, The Netherlands

EVELINE VAN DER SLUIJS, MSc
Department of Periodontology, Academic Centre for Dentistry Amsterdam (ACTA), University of Amsterdam, VU University Amsterdam, Amsterdam, The Netherlands

FRIDUS A. VAN DER WEIJDEN, PhD
Department of Periodontology, Academic Centre for Dentistry Amsterdam (ACTA), University of Amsterdam, VU University Amsterdam, Amsterdam, The Netherlands

JOHN WALTERS, DDS, MMSc
Division of Periodontology, College of Dentistry, The Ohio State University, Columbus, Ohio

HOM-LAY WANG, DDS, MSD, PhD
Director and Professor, Department of Periodontics and Oral Medicine, University of Michigan School of Dentistry, Ann Arbor, Michigan

LUGE YANG, MS
Department of Biostatistics, University at Buffalo, The State University of New York, Buffalo, New York

JIHNHEE YU, PhD
Associate Professor, Department of Biostatistics, University at Buffalo, The State University of New York, Buffalo, New York

HATTAN A.M. ZAKI, BDS
Department of Oral Biology, School of Dental Medicine, University at Buffalo, The State University of New York, Buffalo, New York; Demonstrator, Department of Oral Basic and Clinical Sciences; Faculty of Dentistry, Taibah University, Madinah al Munawwarah, Kingdom of Saudi Arabia

JOSEPH J. ZAMBON, DDS, PhD
Interim Dean and SUNY Distinguished Teaching Professor, Department of Periodontics and Endodontics, School of Dental Medicine, University at Buffalo, The State University of New York, Buffalo, New York

Contents

> Antimicrobial photodynamic therapy (PDT) has attracted much attention for the treatment of pathogenic biofilm associated with peridontitis and peri-implantitis. However, data from randomized controlled clinical studies (RCTs) are limited and, to some extent, controversial, making it difficult to provide appropriate recommendations. Therefore, the aims of the present review article were (a) to provide an overview on the current evidence from RCTs evaluating the potential clinical benefit for the additional use of PDT to subgingival mechanical debridement (ie, scaling and root planing) alone in nonsurgical periodontal therapy; and (b) to provide clinical recommendations for the use of PDT in periodontal practice.

> The mainstay of periodontal assessment is clinical probing. Radiographic assessment provides quantitative information on the status of tooth-supporting bone. This article reviews methods to assess periodontal structures, including basic radiograph acquisition, assessment of alveolar crest levels, and typical patterns of bone loss. Computer technology to objectively assess loss of alveolar crest from radiographs is reviewed. Developments in computer-assisted quantitation of alveolar crest height are described. Although probing measurements continue to be viewed as more practical than radiographic measurements, radiographic assessment can be made quantitative and is likely easier and more precise than probing for routine assessment of periodontal disease activity.

> The impact of tooth mobility and occlusal trauma (OT) on periodontal bone loss and need for therapy has been debated for many years. This article summarizes the relevant literature reported in three *Dental Clinics of North America* articles in the late 1990s, and adds newer information from the 2000s. Principle findings indicate that strong evidence of mobility and OT impacting tooth longevity is lacking, but reducing inflammation in the surrounding periodontium remains a critical treatment. Occlusal therapy when mobility is increasing, comfort or function are compromised, or periodontal regeneration procedures are planned should be considered.

> Periodontal diseases are the most common human diseases globally, with gingivitis affecting up to 90% and periodontitis 50% of adults. Evidence exists that routine, non-surgical periodontal treatment can lead to: 1) improved periodontal health, 2) diminished cumulative bacterial load in

the body, 3) decreased blood levels of glucose and pro-inflammatory and lipids, 4) decreased intima-media thickness of carotid and brachial arteries, 5) improved endothelial function, 6) improvement of rheumatic arthritis signs and symptoms, and 7) prevention of aspiration pneumonia. Hence, scientific evidence supports that such periodontal therapy can prevent or decrease severity of several chronic, inflammation-related diseases, including cerebro-cardiovascular events.

Although scaling and root planing is a cost-effective approach for initial treatment of chronic periodontitis, it fails to eliminate subgingival pathogens and halt progressive attachment loss in some patients. Adjunctive use of systemic antibiotics immediately after completion of scaling and root planing can enhance the degree of clinical attachment gain and probing depth reduction provided by nonsurgical periodontal treatment. This article discusses the rationale for prescribing adjunctive antibiotics, reviews the evidence for their effectiveness, and outlines practical issues that should be considered before prescribing antibiotics to treat chronic periodontitis.

Periodontal regeneration—treatment that results in new alveolar bone, cementum, and a functional periodontal ligament—is successful in class II furcation defects. This article examines one aspect of periodontal regeneration—alveolar bone growth in furcation defects—in trying to answer the question, Can bone lost from furcations be regenerated? The best evidence for bone growth is histology but there is limited histologic evidence for bone growth in human furcation defects. There is more evidence from intraoperative measurements for hard tissue growth in treated furcation defects, but the nature of the hard tissue needs to be determined histologically.

Over the past few decades, dental implants have been found to have high predictability and survival rates because of improvements in knowledge, clinical expertise, and implant designs. As such, dental implants are frequently integrated in the clinical management of fully or partially edentulous patients. It is prudent to realize that despite the high early survival rates, dental implants do have their fair share of long-term esthetic, biological, and mechanical complications. Therefore, this article aims to review the current evidence on the management of peri-implant diseases in an attempt to answer the following question: Can periimplantitis be treated?

Gingival recession represents a clinical condition in adults frequently encountered in the general dental practice. Clinicians often face dilemmas of whether or not to treat such a condition surgically. An initial condensed literature search was performed using a combination of gingival recession and surgery controlled terms and keywords. An analysis of the search results highlights the limited understanding of the factors that guide the treatment of gingival recession. Understanding the cause, prognosis, and treatment of gingival recession continues to offer many unanswered questions and challenges in periodontics as we strive to provide the best care possible for our patients.

DENTAL CLINICS OF NORTH AMERICA

DENTAL CLINICS OF NORTH AMERICA

FORTHCOMING ISSUES

February 2015
Oral Radiology in Interpretation and Diagnostic Strategies
Mel Mupparapu, Editor

April 2015
Clinical Pharmacology for Dentists
Harry Dym, Editor

July 2015
Special Care Dentistry
Burton S. Wasserman, Editor

RECENT ISSUES

July 2014
Modern Concepts in Aesthetic Dentistry and Multi-disciplinary Research and Grand Rounds
John R. Calamia, Richard D. Trushkowsky, Steven B. David, Mark S. Wolff, Editors

April 2014
Implant Procedures for the General Dentist
Harry Dym, Editor

January 2014
Complications of Implant Dentistry
Mohanad Al-Sabbagh, Editor

ISSUE OF RELATED INTEREST

Oral and Maxillofacial Surgery Clinics February 2015 (Vol. 24, No. 1)
Contemporary Assessment of Temporomandibular Joint Disorders
Daniel E. Perez and Larry M. Wolford, Editors
Available at: www.oralmaxsurgery.theclinics.com

Preface

Unanswered Questions in Periodontology

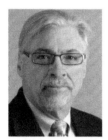

Frank A. Scannapieco, DMD, PhD
Editor

This is now the third issue of *Dental Clinics of North America* I have edited on the subject of periodontology. The first, published in 2005, attempted to provide a broad summary of the state-of-the-art and science of periodontics for the general practitioner as it existed at that moment and included articles on etiology, epidemiology, diagnosis and risk assessment, prevention, systemic impact, and treatment. For the second issue, I thought a focus on the myriad treatment approaches taken to manage periodontal disease would be of interest. Thus, articles were provided on a range of treatment modalities, from simple nonsurgical mechanical treatment strategies, to the use of lasers, various regenerative approaches, implants, nonsurgical chemotherapeutic strategies, as well as nascent treatment approaches that include developing techniques involving gene therapy, RNA interference, and stem cells. For both issues, each article was written by recognized experts who graciously provided their time and skills that culminated in two fairly comprehensive and up-to-date summaries of the discipline of periodontology.

When asked to again edit this issue of *Dental Clinics of North America* on periodontics, I struggled to define a theme that would not simply rehash the previous issues. As a member of the American Academy of Periodontology, I am able to monitor their "Open Forum," an on-line "chat room" that allows members of the Academy to share ideas. Like all chat rooms, the participants are not afraid to offer their opinions on a variety of topics, including the efficacy of various treatment and diagnostic modalities. Over time, it became evident to me that not all practitioners seemed to agree on what strategies work well in the clinical setting. Indeed, what seemed most clear is that we are faced with many unanswered questions regarding the effectiveness of a number of strategies in routine use in clinical practice. Hence, the theme of the present issue, "Unanswered Questions in Periodontology," was born. I made a rather long list of a number of questions for which I did not have an obvious answer. This list was whittled down, and I searched the literature to identify potential authors who seemed most able

Dent Clin N Am 59 (2015) xiii–xiv
http://dx.doi.org/10.1016/j.cden.2015.06.012
0011-8532/15/$ – see front matter © 2015 Published by Elsevier Inc.

dental.theclinics.com

to address the questions posed using the latest evidence. Again, in virtually all cases, the authors agreed to contribute, and the issue came together.

In all, 11 questions are posed. I believe all of the questions are provocative and are answered using the latest evidence. It is my hope that the reader will not only be able to use the information provided to help make more definitive and effective treatment decisions for their patients but also become better educated and knowledgeable about the complex nature of periodontal disease.

It has been a pleasure to work with each of the contributors, and I thank them all for making available their time and talents. I also very much appreciate the support of the editorial staff of *Dental Clinics of North America.* I especially would like to express my gratitude to John Vassallo, who continues to invite me back, and to Kristen Helm, who patiently guided me through the editorial process. Much appreciation to colleagues who generously agreed to provide expert reviews for several articles: Drs. Albert Best, David E. Deas, Jill Bashutski, Peter Polverini, Thomas E. Rams, and Dimitris Tatakis.

Frank A. Scannapieco, DMD, PhD
Department of Oral Biology
School of Dental Medicine
University at Buffalo
The State University of New York
Foster Hall
3435 Main Street
Buffalo, NY 14214, USA

E-mail address:
fas1@buffalo.edu

What is the Contribution of Genetics to Periodontal Risk?

Bruno G. Loos, DDS, MSc, PhD[a],*,
Georgios Papantonopoulos, DDS, MSc[b],
Søren Jepsen, DDS, MSc, PhD[c], Marja L. Laine, DDS, PhD[a]

KEYWORDS

- Periodontitis • Etiology • Complex disease • Multi-causality • Genetics
- Candidate gene • GWAS

KEY POINTS

- Periodontitis is a multicausal disease, with each of the causal factors playing a role but the relative contribution of these vary from case to case.
- The disease behaves in a nonlinear fashion, with periods of aberrant host response and periods of a disease resolving state.
- To date only a few of the multitude of possible genetic factors for periodontitis have been identified.

INTRODUCTION

Periodontitis is a chronic inflammatory disease of the supporting tissues around the teeth, which results in irreversible periodontal attachment loss, alveolar bone destruction, subsequent tooth mobility, and, ultimately, if left untreated, tooth exfoliation. There are 2 main types of periodontitis: aggressive periodontitis (AgP) and chronic periodontitis (CP).[1] Severe periodontitis occurs in approximately 8% to 15% of the

Authors B.G. Loos and M.L. Laine are supported in part by a grant from the University of Amsterdam, the Netherlands, for the focal point 'Oral infection and inflammation'.
Disclosures: No potential conflicts of interests relevant to this review are reported.
[a] Department of Periodontology, Academic Centre for Dentistry Amsterdam (ACTA), University of Amsterdam, VU University Amsterdam, Gustav Mahlerlaan 3004, Amsterdam 1081 LA, The Netherlands; [b] Department of Mathematics, Center for Research and Applications of Nonlinear Systems, University of Patras, Panepistimioupoli Patron 265 04, Patras, Greece; [c] Department of Periodontology, Operative and Preventive Dentistry, Center of Dento-Maxillo-Facial Medicine, Faculty of Medicine, University of Bonn, Regina-Pacis-Weg 3, Bonn 53113, Germany
* Corresponding author.
E-mail address: b.g.loos@acta.nl

population[2,3] depending on the definitions used for severe periodontitis and depending on the specific study population subjected to epidemiologic studies. In countries with a high availability of dental care, with dental and health awareness, and with preventive measures available, the prevalence of severe periodontitis may be less than 10%.[4] In contrast, the prevalence can even be greater than 15% in less developed countries with no dental care.[5] Recent studies suggest that almost half of the population suffers from mild to moderate periodontitis.[6,7] Nevertheless, severe periodontitis is a disease occurring only in a minority of the population (8%–15%)[6,8] and specific susceptibility factors play a role.

This article discusses the multicausal etiology and complexity of periodontitis with emphasis on the genetic risk factors. It is based in part on a recent review.[9]

PERIODONTITIS IS A COMPLEX DISEASE

The current concept of the etiology of periodontitis is that it is a *complex disease*. Complexity of periodontitis means that it is a process involving multiple causal components,[10,11] which interplay with each other simultaneously. Complex systems are almost always *nonlinear*. Nonlinearity in complex systems means that the causes and effects are disproportional so that a small cause may result in a large effect or a large cause may result in a small effect, *and* that the disease progression rate fluctuates, or rather, can move from one state to another and back. Nonlinearity in periodontitis is revealed by heterogeneity in its clinical course; the latter is a common clinical finding by the many periodontal specialists who treat patients with periodontitis.

There are several main causal risk factors: (1) the subgingival bacterial biofilm on both the tooth root surface and on the pocket epithelial lining[12]; (2) genetic risk factors and epigenetic modifications[9,13,14]; (3) lifestyle–related risk factors, such as smoking, stress and poor diet[15–17]; (4) systemic disease, notably diabetes[18]; and (5) other as of yet unknown factors (eg, occlusal disturbances or fremitus, iatrogenic causes)[19] (**Fig. 1**).

The 5 main causal components for periodontitis can be brought together into a pie chart. **Fig. 2** presents a generic multicausality model for periodontitis, where each of the 5 causal components have an equal contribution.

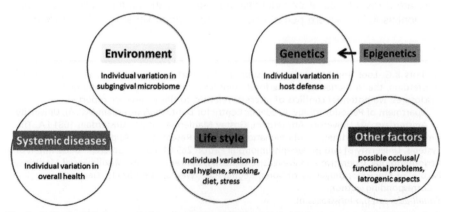

Fig. 1. Periodontitis is a complex disease; multiple causal risk factors act simultaneously in the onset and progression of the disease. Several main causal factors play a role: environmental, (epi)genetics, lifestyle, systemic diseases, and others. (*Data from* Refs.[9,12–19])

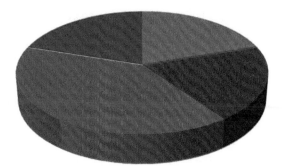

Fig. 2. A generic multicausality model for periodontitis, in which 5 causes are playing a role simultaneously, genetic factors (*blue*), lifestyle factors (*red*), environmental factors (bacterial biofilms) (*yellow*), systemic disease (*orange*), other (unknown) factors (*dark blue*). For each individual patient with periodontitis, the relative contribution of the causal factors varies. (*Adapted from* Heaton B, Dietrich T. Causal theory and the etiology of periodontal diseases. Periodontol 2000 2012;58:26–36; and Rothman K, Greenland S. Causation and causal inference in epidemiology. Am J Public Health 2005;95(Suppl 1):S144–50.)

However, it is important to note that the relative contribution of each of the causal factors varies from patient to patient (**Fig. 3**). In general, older patients with CP are considered to have a major contribution from environmental and lifestyle factors. So, many years of biofilm accumulation and unfavorable lifestyle behaviors like smoking, poor diet, and no or irregular visits to dental professionals, likely make substantial contributions to disease progression (see **Fig. 3**). On the other hand, periodontitis in

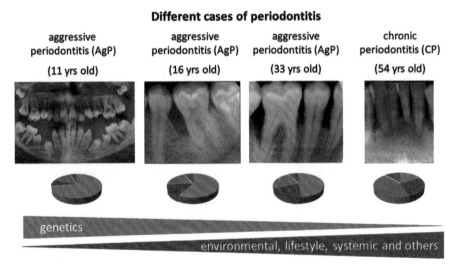

Fig. 3. Genetics contribute more in relatively younger patients with aggressive periodontitis (AgP) than in adults with CP. Conversely, in relatively older patients the microbiological risk factors and lifestyle factors contribute the most to onset and/or progression, whereas genetics plays a smaller role. Multi causal pie charts and the different colored segments are as explained in **Fig 2**. (*Adapted from* Gu Y, Ryan ME, Loos BG. Periodontal disease: classification, epidemiology, pathogenesis, and management. In: Genco RJ, Williams RC, editors. Periodontal disease and overall health: a clinician's guide. 2nd edition. Yardley (PA): Professional Audience Communications, Inc; 2014. p. 6–29; with permission.)

younger patients, for example suffering from AgP, can be caused to a greater extent by genetic factors (see **Fig. 3**).[13,20,21]

Evidence for the role of genetics in periodontitis has been gained from population, family, and twin studies.[22–25] Studies in twins and especially in monozygotic twins are a strong and preferred model to study heritability of a disease. Michalowicz and colleagues[23] studied 110 twin pairs (63 monozygotic and 33 dizygotic twin pairs) with CP and showed that among monozygotic twins a higher concordance of alveolar bone loss patterns was seen than in the dizygotic twins. The heritability estimates for alveolar bone loss among reared-apart monozygotic twins was 38%.[23] For the early-onset form of periodontitis, often equated with AgP, there is only 1 study that has reported on the heritability in twins.[26] The study consisted of a low number of twins (7 monozygotic and 19 dizygotic twin pairs at age 12–17 years) and therefore no clear conclusions could be made on the concordance rate of early-onset periodontitis. Because of a relatively low prevalence of AgP in the general population, it is very difficult to identify enough affected twins to provide sufficient statistical power to test the concordance of this disease phenotype. Nevertheless, because of strong familial aggregation, rapid progression, and early onset of disease, it is clear that genetic factors play a large role in the disease susceptibility of AgP (see **Fig. 3**).[20,21] Thus, the earlier periodontitis manifests itself, the greater the role of genetic factors, which is similar to other complex inflammatory diseases.

PERIODONTITIS DEVELOPMENT AND PROGRESSION

The bacteria in the subgingival biofilms, as well as their toxic and antigenic products (eg, endotoxin, bacterial metabolic components), initiate the inflammatory reactions that recruit polymorphonuclear neutrophilic granulocytes (PMN) and other inflammatory cells into the gingival tissues.[27] Subsequently, the recruited immune cells, in particular PMNs, but also activated pocket epithelial cells and fibroblasts in the underlying matrix, release proinflammatory mediators, including cytokines, prostanoids, and proteolytic enzymes.[28]

The type and severity of the periodontal inflammatory reaction to the dental biofilm is determined by genetic risk factors and the other causal factors named previously. The *disease-type of inflammatory reactions* in the periodontal tissues, results in a white-cell infiltrated connective tissue, loss of periodontal ligament, and resorption of alveolar bone. This destruction is thought to be "collateral damage" due to the inflammatory processes. Collagen and intercellular matrix degradation is thought to be caused by the activity of a large variety of proteolytic enzymes derived from fibroblasts and PMN. Moreover, enhanced osteoclastogenesis and osteoclast activation is initiated by cytokines and prostanoids, like interleukin (IL)-1 and prostaglandin (PG)-E2 respectively,[28,29] resulting in alveolar bone destruction.

The host response (ie, the inflammatory reactions) varies from person to person, and is determined by genetics and other factors known to lower host responses, such as an unfavorable lifestyle and/or systemic disease such as diabetes (gene–lifestyle interactions). The genetic blueprint of an individual is not a black and white deterministic causal factor. It is very dependent on the type and function of variants in multiple genetic loci: (1) multiple genes play a role (polygenic) (gene-gene interactions) and (2) not all cases have the same genetic risk variants and (3) multiple, genetic variations are present at the same time. All these genetic variations essentially *modify* the host response, which is also not set at a constant level. The host response can fluctuate or swing between states. The patient's susceptibility to periodontitis (and many other complex chronic diseases), is determined by the complex interplay between the environment (ie, bacteria) and the host. Here, genetic variations may cause modifications in the immune system, and the immune system is also affected by lifestyle factors such as smoking, stress, and diet, as well as certain systemic diseases (eg, diabetes) (see **Fig. 1**). Furthermore, *epigenetic changes* of DNA and mutations during lifetime may modify an individual's susceptibility to periodontitis.

A depiction of the complex system of periodontitis can be attempted on the basis of the current understanding and interpretation of complexity.[11] Undisturbed subgingival biofilms become maximum climax pathogenic communities as described in the literature,[12] which are considered a state of stable equilibrium. In mathematical terms, the bacteria of the subgingival biofilms come into contact with the host defense elements through random interactions and beyond a criticality in their interaction, the confrontation of bacteria with the host defense can be driven out of equilibrium. Interestingly, it has been proposed that there are keystone pathogens that elevate community virulence and the resulting dysbiotic community targets specific aspects of host immunity promoting an aberrant immune response.[30] At this point, self-organization (SO) of the host defense system occurs.[31] SO represents a spontaneous arrangement of the system from a state of initially separated parts to a final state of joined and tied-up parts. As the term implies, SO is a complex system's evolutionary process without any external factor imposed. SO happens in a space of scale invariance. Such a space is provided by periodontal ligament, which is a scale invariant self-similar object.[32] SO is based on (1) amplification of disease activity by positive feedback, (2) balancing of disease activity by negative feedback, (3) amplification of random fluctuations (all 3 situations are obvious causes of nonlinearity), and (4) on multiple local interactions of the system's components. In other words, periodontitis can fluctuate or move between an aberrant immunologic reaction state and a resolving state (resolution).[33,34]

Fluctuations and chance are parts of a complex system's behavior (mathematical term for host response) and random perturbations ("noise") facilitate the system to make a series of attempts to explore all possibilities and finally make a choice and stabilize at a state for some period; this can be regarded as an order out of "noise." A coherent global behavior appears as SO (eg, the system behaves as AgP [aberrant immune reactions] or CP [minor disease progression or in resolving state, often no differences in immune reactions found between CP cases and healthy controls]). The resultant emergent global behavior offers the ground for predictability out of the system's chaotic (aperiodic, sensitive to initial conditions and therefore unpredictable) behavior.[35] After SO occurrence we can no longer reduce the description of the system to one of its parts: all contributing parts (eg, genetics, environment, lifestyle) are tied up into a collective host defense system.

It is suggested in the literature that even the immune response level mounted at the early stage of gingivitis is the determinant factor of periodontitis progression and not the presence of specific bacteria known for their virulent properties.[33,34] The host response level can vary widely without affecting the SO, and there is no real specific value for the host response level for SO to occur.

Thus, we can formulate the hypothesis that the host response against the subgingival microbiome is a function of host genetics, environmental and lifestyle factors, systemic disease(s), and unknown factors. However, the outcome is not simply a summation. There are no clear-cut borders in the behavior of complex systems; there is always a mixture of regularity, chance, and fluctuations. In most of the population, the host response is basically "normal" regarding the susceptibility to periodontitis. The host response swings like a pendulum, from the aberrant immune response to the resolving state, and it always passes through a settlement or accommodation zone with little disease progression (**Fig. 4**), and where the level of the host response

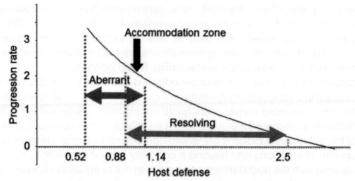

Fig. 4. A recently published mathematical model suggests that there are 2 zones of host defense level that overlap. We indicate the specific zones as on one side an "aberrant" (*red zone*) resulting in a relative fast periodontal progression rate (exponential units, mean local lyapunov exponent) and on the other side a "resolving" (*blue*) zone with minor or minimal progression. The overlap represents an accommodation or settlement zone for most patients with periodontitis (supported by clinical data, where no differences have been found in mean values of immunologic variables among aggressive and CP cases and healthy controls[36]). Thus, we suggest that the host response of AgP cases tends to "swing" into the aberrant zone, whereas the host defense for CP cases might fluctuate mainly in the settlement and resolving zone (on x-axis, the level of host response of periodontitis patients compared with healthy controls, being x-fold times more/less than the "normal healthy" level). Note, with this model, cases can fluctuate from CP to AgP and back also in the resolving zone. We can compare the host response as a pendulum of a clock. (*From* Papantonopoulos G, Takahashi K, Bountis T, et al. Mathematical modeling suggests that periodontitis behaves as a nonlinear chaotic dynamical process. J Periodontol 2013;84(10):e35; with permission.)

is essentially normal, not different from immune parameters in healthy controls.[36] In the light of recent epidemiologic data that point that periodontitis is a pandemic disease,[7,8] we propose the paradigm that the host response is mostly normal and comparable with healthy controls. However, as the system is always in some sort movement, it can swing into an aberrant immune function (one can observe this as an AgP case) or it can swing into a resolving or resolution phase (slow periodontal progression of many CP cases). Both the aberrant and resolution-type host responses for periodontitis have been suggested in the literature.[27,33,34]

SOME THEORETIC BACKGROUND ON GENETICS

Hundreds of thousands genetic loci can be identified in the human genome (ie, the complete set of chromosomes). These are stretches of DNA on the chromosomes with an order, with a start and an end. Many of these genetic regions do not contain a gene proper (a genetic region coding for a protein), rather just regulatory elements or DNA with unknown function (originally called "junk DNA"). There are some 20,000 to 30,000 genetic loci that do contain one or several genes coding for proteins and having flanking regulatory regions.

Genes direct the production of proteins with the assistance of enzymes and messenger molecules. In humans, the genes are located on 23 pairs of chromosomes, 22 pairs of autosomal chromosomes and 1 pair of sex chromosomes (XX for females and XY for males). From each pair, one chromosome is inherited from the father and one from the mother.

In the chromosomes, DNA is arranged in a double helix: 2 polynucleotide chains are associated together by hydrogen bonding between the nitrogenous bases. The pairing of the 2 single-stranded nucleotide chains is complementary: G pairs only with C, and A pairs only with T; these are called base pairs (bp). The sequences of these 4 nucleotides determines the information encoded in the DNA. Every cell in the body contains a complete copy of the approximately 3 billion DNA base pairs that make up the genome.[37]

A genetic locus containing a gene is illustrated in **Fig. 5**. This genetic locus consists of various parts. A *promoter region* is a sequence of nucleotides upstream of the coding region that contains specific sequences of nucleotides that are essential for the regulation and initiation or inhibition of the transcription of the coding region. *Introns* are often relatively large stretches of non–protein coding nucleotides within the gene, which also often participate in the regulation of transcription of DNA into mRNA. Another function of introns may be to help in splicing events of mRNA before the translation step. Introns are surrounded by *exons*, which code for the sequence of amino acids of a protein. For transcription and translation into a protein, the genetic code in such an exon is read in groups of 3 nucleotides; each trinucleotide sequence (triplet) is called a codon, which encodes a specific amino acid. The collection of known exons in our genome is called the *exome*.

Genes can be transcribed in alternative ways, where the regulatory regions play decisive roles; thus with this, each of the estimated 20,000 to 30,000 genes in the human genome code for an average of 3 proteins.[37] Proteins make up all the body structures, and of course are essential for development and function of teeth, oral mucosa, and the periodontium. Proteins also carry signals between cells, code for components of the immune system, serve as enzymes, and control biochemical reactions. If a cell's DNA is mutated, an abnormal protein or abnormal quantities of protein *may* be produced, which can disrupt the body's usual processes and lead to a disease.

Nucleotide sequencing technologies determined the exact orders of the base pairs in the DNA. The international Human Genome Project finished the first working draft sequence of the entire human genome in 2000,[38,39] and a first high-quality reference sequence of the human genome was successfully completed in 2003. In May 2006, the finished high-quality version of the sequences of all human chromosomes was published. It showed that the genomes of any 2 people are more than 99% identical, but variations between the individual genomes exist and differ on average in about 1 in

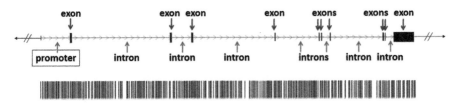

Fig. 5. Schematic drawing of a genetic locus containing a gene (length 63.5 × 10³ bp) that codes for a protein (here in this example for the vitamin D receptor), being flanked by regulatory regions. The genetic locus contains exons (indicated by *red arrows*) and introns (indicated by *blue arrows*). The exons contain the proper DNA coding sequences for the amino acids making up the protein. The vertical "bar code" below the genetic locus indicates all known positions in which 100s of SNPs may exist on basis of genome sequencing of 1000 individuals (**Fig. 6**). Any given individual may have on average an SNP every 1200 bp. A given allele is present (major or minor allele) at each genome position. Many SNPs are inherited "per block," they are linked (LD). (*Courtesy of* Arne Schäfer, PhD Berlin.)

every 1200 bp. Differences in individual bases are by far the most common type of genetic variation, and are known as *single nucleotide polymorphisms (SNPs)* (see **Fig. 5**; **Fig. 6**).

HOW TO IDENTIFY PERIODONTITIS-ASSOCIATED GENETIC MARKERS
Candidate Gene Approach

In general, the genetic loci and the known genetic polymorphisms occurring in such loci, are chosen for *candidate gene association studies* in periodontitis based on their relation with immune responses and/or have previously been associated with other chronic inflammatory diseases, such as rheumatoid arthritis, cardiovascular disease, Crohn disease (CD), type 2 diabetes, and systemic lupus erythematosus. The overlapping genetic risk factors for common chronic inflammatory diseases is called *pleiotropy*.[40,41]

Approximately 11 million SNPs are estimated to occur commonly in the human genome. All known common SNPs are listed in the catalog of common genetic variation, the HapMap, which was generated by the HapMap project and first published in 2005.[42] It describes the characteristics of the variants, where they occur in the DNA, and how they are distributed among people within populations and among populations (www.hapmap.org).

The catalog with the highest coverage of human genetic variation, obtained from population-based sequencing was published in 2010 by the "1000 Genomes Project" (www.1000genomes.org), and reported that each individual differs by more than 11 million often very rare SNPs, and that in each generation greater than 30 de novo mutations arise per individual.[43]

The different variants at a specific genetic position are called *alleles*, and the individual's personal unique collection of alleles in his or her genome makes up the individual's *genotype*. Two or more alleles for a given position may exist in nature, and occur with different frequencies. The *minor allele frequency* (MAF) in a population is the proportion of the least frequent allele at a given chromosomal/genetic position and can range from 0% to 50%. Variants with an MAF greater than 5% in a population are termed common variants. If the MAF of a variant ranges between 1% and 5% it is called a rare variant. Genetic variants with frequencies less than 1% are called mutations.

In candidate gene association studies, allele frequencies of selected SNPs are determined and compared between a well-defined group of cases and controls (**Fig. 7**). Next to the statistical significance, the results are expressed with an odds ratio (OR). The ORs of common gene polymorphisms associated with complex diseases are typically less than or equal to 1.5 (in **Fig. 7** for the purpose of illustration an extreme OR of 3.7 is shown).[44]

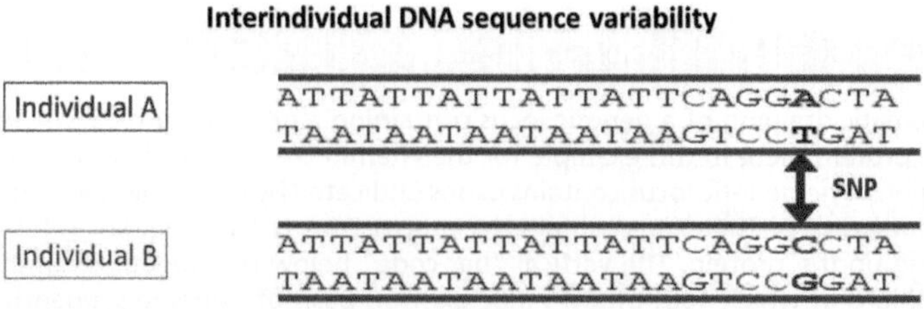

Interindividual DNA sequence variability

Fig. 6. SNP. SNPs occur at random and are mainly "neutral" (ie, without any consequence). There are approximately 11×10^6 SNPs/individual and 30 novel SNPs evolve per generation. (*Courtesy of* Arne Schäfer, PhD, Berlin.)

Example of the prevalence of a given SNP

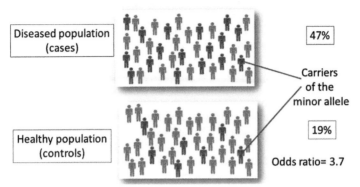

Fig. 7. Case-control studies compare the frequency of selected SNPs, representing alleles, in 2 well-defined groups of nonrelated individuals: controls, who are either known to be unaffected, or who have been randomly selected from the population, and cases with periodontitis. These studies can be used to estimate the disease risk conferred by the allele, which is expressed by the OR. The OR is the ratio of allele carriers to noncarriers in cases compared with that in controls, which gives the increase in disease risk for carriers compared with noncarriers. (*Adapted from* Schäfer A, van der Velden U, Laine ML, et al. Genetic susceptibility to periodontal disease: new insights and challenges. In: Lang NP, Lindhe J, editors. Clinical periodontology and implant dentistry. 6th edition. New York: Wiley-Blackwell; 2015. p. 290–310; with permission.)

A mutation or a genetic variant may have no effects on phenotype, or may have moderate to strong effects. For example, if a transition has taken place within the coding region of a gene, it may result in an amino acid substitution and therefore an altered protein structure, which may affect its function (nonsynonymous SNP). Or, when such mutations have taken place in the promoter region of the gene, it may alter the expression levels of the gene. Accordingly, genotypic differences among individuals can contribute to phenotypic variation, which is termed the genetic variance. How strongly a genetic variant affects the susceptibility to a disease is defined as the genotype relative risk, the ratio of the risk of disease between individuals with and without the genotype. A ratio of 1.1 equates to a 10% increase in risk and is often expressed as the OR. However, carriership of a genetic variant or mutation does not inevitably lead to disease, but only a proportion of individuals with a mutation or risk variant will develop the disease, this is known as *penetrance*. The severity of the disease in individuals who carry the risk variant *and* actually have disease, is described by the expressivity of the variant. As explained previously, factors other than genetic risk factors also *must* play a role in disease expression.

Despite the existence of many genetic variants, only a fraction of the genotypic differences contributes to phenotypic variation. The exact locations where in the chromosomes the true causative variants are located is mostly unknown. Testing all of the several millions of common and rare SNPs in a person's chromosomes would be extremely expensive. But variants that are near each other tend to be inherited together (eg, people who have a nucleotide A rather than a nucleotide G at a particular location in the chromosome can have identical genetic variants at other locations in the chromosomal region surrounding the A). This nonrandom association between alleles at different loci is termed linkage disequilibrium (LD) and the regions of linked variants are known as haplotypes (www.hapmap.ncbi.nlm.nih.gov).[42] Determining the identity of a common SNP in a haplotype, the tag SNP, uniquely identifies all other linked variants on the same haplotype. Testing an individual's tag SNPs, enables the identification of haplotypes in the chromosomes. If patients tend to share a particular haplotype, variants contributing to the disease might be somewhere within or near that haplotype. The number of tag SNPs that contain most of the information about the patterns of genetic variation of a genome is estimated to be 300,000 to 600,000, which is far fewer than 11 million common SNPs, and extremely less expensive to genotype. Thus, the information from the HapMap has been instrumental to map variants associated with various diseases.

The genetic factors associated with or actually contributing to the pathogenesis of periodontitis have been identified to a limited extent. In the past decades research on the genetics of periodontitis has focused on identifying specific SNPs in specific genetic loci as risk factors for AgP and CP. In general, genetic studies using a severe disease phenotype are the most useful to identify the genes involved in the disease. For complex diseases, the strongest phenotypes will be affected most by genetic factors (genetic penetrance is high) and will suffer the least from "noise" from environmental, lifestyle, systemic, and other factors (see **Figs. 1–3**); in other words, there is more genetic homogeneity in such case populations. Therefore studies using AgP study populations may have less genetic heterogeneity than CP study populations. The genetic risk loci identified in AgP can then be carried forward for testing as candidate risk loci in CP. Notably, as stressed previously, the SNPs identified for periodontitis mostly point to a gene locus of importance, where these SNPs serve only as genetic markers and not particularly as the causative variants.

A large number of candidate gene association studies have been performed in periodontitis with varying and often contradictory results.[13,25,45] Small cohort size resulting in lack of power and the lack of replication have been the major problems for most periodontal genetic studies.[46] Further, most of the candidate gene studies in periodontitis have not captured the complete genetic information of a particular region of interest. In almost all studies, only one or a few candidate SNPs instead of complete haplotypes of the genetic locus of interest were genotyped. Furthermore, many studies on genetics in periodontitis are limited because of inadequate phenotype classification of periodontitis and control subjects, as well as not taking into account lifestyle factors, such as smoking, possible differences in allele carriership related to gender, or the presence of other diseases.[46]

The Genomewide Association Study Approach

A genomewide association study (GWAS) is a powerful molecular technique to analyze hundreds of thousands or even millions of variations in genomic DNA simultaneously and to determine if any genetic locus is associated with a certain disease phenotype. It is an open-ended or hypothesis-free approach; no a priori genetic candidate is being investigated. GWAS analyze SNPs covering the entire human genome with the great majority in regulatory regions and a small part in coding regions. Because of the complex structure of the genome (for example LD), associated variants are mostly not the causative variants; however, the associated variants that are identified are expected to be linked with the causative variants. This can be uncovered in subsequent genetic fine mapping experiments.

Because in a GWAS an enormous number of SNPs are determined, it is essential to include large numbers of well-characterized (most preferably strong phenotypes, such as AgP rather than CP) homogeneous patient populations (all the same ethnic background) and as good as possible, matched controls. Importantly, the statistical significance level for P is usually set at less than 5×10^{-8} to correct for extensive multiple testing.[47] Typically, on the basis of a GWAS, novel candidate genetic loci or SNPs can be proposed; importantly, the results of a GWAS need to be further validated by an independent cohort with a candidate gene study. Therefore, GWAS are instrumental in discovering novel candidate genes and their possible roles in biological pathways, especially in diseases in which the genetic basis is not understood.

Today, more than 1300 GWAS have been performed (www.ebi.ac.uk/gwas/), but only 5 GWAS have been performed in association with periodontitis; 1 in AgP and 4 in CP.[48–52] Another GWAS in periodontitis studied SNPs in association with pathologic periodontal pocket depths, rather than in association with a certain form of periodontitis.[53] Furthermore, 1 GWAS examined host genetic risk loci in association with subgingival bacterial colonization.[54] Recently, Rhodin and colleagues[55] reanalyzed the GWAS data of previous studies,[49,54] with a gene-centric and gene set enrichment analyses. We report the validated gene variants associated with periodontitis from these GWAS studies in combination with candidate gene studies later in this article. Notably, the studies differ in methodology and quality, and level of validation.

THE BEST REPLICATED AND VALIDATED GENETIC FACTORS FOR PERIODONTITIS

We have ordered the results from the literature per chromosome.

COX2 on Chromosome 1

Based on robust reasoning on the role of prostaglandins in periodontitis, the gene locus *COX2* (alias prostaglandin-endoperoxide synthase-2 [PTGS2]) was proposed as a candidate gene.[56] The *COX2* SNP rs20417 (haplotype tagged by rs6681231, having near-perfect LD [$r^2 > 0.95$]) was first identified in a Taiwanese AgP cohort (85 cases vs 153 controls)[56] and later also observed in a Dutch-German AgP study population (520 cases vs 1043 controls).[57] So far, these associations have not been replicated in cohorts having the same ethnic background.

The association of *COX2* SNP rs6681231 was also reported to be associated with CP in Taiwanese (343 cases vs 153 controls).[56] Later, Loo and colleagues[58] and Li and colleagues[59] studied the association between CP and the *COX2* SNP rs20417 in Chinese patients (280 cases vs 250 controls, 122 cases and 532 controls, respectively) and both studies also reported on an association of this gene with periodontitis, but the association was in an opposite direction, as previously suggested. This confirms that SNPs in this genetic locus are related to periodontitis, but that the real causative SNP(s) are not yet identified, only tagging SNPs. No association for the *COX2* SNPs has been found in Dutch-German CP patients.[57]

COX-2 converts arachidonic acid into prostaglandin H2, which is the precursor of prostaglandin E2 (PGE2). PGE2 mediates proinflammatory and anti-inflammatory reactions in many tissues and is also partly responsible for the resorption of the periodontal connective tissues and alveolar bone during the pathogenesis of periodontitis.[29] However, whether the identified genetic association is related to altered function of the protein COX-2, and therefore, indirectly could play a role in the pathophysiology of periodontitis is still an open question.

IL10 on Chromosome 1

The involvement of the *IL10* genetic locus has been long proposed.[13] Nevertheless, only recently has this connection been sufficiently validated. The associations of *IL10* SNPs rs61815643 and rs6667202 were identified in a German population of 600 patients with AgP and 1441 controls.[60] The associations were further tested in validation cohorts of 164 Dutch patients with AgP and 1020 controls, and 105

German-Austrian patients with AgP and 482 controls of the same countries. The genetic region was confirmed in the Dutch validation cohort, but not in the German-Austrian cohort.[60] The *IL10* genetic locus as risk factor for CP is currently not yet sufficiently validated.

The *IL10* genetic region is another example of a pleiotropic locus; for example, it has been associated with inflammatory bowel disease and type 1 diabetes.[60,61] The *IL10* gene encodes the anti-inflammatory cytokine interleukin-10 (IL-10). IL-10 can downregulate the proinflammatory immune response of monocytes and macrophages in paracrine and autocrine fashion: IL-10 is produced by monocytes, macrophages, and T cells, and its actions result in reduced expression of the proinflammatory cytokines, such as IL-1 and tumor necrosis factor-α.

IL1 Genes on Chromosome 2

The *IL1* genetic locus encompasses the IL-1 genes *IL1A*, *IL1B*, and *IL1RN*. *IL1A–889* (rs1800587, in linkage with +4845), *IL1B –511* (in linkage with –31), *IL1B+3954* (rs1143634, also mentioned in the literature as +3953), and *IL1RN VNTR* (in linkage with +2018 [rs419598]) have been studied extensively in relation to CP.[13] Kornman and colleagues[62] were the first to report that the combined presence of the minor allele of the *IL1A* gene at position –889 and the minor allele of the *IL1B* gene at position +3954 was associated with severity of CP, in particular in nonsmoking whites; this combination was proposed to be the "*IL1* composite genotype." Carriage rates of the *IL1* composite genotype vary across populations (eg, a low MAF [<5%] was seen in Asian populations as compared with Caucasian populations).[13] The *IL1* composite genotype and the other *IL1* candidate SNPs are not associated with AgP.[60,63,64] *IL1A* and *IL1B* were originally proposed as candidate genes because these genes code for the proinflammatory proteins IL-1alpha and IL-1beta, respectively, which play a major role in upregulation of the immune response and alveolar bone destruction.

Recent systematic reviews on *IL1* gene polymorphisms in CP cases and controls in whites suggest evidence for minor alleles in *IL1A*, in *IL1B*, and the composite genotype to be risk factors for CP.[65–67] However, the results from meta-analyses also demonstrated significant heterogeneity among the included studies, indicating the possibility that some of the included studies may suffer from a type 1 error, a phenomenon that can occur in small studies. In that respect, a recent letter is useful for the evaluation of systematic reviews on genetic risk factors.[68]

DEFB1 on Chromosome 8

The gene *DEFB1* was proposed as a candidate gene for periodontitis and again first investigated in AgP in a cohort of 532 patients and 1472 controls of German-Dutch origin.[69] A suggestive association was found between the *DEFB1* SNP rs1047031 and AgP. This association was not replicated in another Dutch-German AgP study population, but positively in a German-Dutch CP cohort (805 cases vs 1415 controls).[69]

The rare allele of *DEFB1* was predicted to impair a microRNA binding site at the 3′-untranslated region of this locus. *DEFB1* encodes the antimicrobial peptide beta-defensin 1, which plays a pivotal role in maintaining a healthy status of the mucosal epithelia, including pocket and oral epithelium. However, how the beta-defensin 1 plays a role in the pathophysiology of periodontitis, still remains unclear; and similarly it is unclear whether the genetic polymorphism as just a marker or has a functional effect.

ANRIL on Chromosome 9

The associations between AgP and SNPs in the *CDKN2B* antisense RNA 1 (*ANRIL*) locus can be considered as one of the best replicated genetic associations in periodontitis to date.[60,70–72] The interest for the *ANRIL* locus is based on pleiotropy, as this locus was first the best-replicated gene locus for cardiovascular diseases, in particular coronary artery disease in Caucasians.[70] But this locus is also associated with diabetes and some forms of cancer.[72] Thus by a candidate gene approach, *ANRIL* was discovered to be associated with periodontitis.

The first study of the *ANRIL* gene identified a haplotype block tagged by SNP rs1333048 to be associated with generalized AgP (151 cases vs 736 controls) and localized AgP (137 cases vs 368 controls) in a German population.[70] This association was replicated in a German–Northern Irish population (130 cases vs 339 controls).[71] In a follow-up study by Schaefer and colleagues[72] the entire *CDKN2BAS* region was genotyped in Dutch (159 AgP cases vs 421 controls) and German (301 AgP cases vs 962 controls) cohorts, and significant replicated associations were found between AgP and SNPs in the *ANRIL* locus. Thus, the *ANRIL* locus is associated with AgP; however, the causative SNP still needs to be determined.

For the *ANRIL* SNP rs3217992, a trend was found in German CP ($P = .06$)[73]; however, this association has not been replicated in another CP cohort to date. The latter was concluded, despite that the *ANRIL* SNP rs10811658 was associated with CP in Dutch as well as in German cohorts, also after adjustment for smoking, diabetes, gender, and age; however, importantly, after correcting for multiple comparisons the association lost its significance.[72]

Interestingly, the *ANRIL* locus is a regulatory region and does not contain a protein-encoding gene. Further characterization of the molecular function of *ANRIL* showed, a long-distance regulatory effect on the genetic activity of the *CAMTA1/VAMP3* locus, *ADIPOR1* and *C11ORF10*.[73] The *CAMTA1/VAMP3* region has also been shown to be associated with increased periodontal pathogen colonization.[54,73]

GLT6D1 on Chromosome 9

The gene for a glucosyltransferase (*GLT6D1*) on chromosome 9 was discovered in the first periodontitis GWAS for AgP.[48] The GWAS discovery cohort consisted of 141 patients with AgP and 500 controls, and the second GWAS cohort in the same study for replication, consisted of 142 patients with AgP and 479 controls, both cohorts with subjects of German origin. From the first GWAS 197 quality-controlled SNPs and from the second GWAS 244 SNPs passed the threshold for association. Only the *GLT6D1* SNP rs1537415 remained significant in both AgP GWAS cohorts. This association was further validated in a Dutch cohort with localized and generalized AgP (155 cases vs 341 controls).[48]

The *GLT6D1* SNP rs1537415 is located within intron 2 of the glycosyltransferase 6 domain containing 1 (*GLT6D1*) gene. Preliminary functional analyses have shown that the rare allele of SNP rs1537415 results in impaired binding of the transcription factor GATA-3[48]; however, its functional role in AgP is not clear.

Other Suggested Periodontitis Genes Based on Genomewide Association Study

Divaris and colleagues[49] performed the first GWAS in CP. The study included 761 patients with severe and 1920 with moderate CP, and 1823 periodontally healthy controls of European American origin. No genome-wide significant associations were found (P values were not $<5 \times 10^{-8}$). However, 6 genetic loci showed suggestive associations with CP (with P values $<5 \times 10^{-6}$). In a validation cohort of 686 individuals (86 controls, 373 moderate and 197 patients with severe periodontitis), 3 of these loci showed concordance with the GWAS results. Moderate CP was associated with SNPs rs7762544 (chromosome 6, closest gene *NCR2*) and rs3826782 (chromosome 19, closest gene *EMR1*), and severe CP with SNP rs2521634 (chromosome 7, closest gene *NPY*).[49]

Teumer and colleagues[50] also used a GWAS to study genetic loci (17 million genetic variations) in association with CP in 2 German populations. The first cohort consisted of 670 severe and 1188 moderate CP patients and 1507 controls, and the second cohort consisted of 111 severe and 247 moderate CP patients and 309 controls. No genomewide significant association was found for CP (P values were not $<5 \times 10^{-8}$); however, interestingly, they reported that 25% of CP is explained by genetic factors, and even 34% of variance for mean approximal periodontal attachment loss in individuals younger than 60 years old, was explained by genetic factors. This is in agreement with the previous reports estimating heritability for mean attachment loss in patients with CP.[20,23]

Shaffer and colleagues[53] performed a GWAS in non-Hispanic whites adults in association with periodontal pocket depth. No significant genomewide association was found. The latter study made no distinction for their patients having either AgP or CP, which made the study results also difficult to interpret and compare to others. The AgP phenotype is the more severe phenotype of periodontitis, and has a stronger genetic component in its multi-causality.

The most recent GWAS including a validation cohort was performed on 2760 Japanese patients with CP and 15,158 controls.[52] No SNPs passed the high level of significance set for GWAS ($P<5 \times 10^{-8}$), but 2 genetic loci were proposed for further replication and validation studies: KCNQ5 on chromosome 6 and GPRI41-NME8 on chromosome 7.

In another approach, subgingival infection patterns with oral bacterial species in patients with CP and controls have been investigated as outcome parameters in a GWAS.[54] A total of 1020 Caucasian Americans were included: 416 subjects diagnosed with healthy/mild periodontitis, 415 with moderate and 189 with severe periodontitis. Subgingival plaque samples were analyzed by DNA-DNA hybridization. Subjects with "high" bacterial colonization of "red" complex species: *Porphyromonas gingivalis, Tannerella forsythia, Treponema denticola*; "orange" complex species: *Prevotella intermedia, Prevotella nigrescens, Fusobacterium nucleatum, Campylobacter rectus,* and *Aggregatibacter actinomycetemcomitans* were compared with the non-"high" colonizers. No genomewide association with "high" bacterial colonization or CP was found. However, suggestive evidence was found for 13 loci, including *KCNK1, FBXO38, UHRF2, IL33, RUNX2, TRPS1, CAMTA1,* and *VAMP3*[54]; these results could not be validated in an African American replication cohort (n = 123). However, a recent new study with a candidate gene approach, testing possible SNPs in genes associated with coronary artery disease (CAD) in Northern European patients with AgP and controls, validated the involvement of *CAMTA1* and *VAMP3*.[74]

The recent gene-centric and gene set enrichment analyses on existing GWAS data have offered a promising approach to identify novel periodontitis genes with less demanding cutoffs for multiple testing.[53] Four genes (*NIN, ABHD12B, WHAMM,* and *AP3B2*) were associated with severe CP, and two genes (*KCNK1* and *DAB2IP*) with periodontal pathogen colonization. Furthermore, some other genes were proposed for moderate CP. Several of these associations confirmed the suggestive associations of the earlier studies, and need to be replicated in independent cohorts.

Although to date GWAS have not identified any genomewide associations with CP, several suggestive genetic loci have been identified.[48,50,54] These results have created novel candidate genes and advanced our understanding of genetic factors in the pathophysiology of CP. Nevertheless still open questions remain. GWAS have not been able to validate most of candidate gene associations (exception IL-10), contrasting with previous meta-analyses for example on *IL-1* polymorphisms.[59,66]

Other Suggested Periodontitis Genes Based on the Candidate Gene Approach

Many complex diseases, such as rheumatoid arthritis (RA), CD, and ulcerative colitis (UC) (both CD and UC are termed inflammatory bowel disease IBD), type 2 diabetes, cardiovascular diseases, and other inflammatory diseases, share genetic risk factors.[40,61] Pleiotropy has been found for 13.2% to 18.6% of disease-associated genes and in 4.6% to 7.8% of SNPs associated with disease or disease traits (www.genome. gov). The sharing of genetic variants for multiple diseases and phenotypes may generate new candidate genes for other diseases and can also be incorporated into the future research on genetic risk variants in AgP and CP.[41]

With the approach as described previously, new candidate genes for AgP were explored by considering known RA and systemic lupus erythematosus genes.[75] In the latter study, variants within the *IRF5* and *PRDM1* genes were suggested to be associated with AgP, but not robustly validated; the proteins encoded by these genes play a role in interferon-beta signaling.[75] In a similar fashion, recently new candidate genes for AgP were identified by exploring the well-established risk genes for CAD.[74] The CAD-associated gene *PLG* (plasminogen), was significantly associated with AgP in both an explorative cohort and a validation cohort.

Nevertheless, many genetic variants are not shared between inflammatory diseases or possibly not even between AgP and CP. For example, the genomewide association of *GLT6D1* with AgP has not been found in any other genetic disease or trait not even in CP.[41]

DISCUSSION AND CONCLUSIONS

Periodontitis has a multicausal etiology, in which genetic factors play a role. The various proposed causes for periodontitis work simultaneously, but the relative contribution of each of these varies from case to case. In young individuals often with AgP, a stronger contribution from genetic factors is apparent, whereas in older individuals often with CP, the relative contribution of the established subgingival biofilms (environmental factors) and lifestyle factors (eg, smoking, stress, diet) play a more dominant role in the phenotype of the disease. Nevertheless always some genetic susceptibility is present, for CP this is estimated at 25%. Periodontitis is therefore a complex disease (ie, it behaves in a nonlinear fashion). Actually, the disease progression rate fluctuates, where the disease sometimes moves into an aberrant state of host response and then swings back into a resolving state; between these zones, an accommodation (settlement) zone is present in which essentially no differences are found for immunologic parameters between cases with periodontitis and healthy controls. The genotype determines part of this fluctuation described and the extent of it.

Like many chronic complex diseases, a multitude of genes (>100) are most likely involved; the disease is therefore polygenic. Currently, only a fraction of susceptibility genes are robustly identified, namely *GLT6D1, ANRIL* and *COX2, IL1* and *IL10*.[48,56,57,60,66,70–72] Most of the associations have been reported for AgP, emphasizing the importance of genetic factors in the pathobiology of this severe periodontitis phenotype. Interestingly, polymorphisms within *ANRIL* and *COX2* tended to be associated also with CP.[56,58,59,72] Further, SNPs within the regulatory regions of the *IL10* gene have shown suggestive associations with AgP, and SNPs in *DEFB1* with both AgP and CP.[60,69] Probably, the identified SNPs are "genetic markers" and are not the true causative variants for both AgP and CP.

The identified genetic risk variants for periodontitis are all located within introns (*ANRIL* and *GLT6D1*) or regulatory regions (*COX2, IL10* and *DEFB1*).[41] This is in line with other complex diseases; most common human genomic variants that are genomewide associated with more than 400 complex diseases and traits are located within regulatory and intronic regions and not within coding regions.[76] Genetic variations of intronic and regulatory regions may lead to subtle changes in the expression of associated coding regions and may affect the quantity of the transcription and subsequent protein product.

All individuals harbor millions of genetic variants (eg, SNPs, insertions, deletions, repeats). Most of these variants most likely have no effect, whereas the minority may have some function, mainly physiologic and not pathologic, and are mainly responsible for the "normal" phenotypic differences between individuals. However, some combinations of the inherited variants can make individuals susceptible for certain traits or diseases, always in combination with unfavorable environmental, lifestyle, and other factors; in particular if the latter are unfavorable for the host resistance, the genetic penetrance of inherited variants increases[76] and the host defense may move into an aberrant immune state (see **Fig. 4**).

Another important aspect, not addressed in this article, is the potential role of epigenetics, cellular and physiologic trait variations not caused by changes in the DNA sequence, in the pathobiology of periodontitis.[14] This new and emerging field will yield in the years to come new valuable information in relation to the susceptibility of periodontitis.

For periodontitis, the search for genetic risk factors continues. This will help to better understand the disease and identify pathobiological pathways in which genetic factors, environment, lifestyle, and other factors interconnect. To date, there are several modestly large cohorts of patients and controls available (Northern Europe, United States, Japan), future studies need to concentrate on larger sample sizes in multiple ethnic populations for discovery and validation, and to use (mathematical) modeling (for example, Refs.[36,77]) of the various causative factors to further explore the complexity of periodontitis.

REFERENCES

1. Armitage G. Development of a classification system for periodontal diseases and conditions. Ann Periodontol 1999;4:1–6.
2. Albandar J, Rams T. Global epidemiological of periodontal diseases: an overview. Periodontol 2000 2002;29:7–10.
3. Demmer R, Papapanou P. Epidemiologic patterns of chronic and aggressive periodontitis. Periodontol 2000 2010;53:28–44.
4. Hugoson A, Laurell L. A prospective longitudinal study on periodontal bone height changes in a Swedish population. J Clin Periodontol 2000;27:665–74.
5. Axelsson P, Albandar J, Rams T. Prevention and control of periodontal diseases in developing and industrialized nations. Periodontol 2000 2002;29:235–46.
6. Albandar J. Underestimation of periodontitis in NHANES surveys. J Periodontol 2011;82:337–41.
7. Eke P, Dye B, Wei L, et al. Prevalence of periodontitis in adults in the United States: 2009 and 2010. J Dent Res 2012;91:914–20.
8. Eke P, Dye B, Wei L, et al. Update on prevalence of periodontitis in adults in the United States: NHANES 2009-2012. J Periodontol 2015;17:1–18.
9. Laine ML, Jepsen S, Loos BG. Progress in the identification of genetic factors in periodontitis. Current Oral Health Rep 2014;1:272–8.
10. Heaton B, Dietrich T. Causal theory and the etiology of periodontal diseases. Periodontol 2000 2012;58:26–36.
11. Nicolis G, Nicolis C. Foundation of complex systems: emergence, information and prediction. Singapore (Singapore): World Scientific; 2012.

12. Sokransky S, Haffajee A. Periodontal microbial ecology. Periodontol 2000 2005; 38:137–87.
13. Laine ML, Crielaard W, Loos BG. Genetic susceptibility to periodontitis. Periodontol 2000 2012;58(1):37–68.
14. Lindroth A, Park Y. Epigenetic biomarkers: a step forward for understanding periodontitis. J Periodontal Implant Sci 2013;43:111–20.
15. Akcali A, Huck O, Tenenbaum H, et al. Periodontal diseases and stress: a brief review. J Oral Rehabil 2013;40:60–8.
16. Bergström J. Tobacco smoking and risk for periodontal disease. J Clin Periodontol 2003;30:107–13.
17. Van der Velden U, Kuzmanova D, Chapple I. Micronutritional approaches to periodontal therapy. J Clin Periodontol 2011;38(Suppl 11):142–58.
18. Chee B, Park B, Bartold P. Periodontitis and type II diabetes: a two-way relationship. Int J Evid Based Healthc 2013;11:317–29.
19. Gher M. Changing concepts. The effects of occlusion on periodontitis. Dent Clin North Am 1998;42:285–99.
20. Mucci LA, Bjorkman L, Douglass CW, et al. Environmental and heritable factors in the etiology of oral diseases–a population-based study of Swedish twins. J Dent Res 2005;84(9):800–5.
21. Stabholz A, Soskolne WA, Shapira L. Genetic and environmental risk factors for chronic periodontitis and aggressive periodontitis. Periodontol 2000 2010;53:138–53.
22. Van der Velden U, Abbas F, Armand S, et al. Java project on periodontal diseases. The natural development of periodontitis: risk factors, risk predictors and risk determinants. J Clin Periodontol 2006;33(8):540–8.
23. Michalowicz BS, Aeppli D, Virag JG, et al. Periodontal findings in adult twins. J Periodontol 1991;62(5):293–9.
24. Marazita ML, Burmeister JA, Gunsolley JC, et al. Evidence for autosomal dominant inheritance and race-specific heterogeneity in early-onset periodontitis. J Periodontol 1994;65(6):623–30.
25. Laine ML, Loos BG, Crielaard W. Gene polymorphisms in chronic periodontitis. Int J Dent 2010;2010:324719.
26. Ciancio SG, Hazen SP, Cunat JJ. Periodontal observations in twins. J Periodontal Res 1969;4(1):42–5.
27. Nicu EA, Loos BG. PMN numbers and function in periodontitis and possible modulation as therapeutic approach. Periodontol 2000 2015; 67, in press.
28. Graves D. Cytokines that promote periodontal tissue destruction. J Periodontol 2008;79:1585–91.
29. Offenbacher S, Heasman P, Collins J. Modulation of host PGE2 secretion as a determinant of periodontal disease expression. J Periodontol 1993;64:432–44.
30. Lamont RJ, Hajishengallis G. Polymicrobial synergy and dysbiosis in inflammatory disease. Trends Mol Med 2015;21(3):172–83.
31. Bak P, Tang C, Wiesenfeld K. Self organised criticality: an explanation of 1/f noise. Phys Rev Lett 1987;71:4083–6.
32. Papantonopoulos G, Takahashi K, Bountis T, et al. Using cellular automata experiments to model periodontitis: a first theoretical step towards understanding the nonlinear dynamics of periodontitis. Int J Bifurcat Chaos 2013;23(3):1350056, 1–17.
33. Freire MO, Van Dyke TE. Natural resolution of inflammation. Periodontol 2000 2013;63(1):149–64.
34. Bartold P, Van Dyke TE. Periodontitis: a host-mediated disruption of microbial homeostasis. Unlearning learned concepts. Periodontol 2000 2013;62:203–17.

35. Mitchell M. Complexity: a guided tour. New York: Oxford University press; 2009.
36. Papantonopoulos G, Takahashi K, Bountis T, et al. Mathematical modeling suggests that periodontitis behaves as a non-linear chaotic dynamical process. J Periodontol 2013;84(10):e29–39.
37. NHGRI. National Human Genome Research Institute at the US National Institutes of Health [NIH]. Available at: www.genome.gov.
38. Venter JC, Adams MD, Myers EW, et al. The sequence of the human genome. Science 2001;291(5507):1304–51.
39. Baltimore D. Our genome unveiled. Nature 2001;409(6822):814–6.
40. Sivakumaran S, Agakov F, Theodoratou E, et al. Abundant pleiotropy in human complex diseases and traits. Am J Hum Genet 2011;89(5):607–18.
41. Vaithilingam RD, Safii SH, Baharuddin NA, et al. Moving into a new era of periodontal genetic studies: relevance of large case-control samples using severe phenotypes for genome-wide association studies. J Periodontal Res 2014; 49(6):683–95.
42. International HapMap Consortium. A haplotype map of the human genome. Nature 2005;437(7063):1299–320.
43. 1000 Genomes Project Consortium, Abecasis G, Altshuler D, et al. A map of human genome variation from population-scale sequencing. Nature 2010; 467(7319):1061–73.
44. Ioannidis JP. Genetic associations: false or true? Trends Mol Med 2003;9(4): 135–8.
45. Zhang J, Sun X, Xiao L, et al. Gene polymorphisms and periodontitis. Periodontol 2000 2011;56(1):102–24.
46. Schäfer A, Jepsen S, Loos B. Periodontal genetics: a decade of genetic association studies mandates better study designs. J Clin Periodontol 2011;38:103–7.
47. Manolio TA. Genomewide association studies and assessment of the risk of disease. N Engl J Med 2010;363(2):166–76.
48. Schaefer AS, Richter GM, Nothnagel M, et al. A genome-wide association study identifies GLT6D1 as a susceptibility locus for periodontitis. Hum Mol Genet 2010; 19(3):553–62.
49. Divaris K, Monda KL, North KE, et al. Exploring the genetic basis of chronic periodontitis: a genome-wide association study. Hum Mol Genet 2013;22(11): 2312–24.
50. Teumer A, Holtfreter B, Volker U, et al. Genome-wide association study of chronic periodontitis in a general German population. J Clin Periodontol 2013;40(11):977–85.
51. Feng P, Wang X, Casado P, et al. Genome wide association scan for chronic periodontitis implicates novel locus. BMC Oral Health 2014;14:84, 1–8.
52. Shimizu S, Momozawa Y, Takahashi A, et al. A genome-wide association study of periodontitis in a Japanese population. J Dent Res 2015;94:555–61.
53. Shaffer JR, Polk DE, Wang X, et al. Genome-wide association study of periodontal health measured by probing depth in adults ages 18-49 years. G3 (Bethesda) 2014;4(2):307–14.
54. Divaris K, Monda KL, North KE, et al. Genome-wide association study of periodontal pathogen colonization. J Dent Res 2012;91(7 Suppl):21S–8S.
55. Rhodin K, Divaris K, North K, et al. Chronic periodontitis genome-wide association studies: gene-centric and gene set enrichment analyses. J Dent Res 2014; 93:882–90.
56. Ho YP, Lin YC, Yang YH, et al. Cyclooxygenase-2 Gene-765 single nucleotide polymorphism as a protective factor against periodontitis in Taiwanese. J Clin Periodontol 2008;35(1):1–8.

57. Schaefer AS, Richter GM, Nothnagel M, et al. COX-2 is associated with periodontitis in Europeans. J Dent Res 2010;89(4):384–8.
58. Loo WT, Wang M, Jin LJ, et al. Association of matrix metalloproteinase (MMP-1, MMP-3 and MMP-9) and cyclooxygenase-2 gene polymorphisms and their proteins with chronic periodontitis. Arch Oral Biol 2011;56(10):1081–90.
59. Li G, Yue Y, Tian Y, et al. Association of matrix metalloproteinase (MMP)-1, 3, 9, interleukin (IL)-2, 8 and cyclooxygenase (COX)-2 gene polymorphisms with chronic periodontitis in a Chinese population. Cytokine 2012;60(2): 552–60.
60. Schaefer AS, Bochenek G, Manke T, et al. Validation of reported genetic risk factors for periodontitis in a large-scale replication study. J Clin Periodontol 2013; 40(6):563–72.
61. Lees C, Barrett J, Parkes M, et al. New IBD genetics: common pathways with other diseases. Gut 2011;60:1739–53.
62. Kornman KS, Crane A, Wang HY, et al. The interleukin-1 genotype as a severity factor in adult periodontal disease. J Clin Periodontol 1997;24(1):72–7.
63. Yoshie H, Kobayashi T, Tai H, et al. The role of genetic polymorphisms in periodontitis. Periodontol 2000 2007;43:102–32.
64. Fiebig A, Jepsen S, Loos B, et al. Polymorphisms in the interleukin -1 (IL1) gene cluster are not associated with aggressive periodontitis in a large Caucasian population. Genomics 2008;92:309–15.
65. Deng JS, Qin P, Li XX, et al. Association between interleukin-1beta C (3953/4)T polymorphism and chronic periodontitis: evidence from a meta-analysis. Hum Immunol 2013;74(3):371–8.
66. Karimbux NY, Saraiya VM, Elangovan S, et al. Interleukin-1 gene polymorphisms and chronic periodontitis in adult whites: a systematic review and meta-analysis. J Periodontol 2012;83(11):1407–19.
67. Mao M, Zeng XT, Ma T, et al. Interleukin-1alpha -899 (+4845) C–>T polymorphism increases the risk of chronic periodontitis: evidence from a meta-analysis of 23 case-control studies. Gene 2013;532(1):114–9.
68. Nibali L. Suggested guidelines for systematic reviews of periodontal genetic association studies. J Clin Periodontol 2013;40:753–6.
69. Schaefer AS, Richter GM, Nothnagel M, et al. A 3' UTR transition within DEFB1 is associated with chronic and aggressive periodontitis. Genes Immun 2010;11(1): 45–54.
70. Schaefer AS, Richter GM, Groessner-Schreiber B, et al. Identification of a shared genetic susceptibility locus for coronary heart disease and periodontitis. PLoS Genet 2009;5(2):e1000378.
71. Ernst FD, Uhr K, Teumer A, et al. Replication of the association of chromosomal region 9p21.3 with generalized aggressive periodontitis (gAgP) using an independent case-control cohort. BMC Med Genet 2010;11:119.
72. Schaefer AS, Richter GM, Dommisch H, et al. CDKN2BAS is associated with periodontitis in different European populations and is activated by bacterial infection. J Med Genet 2011;48(1):38–47.
73. Bochenek G, Hasler R, El Mokhtari NE, et al. The large non-coding RNA ANRIL, which is associated with atherosclerosis, periodontitis and several forms of cancer, regulates ADIPOR1, VAMP3 and C11ORF10. Hum Mol Genet 2013;22(22): 4516–27.
74. Schaefer AS, Bochenek G, Jochens A, et al. Genetic evidence for PLASMINOGEN as a shared genetic risk factor of coronary artery disease and periodontitis. Circ Cardiovasc Genet 2015;8(1):159–67.

75. Schaefer A, Jochens A, Dommisch H, et al. A large candidate-gene association study suggests genetic variants at IRF5 and PRDM1 to be associated with aggressive periodontitis. J Clin Periodontol 2014;41:1122–31.
76. Manolio TA, Collins FS, Cox NJ, et al. Finding the missing heritability of complex diseases. Nature 2009;461(7265):747–53.
77. Laine ML, Moustakis V, Koumakis L, et al. Modeling susceptibility to periodontitis. J Dent Res 2013;92(1):45–50.

What is the Proper Sample Size for Studies of Periodontal Treatment?

Jihnhee Yu, PhD*, Luge Yang, MS, Alan D. Hutson, PhD

KEYWORDS

- Rules of thumb for the sufficient sample • Exact nonparametric tests
- Bootstrap method • Periodontal treatment • Small sample size

KEY POINTS

- The authors provide some rules of thumb regarding sufficient sample sizes for a few statistical methods.
- The authors examine distributional characteristics of data from periodontal studies and relevant sampling distributions.
- The authors provide some strategies to perform statistically sound data analysis with a small sample size.

INTRODUCTION

A key feature of scientific research activities is the design of an experiment, the collection of data from the realization of the given experiment, and testing of statistical hypotheses based on the accumulated data. The data itself may take a variety of forms. Thus, a broad knowledge of various statistical methods is crucial for performing scientifically sound research. Basic statistics texts well explain appropriate statistical techniques for different characteristics of the data corresponding to the various hypotheses of interests. Less emphasized is whether those statistical methods are suitable regardless of the sample sizes. What needs to be considered are the 2 types of errors involved in statistical testing termed type I and type II errors, as well as the statistical power (1 minus the probability of a type II error). Type I error is the probability of rejecting the statistical hypothesis of interest (termed the null hypothesis) when in fact it is true. Type II error rate is the probability of failing to reject the statistical null

Department of Biostatistics, University at Buffalo, The State University of New York, 706 Kimball Tower, Buffalo, NY 14214-3000, USA
* Corresponding author.
E-mail address: jinheeyu@buffalo.edu

Dent Clin N Am 59 (2015) 781–797
http://dx.doi.org/10.1016/j.cden.2015.06.006
0011-8532/15/$ – see front matter © 2015 Elsevier Inc. All rights reserved.

dental.theclinics.com

hypothesis when in fact it is false. The statistical power is the probability of rejecting the statistical null hypothesis of interest when in fact it is false.

Many scientific studies suffer from a small sample size owing to limitations on available resources or poor planning. Periodontal research outcomes may include outcomes such as bacteria colonization, measure of plaque, pocket depth, and clinical attachment loss.[1] With these types of data, one may ask whether it is appropriate that someone tests the difference between 2 treatments based on only 10 subjects per group. One may also ask whether several predictors can be included in a regression analysis when the total sample size is only, for example, 30. It is possible through trial and error to have a model that incorrectly overfits the data given a large number of covariates or a small sample size. This is due to an inflation of the type I error across multiple tests of multiple models. That is, if we test enough models, by chance alone we are likely to find one that fits the data well even, although there is no relationship. These issues are to be considered before carrying out the data analysis. Many statistical textbooks extensively address the power of hypothesis testing; however, not many statistical textbooks sufficiently address the validity (especially in the context of the type I error) of statistical inference with a small sample size, even though hypothesis testing with a small sample size may be of great interest to many researchers. The concept of the type I error is equivalent to the confidence level in a confidence interval, thus the validity of tests in terms of the type I error is directly addressing the validity of a confidence interval. This article provides some reasonable guidelines for researchers who want to draw statistically sound results and relevant interpretation from studies with small sample sizes.

It is well understood that studies with a small sample size have a low statistical power to detect a true effect. The statistical literature offers a rule of thumb for sample size in the context that the minimum sample size requirement often assures a certain statistical power for detecting a moderate effect size (eg, Refs.[2,3]). The suggested sample sizes based on the statistical power are usually large enough that the accompanying statistical methods are justified in terms of maintaining the desired type I error rate. In practice, the available samples are often limited because of time, budget, or ethical reasons. For researchers with limited resources, the statistical analysis needs to be performed based on the available sample size rather than on the sample size for a certain study power. As a result, the right question to be asked regards the suitability of the statistical methods with a limited sample size. Because many statistical methods rely on so-called large sample properties, a liberal use of statistical tests, regardless of inadequate sample sizes, may lead to inflated statistical type I errors (more detail for this point is given in the section Caution on Using the Bootstrap Method for a Small Sample Size), meaning that nonexistent study effects may too often be declared to be significant. Statistical software packages print out results but in general do not warn users that the results may be inaccurate because of small sample sizes. Inflated type I errors in turn give rise to low reproducibility of the results by future research. The problem of inflated type I error is less commonplace in practice by the incorporation of computationally intensive exact statistical methods (details given in section Alternative Methods for Small Sample Sizes), although the exact methods have a problem to adapt a variety of complex modeling schemes.

This article therefore discusses the sample sizes adequate for several popular statistical methods. It discusses distributional characteristics of the data based on a study to reduce the oral colonization of pathogens in the oral cavity[4] and other periodontal studies, followed by the bootstrap method that can be used to cope with small sample size problems. Alternative statistical methods that can be used with the small sample sizes are also described.

GENERAL REQUIREMENT OF SAMPLE SIZES FOR THE VALIDITY OF STATISTICAL TESTS

Adequate sample sizes are often determined to assure a certain chance to detect the true effect size. For example, analysis of variance (ANOVA) may require 30 observations per cell to detect a medium effect size to have about 80% power.[3] Green[2] suggests that the required sample size is greater than $50 + 8m$ in a regression analysis assuming the medium size association, where m is the number of predictors. These discussions do not answer the questions regarding the minimum sample sizes for the validity of statistical methods besides the use of the target standardized effect sizes, which is difficult to be justified.[5,6] Because the validity of many statistical tests (eg, the likelihood ratio tests) depends on the accuracy of large sample approximations of the true distribution of the test statistic, we discuss how large the sample size should be so that a related inference can be trusted relative to the desired type I error rate in this section. Different statistical approaches may require different sample sizes. Hence, sample sizes for several statistical methods are discussed as follows.

Tests for Categorical Data

Many outcome variables of interest are categorical, that is, either ordinal or nominal. For example,[7] one may want to see an effect of an antibiotic on successful management of harmful microorganisms. The outcome of the microorganisms can be expressed as binary data (ie, successful management or failure). When a study compares effects of k therapies, the binary outcome variable can be summarized by a $k \times 2$ contingency table, and thus the table consists of $2k$ cells. The test statistic for comparing the equality of the response proportions across k therapies can be obtained based on the normal approximation of the binomial distribution or the Poisson distribution. Resulting statistics may have approximately a normal distribution or a χ^2 distribution in a large sample.

A common rule of thumb for the sufficient sample size in normal-based hypothesis testing or constructing confidence intervals is that each cell size should satisfy $pn>5$, where n is the sample size and p is the true or estimated proportion (rate) that corresponds to the cell.[8] Note that pn is the expected cell size. Suppose that one expects that full-mouth disinfectant successfully manages *Porphyromonas gingivalis* infection in 90% of patients. This result also means that the expected rate of management failure is 10%. Then, a study with $n=51$ total subjects would expect to observe 5.1 failures (10% of 51) and 45.9 successes (90% of 50). Notice that this is only for considering one treatment group. If one deals with k different groups, the sample size consideration should address each group separately. A similar calculation finds that the required sample size for the rate of 50% is 11. This fact indicates that the sample size requirements increase drastically for rare events. For outcome variables with more than 2 levels (eg, mild, moderate, and severe), the same argument stated earlier can be applied based on the expected cell size.

In summary, categorical data analysis requires a fairly large sample.

Logistic Regression with Binary Outcomes

Logistic regression is a popular approach for modeling the relationship between a binary outcome and a set of explanatory variables based on the likelihood method. Logistic regression defines the relationship between the binary outcomes and predictors through the log odds or logit function, although a suitable transformation can also express the relationship between the probability of an outcome of interest and the values of the explanatory variables. The method is popular among researchers because it allows investigating multiple factors in predicting a binary outcome. To ensure that the likelihood ratio tests for the model follow a χ^2 distribution, the sample size needs to be sufficiently large. In addition, if the outcome response rate is assumed to be close to the extremes, that is, 0 or 1, the required sample size is even larger for logistic regression.

Some discussions relative to the minimum sample size for logistic regression are found in the related literature. Peduzzi and colleagues[9] and Hosmer and colleagues[10] suggest that the minimum number of events per independent variable is approximately 10. According to these guidelines, if 2 predictors are included, the total number of events is 20. If the event happens about 10% of the time and the other 90% nonevent cases are also taken into account, then the recommended total sample size is 20 + 180 = 200.

In summary, a large sample size is required for proper inferences in logistic regression.

Tests for Numeric Data

Under certain distributional assumptions, some statistical tests are based on exactly correct distributions. These are often called exact tests. One example of an exact test is the t test (or Student's t test). The t statistic follows the t distribution exactly if all observations are independent and from the same normal distribution, and the test is valid even with the sample size as small as 2. But, this also means that the t test is not an exact test when these assumptions are violated. When the underlying distribution is not normal, the t test statistic approximately follows a normal distribution with a sufficiently large sample as dictated by the central limit theorem. Thus, for the t test approximation to be accurate regardless of the underlying distributions, a sufficient sample is required.

A quick rule of thumb indicates 25 to 30 as a sufficient sample size.[11] This criterion is reasonable because the sampling distribution of the sample mean is often well approximated by a normal distribution when the sample size is sufficiently large. Of course, if an underlying distribution of data has a symmetric shape, the approximation to the normal distribution may be achieved much faster than the sample size of 25 to 30. On the other hand, if an underlying distribution is extremely skewed, even much larger sample sizes may not be sufficient for the normal approximation of the summary statistics. For the subsequent discussions, we accept this rule of thumb and consider the sample size of 30 as a general guideline for the large sample for testing based on numeric data.

Now, consider the two-sample t test, the most commonly used test statistic for comparing the mean of 2 independent groups. When the sample size is large, the two-sample t test is well approximated by the standard normal distribution despite nonnormal underlying distributions. First, consider sufficient sample sizes (for a normal approximation) for the t test based on equal variances between the 2 groups. The two-sample t test has the degrees of freedom the total sample size minus 2. The degrees of freedom can be interpreted as the size of independent data. In the degrees of freedom, we subtract 2 from the total sample size because the 2 parameters are estimated, giving rise to the dependence between the summands in the sample variance formula. In this context and also analogously to the 1-sample problem, one may say that the required total sample size is 32 or greater for the 2-group comparison, when the underlying distribution is not normal, which is not larger than 30.

Now, consider the two-sample t test with unequal variances, which can be used when the 2 groups have different variances. Now the value of the degrees of freedom is the function of both the sample sizes and the variances. Suppose that one group variance is k times of the other group variance. Consider a balanced design, that is,

$n_1=n_2=n$ (n_i: the sample size of group i). Then, based on the popular Satterthwaite approximation[12] of the degrees of freedom, the degrees of freedom are $(n-1)(1+k)^2/(1+k^2)$. If $k=2$, one has the degrees of freedom $1.8n$. That is, to achieve the degrees of freedom 30, a sample size of about 17 per group or the total of 34 is needed. A severely unbalanced sample size may require much larger sample sizes. For example, when the sample size of the group with the smaller variance is 2 times larger than that of the group with the larger variance, then the required sample size to have the degrees of freedom 30 is a total of 63 (21 for the larger variance group and 42 for the smaller variance group) with $k=2$.

In summary, based on the sample size 30 as the rule of thumb, the group comparisons based on numeric data may require slightly more than the sample size of 30 with the balanced design or equal variance cases. However, if inequality in variances between the 2 groups is extreme, the sample size requirement may be considerably bigger than the case with equal variances. We again emphasize that this rule of thumb is only a guideline not a definitive number. In some difficult cases, there may not be reasonable performance of the test statistics even with fairly large sample size. This difficult example is dealt with when discussing the bootstrap method. Sufficient sample sizes for ANOVA can be discussed relative to regression.

Regression and Analysis of Variance with Numeric Outcomes

The validity of regression methods depends on assumptions such as normality, constant variance, and the independence of observations. When a numeric predictor is of interest, the t test can be used to show its significance. If a predictor consists of more than 2 categories (eg, ANOVA), the relevant test statistic has the form of F test. These test statistics already take into account the dependence structures of the observations (ie, residuals). Thus, the dependence between residuals may be less of a concern, if the raw observations are independent. Another important question is whether the underlying distribution of the data is a normal distribution because the t statistic and F statistic are based on the normal distribution assumption.

Checking of the underlying distribution can be carried out based on the residuals (this itself can be a problem with a small sample size; please see more detail in section Goodness-of-Fit Testing). If the normal assumption (with equal variances) is met, the t test and F test are exact tests. That is, they provide the promised type I error that users specify under the null hypothesis (ie, coefficient of a predictor $= 0$). If the normal assumption is not met, those tests are not exact, and inferences based on them largely rely on the test statistics' approximation to the normal distribution or χ^2 distributions. For the moment, assume a constant variance of an outcome variable across different predictor values. If the underlying distribution is not normal, analogously to the discussion in section Tests for Numeric Data, the approximation to a normal distribution may require the degrees of freedom of the t test greater than 30. Because the value of the degrees of freedom is given as the sample size minus the number of coefficients in the model (including the intercept), if only 1 numeric predictor is included in the regression model, the approximation requires a total sample size of 32. If the predictor variable is categorical with k levels such as ANOVA, this is counted as equivalent to $k-1$ predictors (excluding the intercept term). If the constant variance assumption is not met, the regression method based on the ordinary least square may not perform well; thus, other techniques such as the generalized least square method[13] need to be considered.

If the number of predictors in the regression model is large, it may be possible that the model itself can be highly significant even if none of the predictors have a relationship with the outcome variable.[14] Freedman and Pee[15] suggest that the ratio of the number of predictors and the observations to be 25% may maintain the desired type I errors in the model. Individually significant predictors that are correlated with each other may lead to so-called multicollinearity issues when combined in a model. In cases of near collinearity, the magnitude of the effect may be reversed or the variables may be no longer significant.

Goodness-of-Fit Testing

Goodness-of-fit tests for distributions quantify the differences between the observations and their expected values under the assumed distribution and are commonly used for evidence that observations have a certain distribution. Many standard statistical programs provide these tests. For example, SAS provides the Shapiro-Wilk test, Kolmogorov-Smirnov test, Anderson-Darling test, and Cramér-von Mises test for testing normality in PROC UNIVARIATE among many distributions.

What is often overlooked is that these tests are subject to sample sizes for their power. For testing normality, these tests use the null hypothesis that the data are normally distributed. When the sample sizes are small, there may not be enough power to reject the null hypothesis even if the data do not follow a normal distribution. Let us consider the Shapiro-Wilk test to investigate its power to detect nonnormality, which, among the goodness-of-fit tests for normality, is known to be the most powerful.[16] In **Table 1**, we generate the random numbers from various distributions with the sample sizes of 5, 10, 20, and 30 (5000 simulations per scenario). The result with the normal distribution is the type I error of the test (the target type I error = 0.05). The result shows that the Shapiro-Wilk test has accurate type I error control even with the sample size of 5. But, with the Gamma (5,1) distribution, the power to detect the nonnormality with the sample size of 20 is only 24%. That is, about 76% of the times, the Shapiro-Wilk test may provide a wrong conclusion. That is, it fails to reject that the data have a normal distribution. The simulation results show that the goodness-of-fit tests may not be a practical approach to show that the data are normally distributed with the small sample sizes. The authors' recommendation is that one needs to apply the valid statistical methods for small samples when the sample sizes are small, rather than using the goodness-of-fit tests to show the normality of the data.

CHARACTERISTIC OF THE DATA IN PERIODONTAL RESEARCH AND THE CORRESPONDING SAMPLING DISTRIBUTIONS

Observed values in the real world rarely have a normal distribution. Note the classic assertion by R. C. Geary: "Normality is a myth; there never was, and never will be, a normal distribution."[17] Most of the distributions that we observe in our collaborations with dental researchers are asymmetric and sometimes discrete. Articles available in the dental literature show a glimpse of the distributions of periodontal outcomes.

Table 1
The simulated power of the Shapiro-Wilk test

Distribution	Sample Size			
	5	10	20	30
Normal (0,1)	0.045	0.048	0.053	0.048
Exponential (1)	0.154	0.458	0.840	0.965
Gamma (5,1)	0.087	0.125	0.242	0.351
Lognormal (0,1)	0.217	0.616	0.933	0.988

Because of diverse outcomes used in periodontal research, it is difficult to specify the overall characteristic of the distributions of the data. For some outcomes, consistent distributional consensus may not be found. For example, the distribution of clinical attachment loss can be moderately skewed to the right (Figure 2 in Rosenberg and colleagues[18]), fairly symmetric (Figure 1 in Zuza and colleagues[19]), or irregular without a specific trend (Box plot 2 in Debnath and colleagues[20]). These different trends of the distribution of clinical attachment may be due to small sample sizes or different treatment/patient characteristics. A sensible strategy for data analysis should be chosen in a way that the analytical approach is acceptable for general scenarios.

Thus, we here investigate some of the characteristics of data and their sampling distributions using data from a study of oral topical chlorhexidine gluconate (CHX) rinse on mechanically ventilated patients in the intensive care unit.[4] In the CHX study, a total of 175 patients were enrolled and randomly assigned to 3 different treatments. Dental plaque samples were collected from patients and sent to a laboratory, where the growth of target microorganisms was assessed. The quantitative cultures were expressed as colony forming units per milliliter. **Fig. 1** describes the histogram of the culture of the target microorganisms (*Staphylococcus aureus*, *Pseudomonas aeruginosa*, *Acinetobacter* spp, and enteric organisms) in baseline. The figure includes patients from all treatment groups because the data were produced before treatment (ie, baseline). Many zeros are prominent in the histogram, suggesting that the distribution is not completely continuous but has a probability mass at 0. **Fig. 1** also shows some sampling distributions based on the distribution of the target microorganisms. For the sampling distribution of the sample mean, we generate 1000 sample means using the samples with sizes of 5, 10, and 30, respectively, assuming that the observed amounts of the microorganism reflect their true distribution. For the sampling distribution of the slope estimate of the simple linear regression, we generate the response variable based on $1+1x+\varepsilon$, where x has the standard normal distribution and ε has the distribution of the target microorganism subtracted by their mean (1000 simulations per scenario). Based on the generated sample means and slope estimates, the density estimates are obtained using the kernel density estimation.[21]

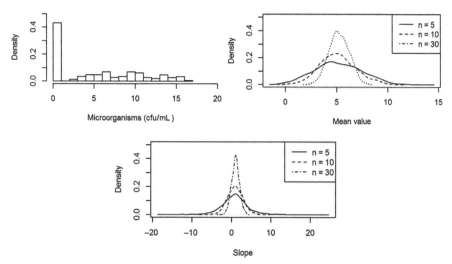

Fig. 1. The histogram of the target microorganisms and the sampling distributions of the sample mean and slope.

With a smaller sample size (eg, 5), the sampling distribution of the sample mean is asymmetric. But, when the sample size approaches 30, the sample mean shows a good approximation of the normal distribution. The slope estimate behaves in a manner similar to the sample mean except it may converge to the normal distribution a little faster. The true normal density is omitted in the figure, as it closely overlaps with the sampling distribution with the sample size 30.

We also examine the ratio of the target microorganisms, that is, the amount of the target microorganisms divided by the total amount of all detected microorganisms. Because this value depends on the total amount of all microorganisms, its distribution does not exactly match with the microorganisms itself. **Fig. 2** shows that the distribution is similar to the distribution of the target microorganisms but the probability at 0 is more amplified. The sampling distributions (see **Fig. 2**) show that the approximation to a normal distribution may not be as good as the sampling distributions of the target microorganisms. But, when the sample size reaches 30, the sampling distributions are almost identical to a normal approximation.

In the CHX study, the plaque index was also measured. The amount of plaque present was discretely scored from 0 (no plaque) to 3 (severe deposit) on up to a total of 6 teeth. **Fig. 3** shows the histogram of the average of the dental scores. The average's denominator is the number of teeth examined considering missing teeth for some patients. The distribution is slightly right skewed but uniform throughout the range of the dental score. Both the sampling distributions of the sample mean and the slope estimate of the simple linear regression approximate well to a normal distribution with increasing sample sizes. In fact it shows reasonable approximation to a normal distribution with the small sample size of 10.

In summary, the sampling distribution of investigated statistics is largely affected by the original underlying distribution. Some may achieve a reasonable approximation to a normal distribution with small sample sizes. But, for a difficult distribution, the approximation may require a large sample. With the data set in the CHX study, it was observed that the sample size of 30 may be a practical and safe rule of thumb to assure a reasonable approximation to the normal distribution of the sample mean and slope of the regression model.

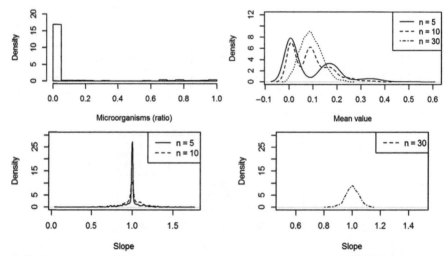

Fig. 2. The histogram of the ratio of microorganisms and the sampling distributions of the sample mean and slope.

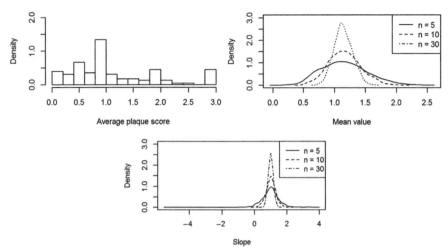

Fig. 3. The histogram of the average plaque score and the sampling distributions of the sample mean and slope.

CAUTION ON USING THE BOOTSTRAP METHOD FOR A SMALL SAMPLE SIZE

The basic concept of the bootstrap method[22] is that the empirical distribution based on the data approximates the true underlying distribution of the data. Hence, one can resample from the approximate distribution as if it were the known distribution to derive quantities such as a variance estimate for a given statistic and approximate confidence intervals, often where analytical formulas do not exist.

One perception of the bootstrap method is that it may be used for data with a small sample size. Is this notion correct? The bootstrap method of a statistic surely works if the statistic behaves well with the small sample with correct variance estimates. But if the statistic has a poor performance with the small sample, the bootstrap method may not improve the statistic's performance much. To explain this point better, we carry out a simulation study. **Table 2** shows that the bootstrap type I errors are based on the simulations (5000 simulations per scenario and 1000 bootstrap samples per simulation). The target type I error in this simulation is 0.05. For each scenario, the data for group 1 and group 2 are generated, whereby each group's data have the distribution described in **Fig. 4**. In **Fig. 4**, the vertical dashed line indicates the common population

Table 2
Comparison of the simulated type I errors between the two-sample *t* test and the bootstrap method using the two-sample *t* test

Distribution	Method	Sample Sizes (n_1,n_2)			
		(10,10)	(15,15)	(20,20)	(30,30)
Gamma vs normal	*t* test	0.066	0.061	0.064	0.064
	Bootstrap	0.057	0.052	0.057	0.058
Gamma vs lognormal	*t* test	0.253	0.235	0.215	0.200
	Bootstrap	0.230	0.202	0.180	0.166
Normal vs lognormal	*t* test	0.051	0.048	0.047	0.048
	Bootstrap	0.042	0.044	0.043	0.044

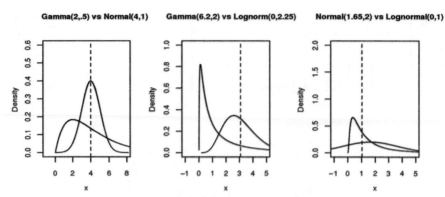

Fig. 4. Illustration of the underlying distributions used in **Table 2**.

mean. We consider these distributions because the distributions are not normal distributions and the densities are different in shape from each other, although they share the common mean. If the test statistic works desirably, the simulated type I error should be close to 0.05. In **Table 2**, the two-sample t test with unequal variances is applied to compare the 2 group means. We also use the bootstrap method on the two-sample t test and obtain the bootstrap P-value. For technical details of this method, we refer to Fox.[23] For cases of gamma versus normal and normal versus lognormal, although their underlying distributions are quite different, the type I errors are satisfactory. For the case of gamma versus normal, the t test's type I error is slightly larger than 0.05, and it seems that the bootstrap method somewhat corrects the type I error toward 0.05, although the correction is not dramatic. For the case of gamma versus lognormal, the type I errors of both the tests are not so close to 0.05. In fact, they are too liberal even with fairly large sample sizes, and the type I errors of the t test and its bootstrap application are similar. Again, the bootstrap method slightly corrects the type I error, but it may only reflect the fact that the bootstrap method may provide slightly more conservative tests than the original test, not the fact that the bootstrap can repair the type I error of the original test. In fact, we also observe a similar characteristic of the bootstrap method for other statistics. Confidence intervals based on the bootstrap methods (eg, BC_a interval[24]) show similar results as well (not presented in this article).

In summary, the bootstrap method may not be a cure for small samples, and its performing characteristic with small or large samples is similar to the original test applied (if available) for the bootstrap method. The bootstrap method is especially useful in case the closed formula for a variance estimate of a statistic is not available. But, the overall performance based on the bootstrap estimate is likely to be affected by the sample size and underlying distributions. Researchers should consider the small sample behavior of a statistic for data analyses before using the bootstrap method for the statistic.

ALTERNATIVE METHODS FOR SMALL SAMPLE SIZES
Categorical Data Analysis

For categorical data analysis, exact nonparametric methods are well developed for the small samples. Exact nonparametric tests (or simply exact tests) are based on the distribution of the test statistic that is obtained empirically rather than its approximated theoretic distributions. Because the exact methods do not depend on an inference on the approximation, they are valid with any sample sizes as far as exact distributions can be obtained. These exact tests are known for guaranteeing the type I error no greater than the user-specified nominal level (eg, 0.05) and thus providing a confidence interval with the designated (or slightly larger) confidence level.[25]

Many exact tests for categorical data analysis use a conditional approach. That is, the exact distribution with the permutation fixing on certain statistics (called as sufficient statistics) is obtained to build the test. Often, this means that the permutation is carried out maintaining the same number of observations in margins of the contingency table. When one considers all the possible values of the fixed statistics as well in the exact distribution, the method is called an unconditional exact test. There are some arguments about the preference between the conditional and unconditional approach. For more detailed discussion, we refer to Agresti.[25]

Many exact tests are readily available in statistical software packages. For instance, SAS offers the exact tests of popular statistics including the Pearson χ^2test, Mantel-Haenszel χ^2test, McNemar test, and Jonckheere-Terpstra test.

Exact Logistic Regression

When the sample size is small or some cells (in the context of contingency tables) have no or few observations, exact logistic regression can be used as an alternative to the maximum likelihood method of logistic regression. Exact logistic regression considers all permutations of the data conditioning on its certain statistics, providing the exact distribution of the parameter of interest. The algorithm to obtain the exact distribution was developed by Hirji and colleagues,[26] which made the exact method to be computationally feasible. The method can be used for small and sparse data sets. Statistical software such as SAS offers this method in their standard package.

For exact logistic regression, the exact distribution of certain sufficient statistics needs to be obtained; this requires that each level of a covariate should have sufficient number of observations. This fact causes that, when the covariate is thoroughly continuous data, exact logistic regression cannot be carried out because of degenerate distributions of the sufficient statistics.[27] When the model cannot be fitted because of a continuous factor, one may consider categorizing the factor to a few levels.

It may be possible that the outcome of interest has more than 2 categories. If a sample size is small, one possible solution can be reducing the number of categories to 2, which allows the use of exact logistic regression. Because collapsing values increases the number of events for each cell, it may provide more reliable results with the small sample size.

Data Analysis with Numeric or Ordinal Data

When the sample values are numeric or ordinal and the sample size is small, suitable exact nonparametric methods[28] are recommended for group comparisons to control the type I error. Examples of some popular nonparametric methods available for exact methods include (but not limited to) the Wilcoxon-Mann-Whitney test and Kruskal-Wallis test. The Wilcoxon-Mann-Whitney test tests that the probability of any elements of one group is greater than the other group. The Kruskal-Wallis test is a nonparametric counterpart of the ANOVA, which carries out the ANOVA based on the ranks of the data. The exact distribution of these statistics can be obtained by permuting the ranks of observations. The statistic obtained from the original observations is compared with the exact distribution, and the P-value can be computed. This P-value does not rely on the approximated distribution of test statistics; thus, the methods are valid for a small sample even with sparse and skewed distributions. These nonparametric exact tests are available in standard statistical software such as SAS.

Table 3 shows that the type I errors of the Wilcoxon-Mann-Whitney test and its exact test are based on the simulations (5000 simulations per scenario). The distributions that we used for this simulation are illustrated in **Fig. 5**. The distributions described in **Fig. 5** satisfy the null hypothesis, whereas the shapes of the distributions are different. A common misunderstanding of the Wilcoxon-Mann-Whitney test is that it tests the equality of the medians. But, as basic statistical books state,[29] the test is equivalent to test of the medians only if they have equal distributions except the location. As stated previously, what the Wilcoxon-Mann-Whitney test tests is more precisely the null hypothesis $P(X>Y)=0.5$, where X and Y represent the observations from 2 different groups. That is, it tests whether it is more likely that the observations from one group are larger than the observations from the other group. The distributions illustrated in **Fig. 5** are well thought out to satisfy the null hypothesis $P(X>Y)=0.5$. **Table 3** shows that the Wilcoxon-Mann-Whitney test has an accurate type I error even with very small sample sizes and underlying distributions far departed from the normal distributions. In these cases, the type I errors of the Wilcoxon-Mann-Whitney test and its exact test are similar. Based on this result, it seems that the nonparametric test may itself satisfactorily address the issue related to the nonnormal distributions. However, because popular statistical software provides the exact test as an option, using the exact test requires hardly any extra effort; thus, we recommend using the exact test unless the sample size is too large so that the calculation of the exact P-value takes too much time. The software R (http://www.r-project.org/) provides the exact test as a default for Wilcoxon-Mann-Whitney test if samples contain less than 50 finite values.

Alternatives to Regression Given Small Sample Sizes

When the residuals of the regression model have a normal distribution with constant variance throughout the range of the predictor, inference based on the normal distribution assumptions are valid. However, those assumptions are difficult to prove as described in the discussion of the goodness-of-fit test, and thus it is always safe to make sure that there is an adequate number of sample sizes as described in section General Requirement of Sample Sizes for the Validity of Statistical Tests.

When the sample size is small, we do not recommend incorporating multiple variables in one model. Inferences based on only small samples generally do not provide conclusive evidence. The results may have limited generalizability unless they are based on diverse observations with enough variability. With a small sample size, model building incorporating more variables may not make a model better because of losing a control of the type I error. Thus, model building with multiple predictors is not an appropriate analytical goal with the small sample. Again, including more

Table 3
Comparison of the simulated type I errors between the Wilcoxon-Mann-Whitney (W-M-W) test and the exact method based on the W-M-W test

Distribution	Method	Sample Sizes (n_1,n_2)			
		(10,10)	(15,15)	(20,20)	(30,30)
Lognormal vs lognormal	W-M-W test	0.048	0.053	0.056	0.060
	Exact test	0.048	0.053	0.056	0.061
Normal vs lognormal	W-M-W test	0.055	0.049	0.058	0.057
	Exact test	0.055	0.049	0.058	0.059
Gamma vs gamma	W-M-W test	0.054	0.052	0.055	0.054
	Exact test	0.054	0.052	0.055	0.056

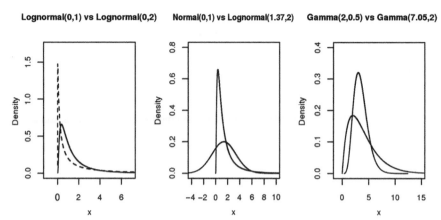

Fig. 5. Illustration of the underlying distributions used in **Table 3.**

variables may end up showing spurious relationship between the outcome and predictors as previously discussed. The results based on the small sample size should be interpreted in the context of hypothesis generation, which can be tested more rigorously later in larger and better designed experiments.

As an alternative to regression with a single predictor, the methods to measure the association between 2 variables can be used, where the exact tests are available. For example, SAS provides the exact tests and confidence intervals for Pearson correlation coefficient, Spearman rank correlation coefficient, and Kendall tau. Pearson correlation coefficient is equal to the coefficient of the predictor (slope) in the simple linear model adjusted by the ratio of the standard deviations of the outcome and the predictor; thus, it can be used as a direct replacement of the slope of the simple linear regression. If someone expects a nonlinear relationship between 2 variables, Spearman rank correlation coefficient or Kendall tau[30] can be better measures of association. Especially, Kendall tau measures the extent of concordance between any 2 pairs of observations.

If there is a categorical predictor, the exact Kruskal-Wallis test can be used rather than a regression model. If there are 2 predictors, say one is of primary interest and the other is a potential confounding factor, one may consider categorizing the confounding factor to 2 or 3 levels. The association can be observed within each level. Different extents of associations between the different levels of the confounding factor may reflect the interaction between the confounder and the primary predictor. This way of doing the analysis may reduce the overall study power, but it also means to reduce the chance of finding a spurious relationship.

Confidence Intervals

Often the confidence interval (for one treatment group) is constructed based on a sample size much smaller than the total sample size of a study (based on multiple treatment groups) unless a model-based approach is used (however, the validity of a model-based approach relies on a large sample). With a small sample size, the normal-distribution-based confidence intervals in general do not provide the nominal confidence level. A simple solution of this is to provide only summary statistics. For example, one may simply provide the sample mean and the standard deviation of each group without attaching any probability claim (ie, confidence level).

One can use a model-based approach (eg, regression using the least square method) to estimate the variance of a statistic, which can be used for construction of a confidence interval. Again, the correct usage of a model relies on certain distributional assumptions of the model. If distributional assumptions are not met and the inference is done based on a large sample property, one should check whether the model is built using a sufficient sample size as seen in section General Requirement of Sample Sizes for the Validity of Statistical Tests.

When the proportion is of interest, there is a more direct solution, that is, the exact confidence intervals.[31] The exact confidence interval of the proportion always guarantees that the confidence level is larger than or equal to its nominal confidence level[32]; thus, it can be safely used for even very small sample sizes.

DISCUSSION

We have discussed the definition of the small sample sizes using several popular statistical analyses and outlined the impact of a small sample size across a few statistical methods. We have shown some examples from the real oral health research. The examples illustrate that some conventionally accepted large sample sizes provide a reasonable approximation to the theoretic distributions in most cases; however, greater care needs to be taken for small sample sizes relative to these same approximations.

Often in dental research, the outcomes consist of repeated measures data. If appropriate, one may use repeated measures data to increase the number of observations for increasing the statistical power.[33] The repeated measures design should be used in a prudent manner that considers the clinical relevance of having repeated observations from the same subjects, particularly relative to the increased complexity of the statistical modeling.

In some scenarios, researchers may consider a transformation of the data, such as a power transformation (a nonlinear transformation), to better account for model assumptions, that is, attempt to transform the data to better meet normality assumptions. For example, the log transformation is a popular power transformation technique for right-skewed data. A nonlinear transformation can change the makeup of data drastically and may result in misleading inferential result[34] because location and scale changes are disproportionate. In the regression setting, which uses the least square method or the likelihood method, a nonlinear transformation of an outcome variable may alter its relationship with covariates drastically.[35] One should be aware that inference based on the transformed data may not be consistent with inference based on the original scale data. To demonstrate this point, we carried out simulations (**Table 4**) of the t test (with unequal variances) comparing 2 groups, whereby 1 group was sampled from an exponential (1) distribution and the other group was sampled from a gamma (10, 10) distribution. In practice, the log transformation may be considered as a reasonable transformation because both the distributions are right skewed. Theoretically, both

Table 4
The simulated type I error rates (target value = 0.05) of the two-sample t test (with unequal variances) of log-transformed data and the data with the original scale

Method	Sample Sizes (n_1, n_2)			
	(10,10)	(20,20)	(50,50)	(100,100)
Log transformation	0.150	0.355	0.824	0.987
Original scale	0.092	0.071	0.062	0.056

The two groups to be compared have the exponential (1) and gamma (10, 10) distributions.

distributions have a true mean of 1; thus, the desirable test of a mean difference (with the target type I error = 0.05) would reject the null hypothesis, that is, incorrectly declaring different means only 5% of times. We carried out the simulations based on data with the original scale and using the log transformation. With the original scale, the type I error is larger than the target type I error 0.05 with the small samples ($n_1 = n_2 = 10$); however, when the sample size increases, the t test with original scale eventually approaches to the desired type I error. On the other hand, the log transformed data have a worse type I error with the small sample size than that of the original scale data, and then the error rate increases more than 90% with an increasing sample size (see **Table 4**). The transformation alone generates false-positive conclusions.

In conclusion, researchers need to use statistics based on the large sample approximation with careful consideration of an adequate sample size. But, this does not mean that researchers are prohibited from offering any statistical analysis when the sample size is small. If the sample size is small, researchers should adapt statistical methods developed for small samples, such as those listed in section Alternative Methods for Small Sample Sizes. Applying a correct statistical method given a small sample size in general reduces the likelihood of a false-positive or nonreproducible results and thus provides more valid and likely reproducible results for the general scientific community; this also means that publication of a study result need not be held because of a small sample size, as long as it applies correct statistical methods rigorously and the result seems to carry valuable information to readers.

REFERENCES

1. Srikanth K, Chandra RV, Reddy AA, et al. Effect of a single session of antimicrobial photodynamic therapy using indocyanine green in the treatment of chronic periodontitis: a randomized controlled pilot trial. Quintessence Int 2015;46(5):391–400.
2. VanVoorhis CW, Morgan BL. Understanding power and rules of thumb for determining sample sizes. Tutor Quant Methods Psychol 2007;3(2):43–50.
3. Green SB. How many subjects does it take to do a regression analysis? Multivariate Behav Res 1991;26(3):499–510.
4. Scannapieco FA, Yu J, Raghavendran K, et al. A randomized trial of chlorhexidine gluconate on oral bacterial pathogens in mechanically ventilated patients. Crit Care 2009;13(4):R117.
5. Lenth RV. Some practical guidelines for effective sample size determination. Am Stat 2001;55:187–93.
6. Hoenig JM, Heisey DM. The abuse of power: the pervasive fallacy of power calculations for data analysis. Am Stat 2001;55:19–24.
7. Preus HR, Gjermo P, Scheie AA, et al. The effect of metronidazole on the presence of *P. gingivalis* and *T. forsythia* at 3 and 12 months after different periodontal treatment strategies evaluated in a randomized, clinical trial. Acta Odontol Scand 2015;73(4):258–66.
8. Brown LD, Cai T, DasGupta A. Interval estimation for a binomial proportion. Stat Sci 2001;16(2):101–33.
9. Peduzzi P, Concato J, Kemper E, et al. A simulation study of the number of events per variable in logistic regression analysis. J Clin Epidemiol 1996;49:1373–9.
10. Hosmer DW, Lemeshow S. Special topics. In: Applied logistic regression. 2nd edition. Hoboken (NJ): John Wiley & Sons; 2004. p. 260–351.
11. Welkowitz J, Ewen RB, Cohen J. Inferences about the mean of a single population. In: Introductory statistics for the behavioral sciences. San Diego (CA): Academic Press Inc; 1971. p. 101–30.

12. Satterthwaite FE. An approximate distribution of estimates of variance components. Biometrics 1946;2(6):110–4.
13. Strutz T. Weights and outliers. In: Data fitting and uncertainty (a practical introduction to weighted least squares and beyond). Germany: Vieweg+Teubner Verlag; 2010. p. 47–104.
14. Freedman DA. A note on screening regression equations. Am Stat 1983;37(2): 152–5.
15. Freedman LS, Pee D. Return to a note on screening regression equations. Am Stat 1989;43(4):279–82.
16. Razali N, Wah YB. Power comparisons of Shapiro–Wilk, Kolmogorov–Smirnov, Lilliefors and Anderson–Darling tests. Journal of Statistical Modeling and Analytics 2011;2(1):21–33.
17. Geary RC. Testing for normality. Biometrika 1947;34:209–42.
18. Rosenberg DR, Andrade CX, Chaparro AP, et al. Short-term effects of 2% atorvastatin dentifrice as an adjunct to periodontal therapy: a randomized double blind clinical trial. J Periodontol 2015;29:1–13.
19. Zuza EP, Vanzato Carrareto AL, Pontes AE, et al. Chronic periodontal disease may influence the pulp sensitivity response: clinical evaluation in consecutive patients. ISRN Dent 2012;2012:246875.
20. Debnath T, Chakraborty A, Pal TK. A clinical study on the efficacy of hydroxyapatite - bioactive glass composite granules in the management of periodontal bony defects. J Indian Soc Periodontol 2014;18(5):593–600.
21. Sheather SJ. The performance of six popular bandwidth selection methods on some real data sets (with discussion). Comput Stat 1992;7:225–50, 271–81.
22. Efron B. Bootstrap methods: another look at the jackknife. Ann Stat 1979;7(1): 1–26.
23. Fox J. Bootstrapping regression models. In: An R and S-PLUS companion to applied regression: a web appendix to the book. Thousand Oaks (CA): Sage; 2002. Available at: http://CRAN.R-project.org/doc/contrib/Fox-Companion/appendix-bootstrapping.pdf.
24. Efron B. Better bootstrap confidence intervals (with discussion). J Am Stat Assoc 1987;82:171–200.
25. Agresti A. Exact inference for categorical data: recent advances and continuing controversies. Stat Med 2001;20(17–18):2709–22.
26. Hirji KF, Mehta CR, Patel NR. Computing distributions for exact logistic regression. J Am Stat Assoc 1987;82:1110–7.
27. Heinze G, Schemper M. A solution to the problem of separation in logistic regression. Stat Med 2002;21(16):2409–19.
28. Weerahandi S. Exact nonparametric methods. In: Exact statistical method for data analysis. New York: Springer-Verlag; 1995. p. 77–107.
29. Ott RL, Longnecker MT. Inferences comparing two population central values. In: An introduction to statistical methods and data analysis. 6th edition. Belmont (CA): Cengage Learning; 2008. p. 290–359.
30. Kendall MA. New measure of rank correlation. Biometrika 1938;30(1–2):81–9.
31. Clopper C, Pearson ES. The use of confidence or fiducial limits illustrated in the case of the binomial. Biometrika 1934;26:404–13.
32. Agresti A, Coull BA. Approximate is better than 'exact' for interval estimation of binomial proportions. Am Stat 1998;52:119–26.
33. Marshall JA, Scarbro S, Shetterly SM, et al. Improving power with repeated measures: diet and serum lipids. Am J Clin Nutr 1998;67(5):934–9.

34. Chatfield C. Analysing the data – 2: the initial examination of data. In: Problem solving: a statistician's guide. 2nd edition. Boca Raton (FL): CRC Press; 1995. p. 37–74.
35. Yu J, Liu L, Collins RL, et al. Analytical problems and suggestions in the analysis of behavioral economic demand curves. Multivariate Behav Res 2014;49(2): 178–92.

Can Chemical Mouthwash Agents Achieve Plaque/Gingivitis Control?

Fridus A. Van der Weijden, PhD[a],*, Eveline Van der Sluijs, MSc[a],
Sebastian G. Ciancio, DDS[b], Dagmar E. Slot, MSc, PhD[a]

KEYWORDS

- Dental plaque • Gingivitis • Mouthwash • Mouthrinse • Systematic review
- Meta-review

KEY POINTS

- Oral health is important since the mouth is the gateway to the human body. Bacteria are always present in the oral cavity and when not frequently removed the dental plaque biofilm leads to the development of oral disease.
- Over the past decades, the use of mouthwashes has become customary, usually following mechanical plaque biofilm control.
- Although people in industrialized countries use various oral hygiene products with the expectation of an oral health benefit, it is important that sufficient scientific evidence exists to support such claims.
- This meta-review summarized and appraised the current state of evidence that was based on systematic reviews, with respect to the efficacy of various active ingredients of over-the-counter chemotherapeutic mouthwash formulations for plaque control and managing gingivitis.
- Evidence suggests that a mouthwash containing chlorhexidine (CHX) is the first choice. The most reliable alternative for plaque control is essential oil (EO). No difference between CHX and EO with respect to gingivitis was observed.

Conflict of Interest and Source of Funding Statement: The authors declare that they have no conflict of interest. This study was self-funded by the authors and their institutions. Ethical approval was not required. D.E. Slot and F.A. Van der Weijden have formerly received external advisor fees, lecturer fees, or research grants from companies that produce mouthwash products. Among these were Colgate, Dentaid, GABA, Lactona, Oral-B, Philips, Procter & Gamble, Sara Lee, Sunstar, and Unilever. Similarly, S.G. Ciancio has interacted with Colgate, Johnson & Johnson, St. Renatus, Phoenix Dental, and Sunstar.
[a] Department of Periodontology, Academic Centre for Dentistry Amsterdam (ACTA), University of Amsterdam, VU University Amsterdam, Amsterdam, The Netherlands; [b] Department of Periodontics and Endodontics, University at Buffalo, The State University of New York, Buffalo, NY, USA
* Corresponding author. Academic Centre for Dentistry Amsterdam (ACTA), Department of Periodontology, Gustav Mahlerlaan 3004, 1081 LA, Amsterdam, The Netherlands.
E-mail address: ga.vd.weijden@acta.nl

Dent Clin N Am 59 (2015) 799–829
http://dx.doi.org/10.1016/j.cden.2015.06.002
0011-8532/15/$ – see front matter © 2015 Elsevier Inc. All rights reserved.

dental.theclinics.com

INTRODUCTION

The need to prevent human disease is well recognized and is related to making the occurrence or progression of a disease process unlikely or impossible. Oral health is important because the mouth is the gateway to the human body. Bacteria are always present in the oral cavity and when not frequently removed, the dental plaque biofilm leads to the development of oral disease. The merits of daily oral hygiene to oral health have long been understood.[1] Studies of tooth cleaning suggest that despite technological innovations, the level of mechanical oral hygiene practice is inadequate.[2–4]

The principle that plaque biofilm is the major etiologic factor causing gingivitis provides the justification for the use of antimicrobial mouth rinses.[5] The practice of mouth rinsing has been in use by humans for more than 2000 years. The first mouthwash advocated for dental plaque reduction seems to be urine from a child or, even better, from a newborn baby.[6] In the 1880s, Willoughby D. Miller (a dentist trained in microbiology) was the first to suggest the use of an antimicrobial mouthwash containing phenolic compounds to combat gingival inflammation.[7] Over the past decades, the use of mouthwashes has become customary, usually following mechanical plaque biofilm control. Mouthwashes are an ideal vehicle in which to incorporate chemicals and are appreciated by the public because of their ease of use, reduction of plaque biofilm, and breath-freshening effect.[8–10]

With keen competition between individual manufacturers vying for a percentage of this market, various claims for efficacy have been made, using numerous terms to describe efficacy. Although people in industrialized countries use various oral hygiene products with the expectation of an oral health benefit, it is important that sufficient scientific evidence exists to support such claims. Dental professionals have choices and make decisions every day as they advise their patients.[11] An evidence-based clinical decision integrates and concisely summarizes all relevant and important research evidence of acceptable quality that examines the same therapeutic question. The model to guide clinical decisions begins with original single random controlled clinical studies at its foundation. Syntheses (systematic reviews) build up from these to integrate the best available evidence from these original studies.[12] At the next level, a synopsis summarizes the findings of high-quality systematic reviews.[13,14] Meta-analyses (meta-review) in particular are appropriate for describing whether the current evidence base is complete or incomplete. The quantitative evidence is synthesized from relevant previous systematic reviews. The reason for including only systematic reviews is because this kind of research generally provides more evidence than separate empirical studies. Also in the presence of a significant increase in systematic reviews, meta-reviews give the dental community better guidance. From this perspective, it is a step forward in the direction of a clinical guideline.[15,16] Meta-reviews are a tool, a form of information, and guidance based on research evidence that assists the clinician in formulating the answer appropriate for each individual patient.[11]

Recently, 2 meta-reviews have been published that evaluate the efficacy of home-care regimens for mechanical plaque removal (toothbrushes and interdental cleaning devices) on plaque and gingivitis in adults.[2,3] The purpose of this article was to prepare a meta-review that summarizes the contemporary synthesized evidence with respect to the efficacy and safety of home-care self-support activities focusing on chemical agents in mouthwashes to manage plaque and gingivitis.

MATERIALS AND METHODS

The protocol of this meta-review detailing the evaluation method was developed using the AMSTAR[17] (a measurement tool to assess systematic reviews) tool to ensure the methodological quality of the review process.

Focused Question

What is the effect of mouthwashes and their various chemical ingredients for plaque biofilm control in managing gingivitis in adults based on evidence gathered from existing systematic reviews?

Search Strategy

For the comprehensive search strategy, several electronic databases were queried. Three Internet sources were used to search for appropriate articles that satisfied the study purpose. These sources included the National Library of Medicine, Washington, DC (MEDLINE-PubMed), the Cochrane Library, which also includes the DARE database of systematic reviews, and the evidence database of the American Dental Association (ADA) Center for Evidence-based Dentistry. All 3 databases were searched for eligible studies up to and including February 2015. The structured search strategy was designed to include any systematic review published on mouthwash products. For details regarding the search terms used, see **Box 1**. All of the reference lists of the selected studies were hand-searched for additional published work that could possibly meet the eligibility criteria of the study. The PROSPERO (2014) database, an international database of prospectively registered systematic reviews, was checked for reviews in progress. Further unpublished work was not sought.

Screening and Selection

Two reviewers (DES and EvdS) independently screened the titles and abstracts for eligible articles. If eligibility aspects were present in the title, the article was selected for further reading. If none of the eligibility aspects were mentioned in the title, the abstract was read in detail to screen for suitability. Inclusion of titles, abstracts, and ultimately full texts was based initially on full agreement between the 2 reviewers (DES and EvdS). In case of discrepancies, the final decision was made following discussion with GAW. No attempt was made to blind the reviewers to names of authors or institutions and journals while making the assessment. Hand searching of reference lists of reviews was conducted to ensure inclusion of additional published and potentially

---

Box 1
Search terms used for PubMed-MEDLINE, Cochrane Library, and American Dental Association Center for Evidence-based Dentistry

The search strategy was customized appropriately according to the database being searched, taking into account differences in controlled vocabulary and syntax rules.

The following strategy was used in the search mouthwashes:

{[MeSH Terms] Mouthwashes OR [text words] Mouthwashes OR Mouthwash OR mouthwash* OR mouthrinses OR mouthrinse}

Used filter/limits: systematic review OR meta-analysis

* Used as a truncation symbol.

relevant articles. When updates of systematic reviews were published, the latest version was selected. At the outset of this meta-review, no attempt was made to separate specific variables associated with mouthwashes.

Inclusion and Exclusion Criteria

The inclusion criteria were as follows:

- Systematic reviews (with or without a meta-analysis)
- Articles written in the English or Dutch language
- Reviews evaluating studies conducted on humans
  - ≥18 years old
  - In good general health
- Intervention: mouthwashes and their various chemical ingredients for plaque control and reducing gingivitis

The exclusion criteria were as follows:

- Orthodontic patients
- Dental implants

Data Extraction and Assessment of Heterogeneity

The articles that fulfilled all of the selection criteria were processed for data extraction. Information extracted from the studies included publication details, focused questions, search results, descriptive or meta-analysis outcomes, and conclusions. Systematic reviews were categorized by 2 authors (DES and EvdS) according to various active ingredients of mouthwashes. Categorization was confirmed with a second author (GAW). Disagreements between the reviewers were resolved by discussion.

The heterogeneity across studies was detailed according to the following factors:

- Study and subject characteristics
- Methodological heterogeneity (variability in review approach and risk of bias)
- Analysis performed (descriptive or meta-analysis)

Heterogeneity within the meta-analysis was tested by χ^2 test and the I^2 statistical. A χ^2 test resulting in a $P<.1$ was considered an indication of significant statistical heterogeneity. As a rough guide for assessing the possible magnitude of inconsistency across studies, an I^2 statistic of 0% to 40% was interpreted as not being important, and with an I^2 statistic higher than 40%, moderate (40%–80%) to considerable (>80%) heterogeneity may be present.[18]

Quality Assessment

Two reviewers (DES and EvdS) estimated the risk of bias by scoring the reporting and methodological quality of the included systematic reviews according to a combination of items described by the PRISMA[19] guideline for reporting systematic reviews and the[17] checklist for assessing the methodological quality of systematic reviews. A list of 27 items was assessed, and if all individual items were given a positive rating by summing these items, an overall score of 100% was obtained. Only systematic reviews including meta-analysis could achieve a full score of 100%.[20] The estimated risk of bias was interpreted as follows: 0% to 40% may represent a high risk of bias, 40% to 60% may represent a substantial risk of bias, 60% to

80% may represent a moderate risk of bias, and 80%–100% may represent a low risk of bias.[3]

Grading the 'Body of Evidence'

The Grading of Recommendations Assessment, Development, and Evaluation (GRADE) system, as proposed by the GRADE working group, was used to grade the evidence emerging from this meta-review of systematic reviews.[21] Two reviewers (DES and GAW) rated the quality of the evidence as well as the strength of the recommendations according to the following aspects: study design, risk of bias, consistency and precision among outcomes, directness of results, detection of publication bias, and magnitude of the effect.

RESULTS

Search and Selection Results

Fig. 1 describes the search process. A total of 306 unique articles were identified, from which 17 full-text articles were obtained and screened to confirm eligibility. One study was excluded because the data were summarized for a large variety of natural compounds and did not allow for an evaluation of individual ingredients.[22] Hand searching of the reference lists from these articles did not reveal any additional suitable systematic reviews. Neither did a search of the PROSPERO (International Prospective Register of Systematic Reviews) database (2014). Two papers by Gunsolley[23,24] provided data on the same meta-analysis. As a result, a final 15 systematic reviews were identified as being eligible for inclusion in this synopsis. Nine articles were identified that evaluated the efficacy of single active ingredients, of which 2 reviewed more than 1 ingredient.[23,24,26] Five studies compared active ingredients, of which 2 also contributed data for the singles active ingredients.[27,28] In one publication, a combination of 2 active ingredients was systematically evaluated.[29]

Study Outcomes and Assessment of Heterogeneity

Considerable heterogeneity was observed in the 15 systematic reviews with respect to the data bases searched, study and subject characteristics of the original individual articles, description of inclusion and exclusion criteria, quality assessment scale used, reporting of effect scores, presence of meta-analysis, and conclusions made. Because of this heterogeneity, a sophisticated level of data combination and analysis was neither possible nor indicated. A meta-analysis was therefore not undertaken. For the purpose of this synopsis, a summary of the selected systematic reviews was categorized and is presented by various chemical ingredients and ordered by common characteristics in **Table 1**.

Quality Assessment

Most reviews were considered to have a low to moderate estimated risk of bias (**Table 2**). Two studies were estimated to have a substantial risk of bias.[23–25] Critical items in this evaluation were the development of a protocol "a priori" and its registration, including non-English literature, contacting authors for additional information, grading obtained evidence, and the assessment of publication bias.

Active Ingredients

For details regarding the extracted data of the meta-analysis, difference of means, P values, 95% confidence intervals, and test of heterogeneity, please see **Table 3** for Plaque Index scores and **Table 4** for Gingival Index scores.

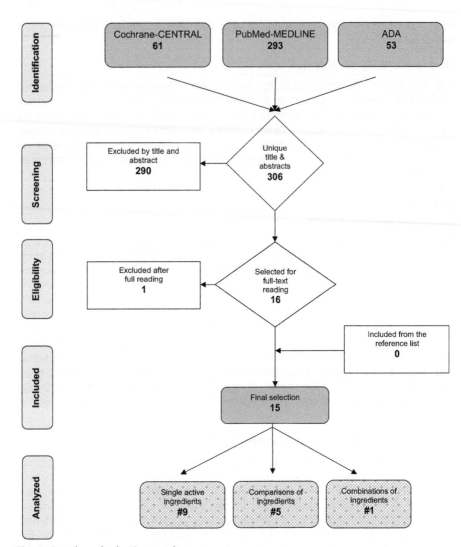

Fig. 1. Search and selection results.

Single Active Ingredients

Alexidine

Alexidine (ALX) is an antimicrobial of the biguanide class, and contains ethylhexyl end groups. This structure favors hydrophobic penetration into membrane lipids and electrostatic adhesion to the negative sites of cell membranes resulting in bactericidal activity. The systematic review by Serrano and colleagues[26] identified 2 articles and evaluated the adjunctive effect of ALX to toothbrushing in the prevention of plaque accumulation and gingival inflammation in studies with duration of 6 months or longer. The study outcome with respect to the Quigley and Hein[36] Plaque Index (PI) scores at the conclusion of the individual studies demonstrated a significant difference of means (DiffM) of −0.16, with nonsignificant heterogeneity ($I^2 = 39.5\%$). Data with respect to

Table 1
Overview of the characteristics of the included systematic reviews processed for data extraction

Author, (Year), Ingredient	Databases Searched	No. of Included Studies/ Trails, No. Involved Participants Base (End)	Leading Mode of Analysis	Original Review Authors' Conclusions	Comments of the Meta-Review Authors
Serrano et al,[26] 2015 Multiple ingredients	• PubMed	? studies ? (?)	Meta-analysis	Formulations with specific agents for chemical plaque control provide statistically significant improvements in terms of gingival bleeding and plaque indices.	TCL was assessed in the meta-analysis as a "pre-rinse" to toothbrushing, which is considered to provide an "indirect" effect because this is not a common daily oral hygiene habit.
Van Leeuwen et al,[30] 2014 EO	• PubMed-Medline • Cochrane-CENTRAL • EMBASE	5 studies 605 (534)	Meta-analysis	EOs produce an effect on plaque and gingivitis that extends beyond the vehicle solution.	Comparisons with vehicle control are frequently done with 5% hydro-alcohol, whereas a true placebo would contain 21.6%–26.9% alcohol.
Van Maanen-Schakel et al,[29] 2012 CHX + H_2O_2	• PubMed-Medline • Cochrane-CENTRAL • EMBASE • Trial registers • Others	4 studies 252 (229)	Meta-analysis	There is moderate evidence that a combination of CHX and an OA reduces tooth staining without interfering with plaque growth inhibition.	Tooth discoloration was considered as the primary outcome variable and plaque and gingivitis as secondary.
Van Strydonck et al,[18] 2012 CHX	• PubMed-Medline • Cochrane-CENTRAL • EMBASE	30 studies 34 experiments 3554 (2965)	Meta-analysis	There is strong evidence for the antiplaque and antigingivitis effects of a CHX rinse as an adjunct to regular oral hygiene in gingivitis patients; however, a significant increase in staining score was seen by CHX mouthrinse.	Staining as a side effect of CHX can affect patient compliance.

(continued on next page)

Table 1
(continued)

Author, (Year), Ingredient	Databases Searched	No. of Included Studies/ Trials, No. Involved Participants Base (End)	Leading Mode of Analysis	Original Review Authors' Conclusions	Comments of the Meta-Review Authors
Van Leeuwen et al,[31] 2011 EO vs CHX	• PubMed-Medline • Cochrane	19 studies 827 (?)	Meta-analysis	Long-term studies showed that CHX mouthwash was statistically more effective than EO with respect to plaque control; however, there was no significant difference with respect to reduction of gingival inflammation. Also, significantly more staining was observed with CHX compared with EO.	The evidence suggests that EO acts primarily through an anti-inflammatory process and is a reliable alternative to CHX for long-term control of gingival inflammation.
Hossainian et al,[28] 2011 H_2O_2	• PubMed-Medline • Cochrane-CENTRAL • EMBASE	10 studies 12 experiments 384 (363)	Descriptive analysis	H_2O_2 mouthwashes do not consistently prevent plaque accumulation when used as a short-term monotherapy. When used as a long-term adjunct to daily oral hygiene, the results of one study indicate that oxygenating mouthwashes reduce gingival redness.	A side effect of painful sensation in the mouth and/or erosive changes of the oral mucosa may occur.
Gunsolley,[23,24] 2006, 2010 Multiple ingredients	• Medline • Unpublished studies	? studies ? (?)	Meta-analysis	The studies provide strong evidence of the antiplaque and antigingivitis effects of multiple agents. It supports the use of mouthwashes as part of a daily oral hygiene.	The review methodology is unclear.

Study	Databases	Studies / Participants	Analysis	Conclusion	Comments
Afennich et al,[27] 2011 HEX	• PubMed-Medline • Cochrane- CENTRAL • EMBASE	6 studies 357 (336)	Descriptive analysis	HEX mouthwashes provide better effects regarding plaque reduction than placebo mouthwashes. They are less effective than CHX.	Higher HEX concentrations cause more side effects compared with lower concentrations.
Berchier et al,[32] 2010 CHX 0.12% vs 0.2%	• PubMed-Medline • Cochrane	8 studies 10 experiments 803 (?)	Meta-analysis	In the comparison, 0.12% and 0.2% CHX information concerning the effect on gingival inflammation was sparse. With respect to plaque inhibition, the results showed a small but significant difference in favor of the 0.2% CHX concentration.	The clinical relevance of the difference between the 2 concentrations was considered negligible. Several subanalyses are performed, such as rinsing duration, mouthwash solution with/without alcohol, manufacturer.
Haps et al,[33] 2008 CPC	• PubMed-Medline • Cochrane	8 studies 867 (?)	Meta-analysis	When used as an adjunct to either supervised or unsupervised oral hygiene, CPC-containing mouth rinses provide a small but significant additional benefit in reducing plaque accumulation and gingival inflammation.	The bioavailability and concentration of the active ingredient may influence its clinical efficacy.
Addy et al,[25] 2007 DEL	• Unknown	8 studies 913 (?)	Pooled weighted point estimate	DEL is effective as an adjunct measure for reducing plaque burden and indices of gingivitis, whether or not it is used under supervision.	No common method for meta-analysis was used.

(continued on next page)

Table 1
(continued)

Author, (Year), Ingredient	Databases Searched	No. of Included Studies/ Trails, No. Involved Participants Base (End)	Leading Mode of Analysis	Original Review Authors' Conclusions	Comments of the Meta-Review Authors
Stoeken et al,[34] 2007 EO	• PubMed-Medline • Cochrane	11 studies 2810 (2515)	Meta-analysis	EO provides an additional benefit to unsupervised oral hygiene with regard to plaque and gingivitis reduction as compared with a placebo or control.	Comparisons are also made to 5% hydro-alcohol, CHX and a group that uses floss.
Paraskevas & van der Weijden,[35] 2006 SnF$_2$	• PubMed-Medline • Cochrane-CENTRAL • EMBASE	3 studies concerning mouthwashes 781 (500)	Descriptive analysis	With regard to SnF$_2$, there is insufficient information on gingivitis and plaque to make any conclusions.	The effect of the combined use of SnF$_2$ dentifrice + SnF$_2$ mouthwash would be of interest.

Abbreviations: ?, unknown; CHX, chlorhexidine; CPC, cetylpyridinium chloride; DEL, delmopinol; EO, essential oils; H$_2$O$_2$, hydrogen peroxide; HEX, hexetidine; OA, oxygenating agents; SnF$_2$, stannous fluoride; TCL, triclosan.

Table 2
Estimated the risk of bias by scoring a list of items related to the reporting and methodological quality of the included systematic reviews

Author, Criteria	Addy et al, 25 2007	Afennich et al, 27 2010	Berchier et al, 32 2010	Gunsolley, 23,24 2006, 2010	Haps et al, 33 2008	Hossainian et al, 28 2011	Paraskevas & van der Weijden, 35 2006	Serrano et al, 26 2015	Stoeken et al, 34 2007	Van Leeuwen et al, 31 2011	Van Leeuwen et al, 30 2014	Van Maanen-Schakel et al, 29 2012	Van Strydonck et al, 18 2012
Defined outcome criteria of interest	+	+	+	+	+	+	+	+	+	+	+	+	+
Describes the rationale	+	+	+	+	+	+	+	+	+	+	+	+	+
Describes the focused (PICO) [S] question/hypothesis	+	+	+	+	+	+	+	+	+	+	+	+	+
Describes if a protocol was developed "a priori"	–	–	–	–	–	–	–	+	–	–	–	–	–
Protocol registration/publication	–	–	–	–	–	–	–	?	–	–	–	–	–
Presented eligibility criteria (in/	+	+	+	+	+	+	+	+	+	+	+	+	+

(continued on next page)

Table 2 *(continued)*

Author, Criteria	Addy et al, 25 2007	Afennich et al, 27 2010	Berchier et al, 32 2010	Gunsolley, 23,24 2006, 2010	Haps et al, 33 2008	Hossinian et al, 28 2011	Paraskevas & van der Weijden, 35 2006	Serrano et al, 26 2015	Stoeken et al, 34 2007	Van Leeuwen et al, 31 2011	Van Leeuwen et al, 30 2014	Van Maanen-Schakel et al, 29 2012	Van Strydonck et al, 18 2012
exclusion criteria)													
Presents the full search strategy	–	+	+	+	+	+	+	–	+	+	+	+	+
Various databases searched	?	+	+	–	+	+	+	+	+	+	+	+	+
Performed (hand) search in additional sources (f.i. grey literature or trial registers)	?	+	+	–	+	+	–	+	+	+	+	+	+
Review selection by more than 1 reviewer	–	+	+	+	+	+	+	+	+	+	+	+	+
Non-English articles included	?	–	–	–	–	–	–	–	–	–	–	+	–
Provide details on the performed	–	+	+	–	+	+	+	+	+	+	+	+	+

study selection process/flow chart											
Report included study characteristics	−	+	+	+	+	+	+	+	+	+	+
Provide data of the selected studies on the outcome measures of interest	+	+	+	+	+	+	+	+	+	+	+
Data were extracted by more than 1 reviewer	?	+	−	+	+	?	+	+	+	?	+
Contacted authors for additional information	+	?	+	?	?	?	+	+	+	?	+
Report heterogeneity of the included studies	−	+	+	+	+	+	+	+	+	+	+
Estimated risk of bias in individual studies	−	+	−	+	+	+	+	+	+	+	+
Performed a meta-analysis	+	−	+	+	−	+	+	+	+	+	+

(continued on next page)

Table 2 (continued)

Author, Criteria	Addy et al, 25 2007	Afennich et al, 27 2010	Berchier et al, 32 2010	Gunsolley, 23,24 2006, 2010	Haps et al, 33 2008	Hossainian et al, 28 2011	Paraskevas & van der Weijden, 35 2006	Serrano et al, 26 2015	Stoeken et al, 34 2007	Van Leeuwen et al, 31 2011	Van Leeuwen et al, 30 2014	Van Maanen-Schakel et al, 29 2012	Van Strydonck et al, 18 2012
Performed a descriptive analysis	–	+	+	+	+	+	+	–	+	+	+	+	+
Described additional subanalyses	+	+	+	–	+	+	–	+	+	+	–	+	+
Grading of the obtained evidence	–	–	–	–	–	–	–	–	–	–	+	+	+
Present limitations of the systematic review	–	–	–	–	–	+	+	+	+	–	+	+	+
Provide a conclusion	+	+	+	+	+	+	+	+	+	+	+	+	+

that respond to the objective												
Publication bias assessed	–	–	–	–	–	–	–	+	+	–	+	+	+
Funding source	–	+	+	+	–	+	–	+	+	+	+	+	+
Conflict of interest statement	+	+	+	+	–	+	–	+	+	+	+	+	+
Original authors estimated level of evidence	NR	NR	NR	NR	NR	NR	NR	NR	NR	NR	Moderate	Moderate	Strong
Current authors estimated quality score	52%	74%	78%	52%	70%	78%	63%	85%	81%	78%	85%	93%	89%
Current authors estimated risk of bias	Substantial	Moderate	Moderate	Substantial	Moderate	Moderate	Moderate	Low	Low	Low	Low	Low	Low

Each of the above items of the reporting and methodological quality item score list was given a rating of a plus (+) for informative description of the item at issue and a study design meeting the quality standard was assigned, plus-minus (±) was assigned if the item was incompletely described, ? when unknown, and minus (–) was used if the item was not described at all.[19]

For the quality assessment score, individual items with a positive rating were summed to obtain an overall percentage score.

Abbreviations: f.i; for instance; NR, not reported.

Table 3
Overview of data extraction of the included systematic reviews regarding plaque index scores

	Source		Outcomes			Heterogeneity	
Ingredient	Systematic Reviews	No. Experiments Included in MA	Difference of Means	95% CI	P	I^2, %	P^a
ALX	Serrano et al,[26] 2015	2	-0.16	-0.25 to -0.08	<.0001	39.5	ns
CPC	Gunsolley,[24] 2006	7	-15.4%	[]		[]	
	Haps et al,[33] 2008	7	-0.35	-0.47 to -0.24	<.00001	71.6	.002
	Serrano et al,[26] 2015	10	-0.39	-0.54 to -0.24	<.0001	93.9	.000
CHX	Gunsolley,[24] 2006	6	-40.4%	[]		[]	
	Van Strydonck et al,[18] 2012	5	-0.68	-0.85 to -0.51	<.00001	60.0	.06
	Serrano et al,[26] 2015	3	-0.64	-0.76 to -0.52	<.0001	47.4	ns
DEL	Addy et al,[25] 2007	8	-0.34	-0.39 to -0.29	<.00001	[]	
	Serrano et al,[26] 2015	3	-0.14	-0.23 to -0.06	.001	0	ns
EO	Gunsolley,[24] 2006	25	-27.0%	[]		[]	
	Stoeken et al,[34] 2007	7	-0.83	-1.13 to -0.53	.00001	96.1	<.00001
	Serrano et al,[26] 2015	9	-0.83	-1.05 to -0.60	.000	97.0	.000
HEX	Afennich et al,[27] 2011	[]	[]	[]		[]	
OA	Hossainian et al,[28] 2011	[]	[]	[]		[]	
SAN	Serrano et al,[26] 2015	1	-12.1%	[]		[]	
SnF$_2$	Paraskevas & van der Weijden,[35] 2006	[]	[]	[]		[]	
	Serrano et al,[26] 2015	2	-0.08	-0.26 to 0.10	ns	60.9	ns
TCL	Serrano et al,[26] 2015	3	-0.68	-0.85 to -0.51	<.0001	68.0	.04
0.12% CHX vs 0.2% CHX	Berchier et al,[32] 2010	9	-0.10	-0.17 to -0.03	.008	0	ns
EO vs CHX	Van Leeuwen et al,[31] 2011	5	-0.19	-0.30 to -0.08	<.0009	0	ns
OA plus CHX	Van Maanen-Schakel et al,[29] 2012	3	-0.10	-0.17 to -0.04	.003	0	.97

Abbreviations: [], no data available; ALX, alexidine; CHX, chlorhexidine; CPC, cetylpyridinium chloride; DEL, delmopinol; EO, essential oils; H_2O_2, hydrogen peroxide; HEX, hexetidine; MA, meta analyzis; OA, oxygenating agents; SAN, sanguinarine; SnF$_2$, stannous fluoride; TCL, triclosan.
[a] *P*>.1 is not significant (NS).

Table 4
Overview of data extraction of the included systematic reviews regarding the Gingival Index scores

Ingredient	Source		Outcomes			Heterogeneity	
	Systematic Reviews	No. Experiments Included in MA	Difference of Means	95% CI	P	I^2, %	P^a
ALX	Serrano et al,[26] 2015	1	−0.09	−024 to 0.07	ns	[]	[]
CPC	Gunsolley,[24] 2006	6	**−13.4%**	[]	[]	[]	[]
	Haps et al,[33] 2008	7	−0.15	−0.23 to −0.07	.0003	87.0	<.0001
	Serrano et al,[26] 2015	4	−0.33	−0.53 to −0.12	.002	95.3	.000
CHX	Gunsolley,[24] 2006	6	**−28.7%**	[]	[]	[]	[]
	Van Strydonck et al,[18] 2012	3	−0.24	−0.29 to −0.20	<.00001	87.0	.0005
	Serrano et al,[26] 2015	6	−0.17	−0.25 to −0.08	<.0001	59.5	.03
DEL	[]	[]	[]	[]	[]	[]	[]
EO	Gunsolley,[24] 2006	24	**−18.2%**	[]	[]	[]	[]
	Stoeken et al,[34] 2007	8	−0.14	−0.25 to −0.03	<.00001	75.4	.02
	Serrano et al,[26] 2015	2	−0.13	−0.19 to −0.07	<.0001	45.1	ns
HEX	Affenich et al,[27] 2011	[]	[]	[]	[]	[]	[]
OA	Hossainian et al,[28] 2011	[]	[]	[]	[]	[]	[]
SAN	Serrano et al,[26] 2015	1	**−2.8%**	[]	[]	[]	[]
SnF$_2$	Paraskevas & van der Weijden,[35] 2006	[]	[]	[]	[]	[]	[]
	Serrano et al,[26] 2015	2	−0.25	−0.43 to −0.07	.007	54.2	ns
TCL	Serrano et al,[26] 2015	3	−0.27	−0.31 to −0.24	<.0001	41.0	ns
0.12% CHX vs 0.2% CHX	Berchier et al,[32] 2010	[]	[]	[]	[]	[]	[]
EO vs CHX	Van Leeuwen et al,[31] 2011	4	−0.03	−0.16 to 0.09	ns	62.0	.05
OA plus CHX	Van Maanen-Schakel et al,[29] 2012	[]	[]	[]	[]	[]	[]

Abbreviations: [], no data available; ALX, alexidine; CHX, chlorhexidine; CPC, cetylpyridinium chloride; DEL, delmopinol; EO, essential oils; H_2O_2, hydrogen peroxide; HEX, hexetidine; MA, meta analyzis; OA, oxygenating agents; SAN, sanguinarine; SnF$_2$, stannous fluoride; TCL, triclosan.
[a] P>.1 is not significant (NS).

the Gingival Index (GI[37]) were based on one study and showed a nonsignificant mean difference of −0.09 as compared with the control group.

Cetylpyridinium chloride

Cetylpyridinium chloride (CPC) is a cationic quaternary ammonium compound with surface-active properties. Its mechanism of action relies on the hydrophilic part of the CPC molecule interacting with the bacterial cell membrane leading to loss of cell components, disruption of cell metabolism, inhibition of cell growth, and finally cell death. It has a broad antimicrobial spectrum, with rapid killing of gram-positive pathogens and yeast in particular. CPC may cause brown staining of teeth. The search retrieved 3 systematic reviews concerning the efficacy of CPC evaluating the adjunctive effect to toothbrushing in the prevention of plaque accumulation and gingival inflammation. The systematic review by Gunsolley[23,24] identified 7 articles in studies with a duration of 6 months or longer. The study outcome with respect to the PI at the finish of the individual studies demonstrated a weighted mean percentage reduction of 15.4% (SD 7.6). Data with respect to the GI showed weighted mean percentage reduction of 13.4% (SD 8.7).

The systematic review by Haps and colleagues[33] identified 8 articles in studies of 4 or more weeks' duration. The meta-analysis of PI scores at the end of the individual studies demonstrated a significant DiffM of −0.35, with moderate heterogeneity (I^2 = 71.6%). Data with respect to the GI showed a significant DiffM of −0.15 in favor of CPC as compared with the control group (considerable heterogeneity, I^2 = 87%). The most recent systematic review by Serrano and colleagues[26] identified 10 articles in studies of 6 or more months' duration. The study outcome with respect to the PI scores at the finish of the individual studies demonstrated a significant DiffM of −0.39, with considerable heterogeneity (I^2 = 93.9%). Data with respect to the GI showed a significant DiffM of −0.33 in favor of CPC as compared with the control group (considerable heterogeneity, I^2 = 95.3%).

Chlorhexidine

Chlorhexidine (CHX) is a cationic bisbiguanide that is active against gram-positive and gram-negative organisms, facultative anaerobes, aerobes, and yeasts. CHX lasts longer in the mouth than other mouthwashes (substantivity) and can cause stains on teeth, tongue, gingiva, and resin restorations. Prolonged use also can reduce bitter and salty taste sensations. CHX was first investigated more than 50 years ago and is currently one of the most widely used and thoroughly evaluated oral topical antiseptics.

The search retrieved 3 systematic reviews concerning the efficacy of CHX evaluating the adjunctive effect against toothbrushing in the prevention of plaque accumulation and gingival inflammation. The systematic review by Gunsolley[23,24] identified 6 articles in studies of 6 or more months' duration. The study outcome with respect to the PI at the finish of the individual studies demonstrated a weighted mean percentage reduction of 40.4% (SD 11.5). Data with respect to the GI[37] showed weighted mean percentage reduction of 28.7% (SD 6.5).

The systematic review by Van Strydonck and colleagues[18] identified 30 articles and evaluated the adjunctive effect of CHX to toothbrushing in the prevention of plaque accumulation and gingival inflammation in patients with gingivitis, including studies of 4 or more weeks' duration.

The meta-analysis of PI scores at the finish of the individual studies considered by the authors to be at "low risk" demonstrated a DiffM of −0.68, heterogeneity was not significant (I^2 = 60%). Data with respect to the GI showed a DiffM of −0.24, in favor of

CHX as compared with the control rinse (considerable heterogeneity, $I^2 = 87\%$). Relative to control, the reduction with CHX for plaque was calculated to be 33% and for gingivitis 26%. The CHX rinsing groups demonstrated significantly more staining.

The most recent systematic review by Serrano and colleagues[26] identified 14 articles in studies of 6 or more months' duration. The study outcome with respect to the PI scores at the finish of the individual studies demonstrated a significant DiffM of −0.64, with nonsignificant heterogeneity ($I^2 = 47.4\%$). Data with respect to the GI showed a significant DiffM of −0.17, in favor of CHX as compared with the control group (considerable heterogeneity, $I^2 = 95.3\%$).

Delmopinol

Delmopinol, an amino alcohol, is a third-generation antiplaque agent used as a mouthwash to reduce plaque and alleviate gingivitis. It has surface-active properties and creates an environment that will not allow plaque biofilm and bacteria to adhere.

The search retrieved 2 systematic reviews concerning the efficacy of CHX evaluating the adjunctive effect to toothbrushing in the prevention of plaque accumulation and gingival inflammation. The systematic review by Addy and colleagues[25] identified 8 studies with durations ranging from 8 to 24 weeks. Analyses for plaque and gingivitis based on aggregated data confirm the efficacy of delmopinol 0.2% over the placebo for PI scores, demonstrating a significant DiffM of −0.34. Data with respect to the GI were not available. Modified gingival index[38] scores and bleeding on probing (BOP) scores also showed a significant effect on gingivitis. Analysis also revealed no sustained heterogeneity of outcome, although the variable of BOP ranged considerably across the studies from less than 10% to greater than 30% (DiffM −2.8%).

The most recent systematic review by Serrano and colleagues[26] identified 3 articles in studies of 6 or more months' duration. The study outcome with respect to the PI scores at the finish of the individual studies demonstrated a significant DiffM of −0.14, with nonsignificant heterogeneity ($I^2 = 0\%$). Data with respect to the GI were not available. Modified GI[38] scores and BOP scores indicate a nonsignificant effect on gingivitis.

Essential oils

Essential oils (EOs) are used in an over-the-counter mouthwash containing a fixed formula of 2 phenol-related EOs, thymol 0.064% and eucalyptol 0.092%, mixed with menthol 0.042% and methyl salicylate 0.060% in a 22% alcohol vehicle. The antimicrobial mechanisms of action of EO against bacteria are complex. At high concentrations, there is disruption of the cell wall and precipitation of cell proteins, whereas at lower concentrations, there is inactivation of essential enzymes. Also, anti-inflammatory action has been proposed based on antioxidant activity. EOs also may cause staining of teeth.[39,40] The search retrieved 3 systematic reviews concerning the efficacy of EO evaluating the adjunctive effect to toothbrushing in the prevention of plaque accumulation and gingival inflammation. The systematic review by Gunsolley[23,24] identified 20 articles with a study duration of 6 or more months including unpublished data. The study outcome with respect to the PI at the finish of the individual studies demonstrated a weighted mean percentage reduction of 27% (SD 11.0). Data with respect to the GI showed weighted mean percentage reduction of 18.2% (SD 9.0).

The systematic review by Stoeken and colleagues[34] identified 11 studies with durations of 6 or more months. The study outcome with respect to the PI scores at the finish of the individual studies demonstrated a significant DiffM of −0.83, with considerable heterogeneity ($I^2 = 96.1\%$). Data with respect to the (modified) GI showed a significant DiffM of −0.14 in favor of CHX as compared with the control group (moderate heterogeneity, $I^2 = 75.4\%$). The most recent systematic review by Serrano and colleagues[26] identified 15 articles including studies of 6 or more months' duration. The study outcome with respect to the PI scores at the finish of the individual studies demonstrated a significant DiffM of −0.14, with nonsignificant heterogeneity ($I^2 = 0\%$). Data with respect to the GI showed a significant ($P<.0001$) DiffM of −0.13 in favor of CHX as compared with the control group (nonsignificant heterogeneity, $I^2 = 45.1\%$). Differences in modified GI scores also were significant and more pronounced (DiffM −0.54, 95% CI −0.76 to −0.31).

Hexetidine

Hexetidine (HEX) belongs to the group of pyrimidine derivatives. It is a broad-spectrum antiseptic, active in vitro and in vivo against gram-positive and gram-negative bacteria as well as yeast. However, oral retention appears to be limited so that the antimicrobial activity does not last long. The systematic review by Afennich and colleagues[27] identified 6 articles and evaluated the adjunctive effect of HEX to toothbrushing in the prevention of plaque accumulation and gingival inflammation in short-term (≤ 4 weeks) and long-term (≥ 4 weeks) study designs. The data that were retrieved did not allow for a meta-analysis. Therefore, a descriptive analysis was presented that showed that both in the short and long term, antiplaque effects can be expected; however, no concomitant effect on GI scores was observed.

Oxygenating agents

Oxygenating agents (OAs), such as hydrogen peroxide (H_2O_2), buffered sodium peroxyborate, and peroxycarbonate, have been recommended for short-term use as disinfectants. They exert antimicrobial effects through the release of oxygen. The systematic review by Hossainian and colleagues[28] identified 10 articles and evaluated the adjunctive effect of OA to toothbrushing in the prevention of plaque accumulation and gingival inflammation in short-term (≤ 4 weeks) and long-term (≥ 4 weeks) study designs. The data that were retrieved did not allow for a meta-analysis. Therefore, a descriptive analysis was presented that showed that OA mouthwashes do not consistently prevent plaque accumulation when used as a short-term monotherapy. When used as a long-term adjunct to daily oral hygiene, the results of one study indicate that OA mouthwash reduces gingival redness.

Sanguinarine

Sanguinarine (SAN) is a (toxic) quaternary ammonium salt from the group of benzylisoquinoline alkaloids. It is extracted from some plants, including bloodroot (*Sanguinaria canadensis*). It is also found in the root, stem, and leaves of the opium poppy. The systematic review by Serrano and colleagues[26] identified 1 article evaluating the adjunctive effect of SAN to toothbrushing in the prevention of plaque accumulation and gingival inflammation with 6 months' duration. The study outcome with respect to the PI at the finish of the study demonstrated a significant mean difference of 12.1% versus placebo and data with respect to the GI showed a nonsignificant mean difference of 2.8%.

Stannous fluoride

Tin fluoride, commonly referred to commercially as stannous fluoride (SnF_2) is a well-known agent that has been used in dentifrice formulations as early as the beginning of the 1940s. Apart from reducing the incidence of dental caries, it has antimicrobial effects and as such has been formulated in mouthwashes. The combination of tin and fluoride is difficult to formulate because of limited stability in an aqueous solution.

SnF_2 may cause a yellowish-brown staining of teeth. The search retrieved 2 systematic reviews concerning the efficacy of SnF_2 evaluating the adjunctive effect to toothbrushing in the prevention of plaque accumulation and gingival inflammation. The systematic review by Paraskevas and van der Weijden[35] identified 2 articles evaluating mouthwashes in studies with a duration of 6 or more months. The data that were retrieved did not allow for a meta-analysis. Therefore, a descriptive analysis was presented that showed that SnF_2 mouthwashes do not consistently prevent plaque accumulation or prevent gingivitis. The most recent systematic review by Serrano and colleagues[26] identified 3 articles in studies of 6 or more months' duration. The study outcome with respect to the PI scores at the finish of the individual studies demonstrated a nonsignificant DiffM of −0.08, with nonsignificant heterogeneity ($I^2 = 60.9\%$). Data with respect to the GI showed a significant DiffM of −0.25 in favor of CHX as compared with the control group (nonsignificant heterogeneity, $I^2 = 54.2\%$).

Triclosan
Triclosan (TCL) is a nonionic chlorinated aromatic compound that has functional groups representative of both ethers and phenols. It has antibacterial and antifungal properties and is applied in consumer products, including soaps and detergents. In mouthwash products it is combined with either zinc sulfate or a copolymer. The systematic review by Serrano and colleagues[26] identified 4 articles that evaluated the adjunctive effect of TCL as pre-rinse to toothbrushing in the prevention of plaque accumulation and gingival inflammation in studies of 6 or more months' duration. The study outcome with respect to the PI scores at the finish of the individual studies demonstrated a significant DiffM of −0.68, with moderate heterogeneity ($I^2 = 68\%$). Data with respect to GI showed a significant DiffM of −0.27 in favor of TCL as compared with the control group (nonsignificant heterogeneity, $I^2 = 41.0\%$).

Comparisons of Active Ingredients

Chlorhexidine 0.12% versus chlorhexidine 0.2%
In their systematic review, Berchier and colleagues[32] identified 8 articles evaluating the 2 CHX concentrations in relation to the prevention of plaque accumulation and gingival inflammation with no limits to study duration. With respect to the PI scores at the finish of the individual studies demonstrated a significant ($P = .008$) DiffM of −0.10 (95% CI −0.17 to −0.03), in favor of 0.2% CHX with nonsignificant heterogeneity ($I^2 = 0\%$). The investigators considered the clinical relevance of this difference likely to be negligible. Information concerning the effect on gingival inflammation was sparse. Descriptive analysis tended to show that there was no difference.

Essential oils versus chlorhexidine
The systematic review by Van Leeuwen and colleagues[31] identified 19 articles that evaluated the adjunctive effect of EO mouthwash against CHX in short-term (≤ 4 weeks) and long-term (≥ 4 weeks) study designs. Long-term studies evaluating the adjunctive effect to toothbrushing showed that, at the end of the studies, PI scores were reduced significantly ($P<.0009$) with DiffM of −0.19 (95% CI −0.30 to −0.08), in favor of CHX as compared with the EO group with nonsignificant heterogeneity ($I^2 = 0\%$). Data with respect to GI showed a nonsignificant DiffM of −0.03 (95% CI −0.16–0.09) with moderate heterogeneity ($I^2 = 62\%$, $P = .05$).

Essential oil versus alcohol solution
The systematic review by Van Leeuwen and colleagues[30] identified 5 articles that evaluated the adjunctive effect of EO mouthwash against an alcohol vehicle solution of 21.6 or 26.9% hydro-alcohol (V-Sol) in short-term (≤ 4 weeks) and long-term

(≥4 weeks) study designs. Long-term studies evaluating the adjunctive effect to tooth-brushing showed with respect to the PI scores at the finish of the individual studies a significant (P<.00001) DiffM of −0.39 (95% CI −0.47 to −0.30), in favor of EO with nonsignificant heterogeneity (I^2 = 0%). Data with respect to GI showed, in favor of EO, a significant (P<.00001) DiffM of −0.36 (95% CI −0.62 to −0.26), with consider-able heterogeneity (I^2 = 92%, P<.00004).

Hexetidine versus chlorhexidine
In their systematic review Afennich and colleagues[27] (see earlier in this article) showed in their descriptive analysis that HEX is consistently less effective in plaque reduction than a CHX mouthwash and also less effective in reducing gingival inflammation than a CHX mouthwash.

Oxygenating agents versus chlorhexidine
In their systematic review, Hossainian and colleagues[28] (see earlier in this article) showed in their descriptive analysis that OAs are consistently less effective in plaque reduction than a CHX mouthwash.

Combination of Active Ingredients

Chlorhexidine and oxygenating agents
In their systematic review, Van Maanen-Schakel and colleagues[29] identified 4 articles that evaluated the adjunctive effect of OA in combination with CHX in relation to the prevention of plaque accumulation and gingival inflammation with no limits to study duration. In their descriptive analysis, CHX in combination with OA showed no consis-tent difference in plaque or gingivitis reduction as compared with CHX mouthwash alone. Meta-analysis concerning the Silness and Löe PI (1964) showed a significant DiffM in favor of the combination (DiffM −0.10, 95% CI −0.17 to −0.04) with nonsig-nificant heterogeneity (I^2 = 0%). However, a significant (P = .02) reduction in staining was observed in the combination with OA (DiffM −0.27, 95% CI −0.49 to −0.05]), with nonsignificant heterogeneity (I^2 = 38%, P = .20).

Evidence Profile

Table 5 shows a summary of the various factors used to rate the body of evidence and strength of recommendations according to GRADE. There is strong evidence in sup-port of the efficacy of both CHX and EO that have a large beneficial effect on plaque reduction and a moderate effect on gingivitis. There is also strong evidence in support of the efficacy of CPC, which has a moderate beneficial effect on both plaque and gingivitis scores. There is moderate evidence for a small effect of ALX and for a large effect of TCL when used as pre-rinse before toothbrushing. Weak evidence emerged for small or indistinct effects of HEX, OA, SAN, and SnF_2.

DISCUSSION

This meta-review summarized the available evidence as was present in the form of systematic reviews with respect to the efficacy of mouthwash for plaque control in managing gingivitis. We included only systematic reviews because there are many such reviews available and this type of research generally provides more evidence than separate empirical studies taken alone.[15] There was strong consistent evidence emerging from 3 systematic reviews that evaluated CHX and EO showing that these ingredients are effective in plaque reduction. However, the evidence also shows mod-erate to considerable heterogeneity in the meta-analysis. In cases in which heteroge-neity is obvious, readers should exercise caution, as the DiffM may not provide an

Table 5
Estimated evidence profile[21] for the effect of various active ingredients of mouthwashes on dental plaque and gingival health

GRADE	ALX	CPC	CHX	DEL	EO	HEX	OA	SAN	SnF$_2$	TCL
Study Designs	Systematic Review n = 1	Systematic Review n = 3	Systematic Review n = 3	Systematic Review n = 2	Systematic Review n = 3	Systematic Review n = 1	Systematic Review n = 1	Systematic Review n = 1	Systematic Review n = 2	Systematic Review n = 1
Reporting and methodological estimated potential risk of bias	Low	Low to Substantial	Low to Substantial	Substantial	Low to Substantial	Moderate	Moderate	Low	Low to Moderate	Low
Consistency	Inconsistent	Consistent	Consistent	Fairly consistent	Consistent	Inconsistent	Inconsistent	Inconsistent	Inconsistent	Consistent
Heterogeneity	ND	Considerable	Considerable	ND	Considerable	ND	ND	ND	Moderate	Moderate
Directness	Direct	Direct	Direct	Direct	Direct	Indirect	Indirect	Direct	Direct	Indirect
Precision	Precise	Precise	Precise	Imprecise	Precise	Imprecise	Imprecise	Imprecise	Imprecise	Precise
Publication bias	Possible	Possible	Possible	Possible	Possible	Possible	Possible	Possible	Possible	Possible
Magnitude of the effect	Small	Moderate	Large	Small	Large	Indistinct	Indistinct	Small	Small	large
Body of evidence	Moderate	Strong	Strong	Weak	Strong	Weak	Weak	Weak	Weak	Moderate

Abbreviations: ALX, alexidine; CHX, chlorhexidine; CPC, cetylpyridinium chloride; DEL, delmopinol; EO, essential oils; HEX, hexetidine; ND, not determinable; OA, oxygenating agents; SAN, sanguinarine; SnF$_2$, tin (stannous) fluoride; TCL, triclosan.

exact measure of the results. It is therefore difficult to compare these 2 chemical agents based on the DiffM or make inferences that one ingredient would be more effective than the other. Only one review emerged that compared mouthwash ingredients[31] with a moderate estimated risk of bias and a quality score of 78%. It showed that in comparison to EO, CHX provided better results for plaque control. For the long-term control of gingival inflammation, EO was not different from CHX.

Grading

The steps toward guideline development involve formulating recommendations that clinicians and their patients should follow.[41] A variety of systems are used to rate the quality of the evidence underlying their recommendations. The GRADE working group has developed a common, sensible, and transparent approach to grading quality of evidence and strength of recommendations. Many international organizations have provided input into the development of the approach and have started using it. The strength of a recommendation indicates the extent to which one can be confident that the desirable effects of an intervention outweigh its undesirable effects. When a recommendation is weak, clinicians and other health care providers need to devote more time to the process of shared decision-making by which they ensure that the informed choice reflects individual values and preferences. This is likely to involve ensuring patients understand the implications of the choices they are making, possibly by using a formal decision aid. When recommendations are strong, clinicians may spend less time on the process of making a decision, and focus efforts on overcoming barriers to implementation or adherence. However, the strength of a recommendation may not be directly correlated with its priority for implementation.[42] Alternatively, in considering 2 or more possible management strategies, a recommendation's strength represents the confidence that the net benefit clearly favors one alternative or another. From this meta-review, 2 chemical agents emerged for which strong evidence with a large effect was available to recommend their use in mouthwash products. These were CHX and EO.

Side Effects

Various side effects have been reported for mouthwash products of which staining is a more common complaint following use of CHX, CPC, delmopinol (DEL) EO, and SnF_2. The staining can become worse when other products that are known to cause staining, such as tea, coffee, wine, and cigarettes, are consumed at the same time. One systematic review included in this meta-analysis showed that there is moderate evidence that a combination of CHX and an OA reduces tooth staining and also showed that it slightly but significantly increases inhibition of plaque growth.[29] Another issue is taste disturbance, which has been attributed to CHX, CPC, DEL EO, SAN, and HEX. For instance CHX, which tastes bitter, greatly reduces the perceived intensity of the salt.[43] The development of taste disturbance and tooth staining and the promotion of calculus formation does not permit the widespread long-term use of CHX as a daily adjunct to normal oral hygiene procedures.[18] CHX is therefore rather restricted to short-term to moderate-term use and in special clinical situations. A rare side effect that can be disturbing to the patient is parotid swelling, which has been reported after the use of both HEX and CHX.[44] The investigators of this case report concluded that parotid swelling may not be related to the type of mouthwash used, but may instead be a consequence of the rinsing action itself. Another potential adverse effect is a shift in the type or quantity of oral commensals. Virtually all of the main chemical plaque-control agents do not produce major shifts or development of resistant strains. When, on rare occasion, adverse effects on the oral microflora emerge, these effects quickly disappear when the chemical is discontinued.[8,45] Tissue disturbance has been reported for SAN, which is suspect for causing the formation of white lesions.[46] Although the available clinical and animal data provide no support that the use of a SAN mouthwash is causally associated,[47] its production has been discontinued.[48]

Chlorhexidine and sodium lauryl sulfate

Chemicals in mouthwash and dentifrice formulations can result in antagonism with reduction or negation of activity of one or both chemicals. In the broad search, 2 systematic reviews surfaced concerning the negative impact dentifrices containing sodium lauryl sulfate (SLS) may have on the efficacy of CHX mouthwash on the prevention of plaque accumulation and gingival inflammation. This interaction is not restricted to just CHX but any cationic antiseptic-containing mouthwash, such as CPC, making it essential that active mouthwash ingredients are evaluated for bioavailability under normal use. SLS is the most commonly used surfactant in dentifrices that, in addition to other properties, enhance the dentifrice foaming action. In their systematic review Kolahi and Soolari[49] identified an unclear number of articles that evaluated the effect of SLS in combination with CHX in relation to the prevention of plaque accumulation and gingival inflammation with no limits to study duration. There was not sufficient similarity between the included trails to combine them in a formal meta-analysis. Hence, the investigators declare that they used best evidence synthesis as an intelligent alternative for meta-analysis. They concluded that there are adequate reasons to believe CHX and SLS dentifrices are not compatible. Also, besides SLS, CHX may not be compatible with many anionic compounds found in dentifrices.[50]

More recently, Elkerbout and colleagues[51] also evaluated the effect of SLS in combination with CHX in relation to the prevention of plaque accumulation and gingival inflammation with no limits to study duration and identified 4 articles. The study outcome with respect to the PI scores at the finish of the individual studies demonstrated a nonsignificant DiffM of -0.08 (95% CI -0.26–0.11), with nonsignificant heterogeneity ($I^2 = 0\%$). No analysis with respect to gingivitis scores could be performed. The investigators concluded that there is moderate evidence to state that SLS dentifrice can be freely used in combination with CHX. Van Strydonck and colleagues[18] also noted that in most of the studies in their review CHX was always combined with regular oral hygiene procedures. However, this usage still showed a beneficial effect on oral health, which indicates that the impact of SLS may not be clinically relevant.

Substantivity and bioavailability

Mouthwashes are simply a means for delivery of active substances in the oral cavity where, after 20 to 30 seconds of rinsing, all surfaces of the dentition have come into contact with the mouthwash.[52] Most are composed of a water or water-alcohol base, with flavor, surfactant, and humectant added for their cosmetic properties. Mouthwashes and their active ingredients are exposed to the mouth for a relatively short period of time before expectoration from the mouth. In addition, the proteins present in saliva may reduce the activity of some substances.[53] The property of substantivity ensures that, at least for some chemicals (such as CHX), possible antibacterial effects are sustained for much longer periods of time.[45] Substantivity refers to the ability of an agent to be retained in the oral cavity and to be released over an extended period of time with retention of potency. The overall oral retention of an antiplaque agent is determined by the strength and rate of association of the agent with its receptor sites and the accessibility of these sites. The substantivity of an antiplaque agent and its clearance from the oral cavity are determined by the rate of dissociation of the agent from the receptor sites and the salivary composition and flow rate.[9] CHX is well known for its substantivity being retained in supragingival plaque, the tooth pellicle, and the oral soft tissues from where it exerts a plaque inhibitory effect that, within the oral cavity, may last up to 12 hours.[54]

It is noteworthy that the inclusion of a known active agent in a formulation does not guarantee efficacy, although it is often used to make piggy-back claims for new products. For instance, 2 recent systematic reviews have shown that CHX can be successfully formulated into a dentifrice/gel and will inhibit plaque growth to some degree, but not to the same extent as CHX incorporated into a mouthwash.[55,56] Many oral hygiene products are complex formulations, and the potential for ingredient interactions is great. Bioavailability is an issue that deserves attention when formulating a mouthwash. Formulations with high bioavailable CPC are associated with greater biological activity and therefore suggest an increased probability for clinical efficiency.[57]

Alcohol

Alcohol in mouthwashes is used to enhance flavor impact, to solubilize the flavor and some active ingredients, to provide some preservative power, and improve the transport of active ingredients into the dental plaque biofilm. The systematic review by Van Leeuwen and colleagues[30] indicated that the alcohol vehicle solution does not contribute to the efficacy of the mouthwash. Although the accumulated effects of mouthrinse usage with a high percentage of alcohol and ingestion of alcohol could theoretically predispose toward oral or pharyngeal carcinoma, the contributory effects of alcohol in these rinses are unclear and not considered proven[58] by most national regulatory organizations, including the US Food and Drug Administration.[59]

More recently, for various reasons, there has been an increase in the demand for alcohol-free mouthwashes.[60] An important determination is whether the inclusion or exclusion of alcohol could affect the activity of the mouthwashes. In the meta-analysis of Serrano and colleagues,[26] 10 studies evaluating EO included 9 mouthwash products that contained alcohol and 1 that did not. Based on this limited evidence, no major difference was observed (DiffM for alcohol -0.827 and mean difference alcohol free -0.746). Berchier and colleagues,[32] in their 0.12% versus 0.2% CHX article, performed a subanalysis on 0.12% CHX with/without alcohol as compared with 0.2% CHX with alcohol. The data show a trend that the nonalcohol product was slightly less effective.

There has been concern that alcohol from mouthwash products is being converted to acetaldehyde in the oral cavity, which then may cause DNA damage and lead to mutations. A meta-analysis of epidemiologic studies concerning mouthwash and oral cancer also specifically evaluating mouthwash products containing greater than 25% alcohol was performed by Gandini and colleagues.[61] The meta-analysis included 18 studies. No statistically significant associations (relative risk [RR]) were found between regular use of mouthwash and risk of oral cancer (RR 1.13; 95% CI 0.95–1.35). There was also no association reported use of mouthwash specifically containing alcohol and risk of oral cancer (RR 1.16; 95% CI 0.44–3.08). Based on their observations, the investigators came to the conclusion that based on the quantitative analysis of mouthwash use and oral malignancy, no statistically significant associations were revealed between mouthwash use and risk of oral cancer, nor was any significant trend observed in risk with increasing daily use, nor association between use of mouthwash containing alcohol and oral cancer risk.

Rinse Duration and Volume

The manufacturers of mouthwash products recommend different durations for the rinsing procedure. Keijser and colleagues[62] compared mouthwashes with various rinsing times. Results of the questionnaire indicated that the subjects preferred the shorter rinsing time, which raises the question of whether shorter rinsing times can be sufficient for effective plaque control. Another study assessed the plaque-inhibiting effect of a 0.2% CHX solution with 3 different rinsing times following a 72-hour nonbrushing period, this being 60 seconds as proposed by the manufacturer, and 2 shorter rinsing times of 30 seconds and 15 seconds.[63] The outcome did not reveal a significant difference in plaque development whether the subjects rinsed for 60, 30, or 15 seconds, which suggests that even 15 seconds may be long enough to reduce plaque levels. Berchier and colleagues[32] also showed that there is minimal difference between rinsing for 30 or 60 seconds on plaque scores. Further studies are needed to establish whether shorter rinsing times will be sufficient for effective gingivitis control. A consideration is that a shorter rinsing time could have a positive effect on compliance. Manufacturers also recommend different volumes, ranging from 10 to 20 mL. It seems relevant to have information about the mouthwash volume that is understood by the patient to ensure optimal compliance. One study assessed the volume of mouthwash with respect to patients' perceptions of comfort.[64] This study investigated volunteers' subjective perceptions to different volumes of mouthwash (volumes of 5, 10, 15, 20, and 30 mL) to establish the most comfortable volume of mouthwash with which to rinse. Based on the results of this experiment with a nonfoaming mouthwash, it was concluded that the most pleasant volume of mouthwash is 15 mL. This volume had a mean visual analogue scale (VAS) score that was closest to the optimal score. The differences between the mean VAS scores of rinsing with 15 mL and other volumes were statistically significant ($P<.001$).

Limitations of mouthwashes in the prevention of dental plaque formation

- The oral biofilm produces an encased and highly protective community of cells that acts as a barrier and as a result is much less influenced by its environment, including the introduction of chemical agents.[65] This aspect has received little attention in mouthwash studies.
- There appears to be a consensus that mouthwashes with antiplaque agents are not designed to be used in isolation and should be used in combination with mechanical cleaning.[8]
- For individuals with existing disease with frank periodontal pocketing, the use of vehicles such as mouthwash or dentifrice to deliver antimicrobial and antiplaque agents has only limited or no effects on the subgingival flora.[8,45] In these cases, chemical agents need to be placed directly into the subgingival environment by subgingival irrigation or by some alternative drug-release device. However, within minutes, gingival crevicular fluid outflow will dilute subgingivally applied antiseptics.[66]
- Only sparse information is available with respect to the efficacy of chemotherapeutic agents on biofilm-contaminated titanium surfaces.[67]
- Mouthwashes can also act as a vehicle in which to incorporate chemicals that promote fresh breath and help alleviate the problem of oral malodor. This aspect was not addressed by this meta-analysis. Systematic reviews have shown that due to very limited evidence, the potential effect of a specifically formulated mouthwash for treating oral malodor is, in general, unclear.[68,69]
- Publication bias cannot be ruled out. The results as presented in this meta-review may therefore provide a biased estimate of the true effect (overestimation) because there is a tendency to publish mainly positive studies.

Cost-effectiveness

The long-term adjunctive use of antiplaque agents in any vehicle other than dentifrice would have significant cost implications to the average family. At present prices, the cost of mouthwashes would be far greater than that of toothbrushes and dentifrice. This may be prohibitive for many individuals, and dentifrice is thus still the best vehicle for delivering antiplaque agents. Nonetheless, if a mouthwash is highly effective in terms of oral health gain, the additional cost of its use may be a price worth paying.[8] As emerged out of this review, this would apply particularly to CHX and EO mouthwashes.

SUMMARY

This meta-review summarized and appraised the current state of evidence based on systematic reviews, with respect to the efficacy of various active ingredients of over-the-counter chemotherapeutic mouthwash formulations for plaque control in managing gingivitis. Evidence suggests that a mouthwash containing CHX is the first choice. The most reliable alternative for plaque control is EO. No difference between CHX and EO with respect to gingivitis was observed.

ACKNOWLEDGMENTS

Because this is a synopsis of earlier work, parts of this article have been published before and therefore some duplication is inevitable. The authors thank Spiros Para-skevas for providing additional data concerning Stoeken and colleagues.[34]

REFERENCES

1. Axelsson P, Nyström B, Lindhe J. The long-term effect of a plaque control pro-gram on tooth mortality, caries and periodontal disease in adults. Results after 3 years of maintenance. J Clin Periodontol 2004;31:749–57.
2. Sälzer S, Slot DE, Van der Weijden FA, et al. Efficacy of inter-dental mechanical plaque control in managing gingivitis—a meta-review. J Clin Periodontol 2015; 42:S92–105.
3. Van der Weijden FA, Slot DE. Efficacy of homecare regimens for mechanical plaque removal in managing gingivitis: a meta review. J Clin Periodontol 2015;42:S77–91.
4. Van der Weijden F, Slot DE. Oral hygiene in the prevention of periodontal dis-eases: the evidence. Periodontol 2000 2011;55:104–23.
5. Löe H, Theilade E, Jensen SB. Experimental gingivitis in man. J Periodontol 1965; 36:177–87.
6. Weinberger B. Introduction to the history of dentistry. St Louis (MO): Mosby; 1948.
7. Jackson RJ. Metal salts, essential oils and phenols–old or new? Periodontol 2000 1997;15:63–73.
8. Moran JM. Chemical plaque control–prevention for the masses. Periodontol 2000 1997;15:109–17.
9. Cummins D, Creeth JE. Delivery of antiplaque agents from dentifrices, gels, and mouthwashes. J Dent Res 1992;71(7):1439–49.
10. Cummins D. Vehicles: how to deliver the goods. Periodontol 2000 1997;15:84–99.
11. Suvan JE, D'Aiuto F. Progressive, paralyzed, protected, perplexed? What are we doing? Int J Dent Hyg 2008;6:251–2.

12. Shea BJ, Grimshaw JM, Wells GA, et al. Development of AMSTAR: a measurement tool to assess the methodological quality of systematic reviews. BMC Med Res Methodol 2007;7:10.
13. Dicenso A, Bayley L, Haynes RB. Accessing pre-appraised evidence: fine-tuning the 5S model into a 6S model. Evid Based Nurs 2009;12(4):99–101.
14. Smith V, Devane D, Begley CM, et al. Methodology in conducting a systematic review of systematic reviews of healthcare interventions. BMC Med Res Methodol 2011;11:15–21.
15. Francke AL, Smit MC, de Veer AJ, et al. Factors influencing the implementation of clinical guidelines for health care professionals: a systematic meta-review. BMC Med Inform Decis Mak 2008;12:38.
16. Sarrami-Foroushani P, Travaglia J, Debono D, et al. Scoping meta-review: introducing a new methodology. Clin Transl Sci 2015;8:77–81.
17. AMSTAR tool 2007. A measurement tool to assess systematic reviews. Available at: http://amstar.ca/index.php. Accessed April 30, 2015.
18. Van Strydonck DA, Slot DE, Van der Velden U, et al. Effect of a chlorhexidine mouthrinse on plaque, gingival inflammation and staining in gingivitis patients: a systematic review. J Clin Periodontol 2012;39:1042–55 [studies selected for this meta-review].
19. PRISMA statement, Preferred Reporting Items for Systematic Reviews and Meta-Analyses. Available at: http://www.prismastatement.org/. Accessed April 30, 2015.
20. Hidding JT, Beurskens CH, van der Wees PJ, et al. Treatment related impairments in arm and shoulder in patients with breast cancer: a systematic review. PLoS One 2014;9:e96748.
21. GRADE Working Group. Grading of recommendations assessment, development and evaluation. 2011. Available at: http://www.gradeworkinggroup.org/. Accessed April 30, 2015.
22. Chen Y, Wong RW, McGrath C, et al. Natural compounds containing mouthrinses in the management of dental plaque and gingivitis: a systematic review. Clin Oral Investig 2014;18:1–16.
23. Gunsolley JC. Clinical efficacy of antimicrobial mouthrinses. J Dent 2010;38: S6–10 [studies selected for this meta-review].
24. Gunsolley JC. A meta-analysis of six-month studies of antiplaque and antigingivitis agents. J Am Dent Assoc 2006;137:1649–57 [studies selected for this meta-review].
25. Addy M, Moran J, Newcombe RG. Meta-analyses of studies of 0.2% delmopinol mouth rinse as an adjunct to gingival health and plaque control measures. J Clin Periodontol 2007;34:58–65 [studies selected for this meta-review].
26. Serrano J, Escribano M, Roldán S, et al. Efficacy of adjunctive anti-plaque chemical agents in managing gingivitis: a systematic review and meta-analysis. J Clin Periodontol 2015;42:S106–38 [studies selected for this meta-review].
27. Afennich F, Slot DE, Hossainian N, et al. The effect of hexetidine mouthwash on the prevention of plaque and gingival inflammation: a systematic review. Int J Dent Hyg 2011;9:182–90 [studies selected for this meta-review].
28. Hossainian N, Slot DE, Afennich F, et al. The effects of hydrogen peroxide mouthwashes on the prevention of plaque and gingival inflammation: a systematic review. Int J Dent Hyg 2011;9:171–81 [studies selected for this meta-review].
29. Van Maanen-Schakel NW, Slot DE, Bakker EW, et al. The effect of an oxygenating agent on chlorhexidine-induced extrinsic tooth staining: a systematic review. Int J Dent Hyg 2012;10:198–208 [studies selected for this meta-review].

30. Van Leeuwen MP, Slot DE, Van der Weijden GA. The effect of an essential-oils mouthrinse as compared to a vehicle solution on plaque and gingival inflammation: a systematic review and meta-analysis. Int J Dent Hyg 2014;12:160–7 [studies selected for this meta-review].
31. Van Leeuwen MP, Slot DE, Van der Weijden GA. Essential oils compared to chlorhexidine with respect to plaque and parameters of gingival inflammation: a systematic review. J Periodontol 2011;82:174–94 [studies selected for this meta-review].
32. Berchier CE, Slot DE, Van der Weijden GA. The efficacy of 0.12% chlorhexidine mouthrinse compared with 0.2% on plaque accumulation and periodontal parameters: a systematic review. J Clin Periodontol 2010;37:829–39 [studies selected for this meta-review].
33. Haps S, Slot DE, Berchier CE, et al. The effect of cetylpyridinium chloride-containing mouth rinses as adjuncts to toothbrushing on plaque and parameters of gingival inflammation: a systematic review. Int J Dent Hyg 2008;6:290–303 [studies selected for this meta-review].
34. Stoeken JE, Paraskevas S, van der Weijden GA. The long-term effect of a mouthrinse containing essential oils on dental plaque and gingivitis: a systematic review. J Periodontol 2007;78:1218–28 [studies selected for this meta-review].
35. Paraskevas S, van der Weijden GA. A review of the effects of stannous fluoride on gingivitis. J Clin Periodontol 2006;33:1–13 [studies selected for this meta-review].
36. Quigley GA, Hein JW. Comparative cleansing efficiency of manual and power brushing. J Am Dent Assoc 1962;65:26–9.
37. Löe H, Silness J. Periodontal disease in pregnancy. I. Prevalence and severity. Acta Odontol Scand 1963;21:533–51.
38. Lobene RR. A clinical study of the anticalculus effect of a dentifrice containing soluble pyrophosphate and sodium fluoride. Clin Prev Dent 1986;8:5–7.
39. Addy M, Moran J, Newcombe R, et al. The comparative tea staining potential of phenolic, chlorhexidine and anti-adhesive mouthrinses. J Clin Periodontol 1995;22:923–8.
40. Grossman E, Meckel AH, Isaacs RL, et al. A clinical comparison of antibacterial mouthrinses: effects of chlorhexidine, phenolics, and sanguinarine on dental plaque and gingivitis. J Periodontol 1989;60:435–40.
41. Jaeschke R, Guyatt GH, Dellinger P, et al. Use of GRADE grid to reach decisions on clinical practice guidelines when consensus is elusive. BMJ 2008;337:a744.
42. Andrews J, Guyatt G, Oxman AD, et al. GRADE guidelines: 14. Going from evidence to recommendations: the significance and presentation of recommendations. J Clin Epidemiol 2013;66:719–25.
43. Frank ME, Gent JF, Hettinger TP. Effects of chlorhexidine on human taste perception. Physiol Behav 2001;74:85–99.
44. Van der Weijden GA, Ten Heggeler JM, Slot DE, et al. Parotid gland swelling following mouthrinse use. Int J Dent Hyg 2010;8:276–9.
45. Moran JM. Home-use oral hygiene products: mouthrinses. Periodontol 2000 2008;48:42–53.
46. Mascarenhas AK, Allen CM, Loudon J. The association between Viadent use and oral leukoplakia. Epidemiology 2001;12:741–3.
47. Munro IC, Delzell ES, Nestmann ER, et al. Viadent usage and oral leukoplakia: a spurious association. Regul Toxicol Pharmacol 1999;30:182–96.
48. Vlachojannis C, Magora F, Chrubasik S. Rise and fall of oral health products with Canadian bloodroot extract. Phytother Res 2012;26:1423–6.
49. Kolahi J, Soolari A. Rinsing with chlorhexidine gluconate solution after brushing and flossing teeth: a systematic review of effectiveness. Quintessence Int 2006;37:605–12.

50. Sweetman SC, editor. Martindale: the complete drug reference. 33rd edition. London: PhP Pharmaceutical Press; 2002. p. 1138–40.
51. Elkerbout TA, Slot DE, Bakker E, et al. Chlorhexidine mouthwash and sodium lauryl sulphate dentifrice: do they mix effectively or interfere? Int J Dent Hyg 2015. [Epub ahead of print].
52. Paraskevas S, Danser MM, Timmerman MF, et al. Optimal rinsing time for intra-oral distribution (spread) of mouthwashes. J Clin Periodontol 2005;32:665–9.
53. Asadoorian J. Canadian Dental Hygienists Association position paper on commercially available, over-the-counter oral rinsing products. Can J Dent Hyg 2006;40(4):1–13.
54. Tomás I, Cousido MC, García-Caballero L, et al. Substantivity of a single chlorhexidine mouthwash on salivary flora: influence of intrinsic and extrinsic factors. J Dent 2010;38:541–6.
55. Slot DE, Berchier CE, Addy M, et al. The efficacy of chlorhexidine dentifrice or gel on plaque, clinical parameters of gingival inflammation and tooth discoloration: a systematic review. Int J Dent Hyg 2014;12:25–35.
56. Supranoto SC, Slot DE, Addy M, et al. The effect of chlorhexidine dentifrice or gel versus chlorhexidine mouthwash on plaque, gingivitis, bleeding and tooth discoloration: a systematic review. Int J Dent Hyg 2015;13:83–92.
57. Versteeg PA, Rosema NA, Hoenderdos NL, et al. The plaque inhibitory effect of a CPC mouthrinse in a 3-day plaque accumulation model – a cross-over study. Int J Dent Hyg 2010;8:269–75.
58. Elmore JG, Horowitz RI. Oral cancer and mouthwash use: evaluation of the epidemiological evidence. Otolaryngol Head Neck Surg 1995;113:253–61.
59. FDA. Oral health care drug products for over-the-counter human use: tentative final monograph for oral antiseptic drug products. Fed Regist 1994;59:6084–124.
60. Pereira EM, da Silva JL, Silva FF, et al. Clinical evidence of the efficacy of a mouthwash containing propolis for the control of plaque and gingivitis: a phase II study. Evid Based Complement Alternat Med 2011;2011:750249.
61. Gandini S, Negri E, Boffetta P, et al. Mouthwash and oral cancer risk quantitative meta-analysis of epidemiologic studies. Ann Agric Environ Med 2012;19:173–80.
62. Keijser JA, Verkade H, Timmerman MF, et al. Comparison of 2 commercially available chlorhexidine mouthrinses. J Periodontol 2003;74:214–8.
63. Van der Weijden GA, Timmerman MF, Novotny AG, et al. Three different rinsing times and inhibition of plaque accumulation with chlorhexidine. J Clin Periodontol 2005;32:89–92.
64. Keukenmeester RS, Slot DE, Rosema NA, et al. Determination of a comfortable volume of mouthwash for rinsing. Int J Dent Hyg 2012;10:169–74.
65. Auschill TM, Hein N, Hellwig E, et al. Effect of two antimicrobial agents on early in situ biofilm formation. J Clin Periodontol 2005;32(2):147–52.
66. Binder TA, Goodson JM, Socransky SS. Gingival fluid levels of acid and alkaline phosphatase. J Periodontal Res 1987;22:14–9.
67. Ntrouka VI, Slot DE, Louropoulou A, et al. The effect of chemotherapeutic agents on contaminated titanium surfaces: a systematic review. Clin Oral Implants Res 2011;22:681–90.
68. Blom T, Slot DE, Quirynen M, et al. The effect of mouthrinses on oral malodor: a systematic review. Int J Dent Hyg 2012;10:209–22.
69. Slot DE, De Geest S, van der Weijden FA, et al. Treatment of oral malodour. Medium-term efficacy of mechanical and/or chemical agents: a systematic review. J Clin Periodontol 2015;42:S303–16.

Is Photodynamic Therapy an Effective Treatment for Periodontal and Peri-Implant Infections?

Anton Sculean, DMD, Dr med dent, MS, PhD[a],*, Akira Aoki, DDS, PhD[b],
George Romanos, DDS, PhD, Prof Dr med dent[c], Frank Schwarz, Prof Dr med dent[d],
Richard J. Miron, DDS, MS, PhD[a], Raluca Cosgarea, DDS, Dr med dent[e,f]

KEYWORDS

- Photodynamic therapy • Chronic periodontitis • Aggressive periodontitis
- Peri-implantitis • Bacterial biofilm

KEY POINTS

- Antimicrobial photodynamic therapy (PDT) has lately attracted much attention among clinicians for the treatment of pathogenic biofilm associated with peridontitis and peri-implantitis.
- At present, the data from randomized controlled clinical studies (RCTs) are still limited and, to some extent, controversial, which makes it difficult to provide appropriate recommendations for the clinician.
- The aims of the present study were: (a) to provide an overview on the current evidence from RCTs evaluating the potential clinical benefit for the additional use of PDT to subgingival mechanical debridement (ie, scaling and root planing [SRP]) alone in nonsurgical periodontal therapy; and (b) to provide clinical recommendations for the use of PDT in periodontal practice.
- In patients with chronic periodontitis (ChP), the combination of SRP and PDT may result in substantially higher short-term clinical improvements evidenced by probing depth or bleeding on probing reductions compared with SRP alone.
- In patients with aggressive periodontitis, the use of PDT cannot replace the systemic administration of amoxicillin and metronidazole. Because of the lack of data, no conclusions can be made to what extent PDT may replace the use of systemic antibiotics in patients with ChP.
- Limited evidence from one study indicates that PDT may represent a possible alternative to local antibiotics in patients with incipient peri-implantitis.

---

[a] Department of Periodontology, School of Dental Medicine, University of Bern, Freiburgstr. 7, 3010 Bern, Switzerland; [b] Department of Periodontology, Graduate School of Medical and Dental Sciences, Tokyo Medical and Dental University (TMDU), 1-5-45 Yushima, Bunkyo-ku, Tokyo 113-8510, Japan; [c] Department of Periodontology, School of Dental Medicine, Stony Brook University, Stony Brook, NY 11794, USA; [d] Department of Oral Surgery, Heinrich Heine University, Moorenstr. 5, 40225 Düsseldorf, Germany; [e] Department of Periodontology, Philipps University Marburg, Georg-Voigt-Str. 3, 35039 Marburg, Germany; [f] Department of Prosthodontics, Iuliu Hatieganu University, Clinicilor str. 32, 400506 Cluj-Napoca, Romania
* Corresponding author. Department of Periodontology, School of Dental Medicine, University of Bern, Freiburgstrasse 7, Bern 3010, Switzerland.
E-mail address: anton.sculean@zmk.unibe.ch

Dent Clin N Am 59 (2015) 831–858
http://dx.doi.org/10.1016/j.cden.2015.06.008
0011-8532/15/$ – see front matter © 2015 Elsevier Inc. All rights reserved.

dental.theclinics.com

BIOLOGICAL RATIONALE

Periodontitis is a multifactorial disease that is associated with loss of the supporting tissues (ie, periodontal ligament and alveolar bone) around the tooth.[1] A major objective of periodontal therapy is to remove soft and hard, supragingival and subgingival deposits from the root surface in order to stop disease progression.[2] Numerous studies have reported significant improvements of clinical and microbial parameters following nonsurgical periodontal therapy.[3–6]

Despite that nonsurgical periodontal treatment may result in significant clinical improvements in the great majority of cases, evidence indicates that none of the currently available instrumentation techniques are effective in completely eliminating subgingival bacterial biofilm.[7] These limitations may be attributed to several factors, such as the complex anatomy of teeth (ie, furcation involvements, root invaginations); the presence of intrabony defects, and others; mechanical limitations related to the size of instruments, or invasion of periodontal pathogens into the surrounding soft tissues, or possible recolonization of periodontal pockets from other diseased sites or intraoral niches.[8] Power-driven instruments (ie, sonic and ultrasonic scalers) have been introduced to further enhance the effectiveness of scaling and root planing (SRP). However, findings from clinical studies have also shown comparative outcomes following power-driven and manual instrumentation.[9] Thus, the current evidence indicates that nonsurgical periodontal treatment may result in substantial clinical improvements in most cases, but none of the currently available instrumentation techniques are able to completely eliminate subgingival bacteria and calculus.[7]

Photodynamic therapy (PDT), also called photoradiation therapy, phototherapy, photochemotherapy, photo-activated disinfection (PAD), or light-activated disinfection (LAD), was introduced in medical therapy in 1904 as the light-induced inactivation of cells, microorganisms, or molecules and involves the combination of visible light, usually through the use of a diode laser and a photosensitizer.[10] The photosensitizer (**Fig. 1**) is a substance that is capable of absorbing light of a specific wavelength and transforming it into useful energy. Each factor is harmless by itself, but when combined, can produce lethal cytotoxic agents that can selectively destroy cells.[11] Thus, PDT has been proposed as a modality to reduce bacterial load or even to eliminate periodontal pathogens.[12,13]

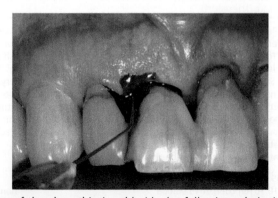

Fig. 1. Application of the phenothiazine chloride dye following subgingival SRP.

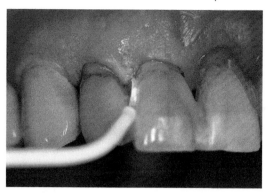

Fig. 2. Application of the low-level laser light into the pocket.

The action mechanism of PDT has been extensively described previously.[14] Briefly, on illumination (**Fig. 2**), the photosensitizer (See **Fig. 1**) is excited from the ground state to the triplet state. The longer lifetime of the triplet state enables the interaction of the excited photosensitizer with the surrounding molecules. It is anticipated that the generation of the cytotoxic species produced during PDT occurs while in this state.[15,16] The cytotoxic product, usually singlet oxygen ($^1O_2$), cannot migrate at a distance more than 0.02 μm after its formation, thus making it ideal for local application of PDT, without endangering distant molecules, cells, or organs.[16]

In vitro studies have revealed that light from a Helium/Neon (He/Ne) laser or a Gallium-Aluminum-Arsenide (GaAlAs) laser, in combination with appropriate photosensitizers, can achieve a significant reduction in the viability of both aerobic and anaerobic bacteria in a solution of subgingival plaque from patients with chronic periodontitis (ChP).[17,18] Dobson and Wilson[19] have shown that bacteria associated with periodontal disease can be killed through photosensitization with Toluidine blue–O and irradiation with a He/Ne soft laser. Subsequent studies in animals have shown PDT was distinctly advantageous in reducing the periodontal signs of redness and bleeding on probing (BOP), and significantly suppressed *Porphyromonas gingivalis*.[20]

During the last decade, considerable interest has evolved in evaluating the use of PDT in the treatment of periodontal and peri-implant infections. However, despite the relatively abundant literature, the data on the clinical relevance of PDT when used in conjunction with mechanical therapy are still controversial and difficult to interpret for the clinician. Therefore, the aims of this review article are (a) to provide an overview of the current evidence from randomized controlled clinical studies (RCTs) evaluating the potential clinical benefit for the additional use of PDT to mechanical debridement alone in nonsurgical periodontal therapy; and (b) to provide clinical recommendations for the use of PDT in periodontal practice.

USE OF PHOTODYNAMIC THERAPY AS ADJUNCT TO NONSURGICAL PERIODONTAL THERAPY IN PATIENTS WITH UNTREATED CHRONIC PERIODONTITIS

A total of 18 RCTs have compared the potential additional benefit of PDT to SRP with the use of SRP alone in untreated periodontitis patients (**Table 1**). Eight of the 18 studies have reported statistically significantly higher improvements in probing depth (PD) reduction and clinical attachment (CAL) gain following SRP + PDT compared with SRP alone,[21–28] whereas the rest of 10 studies have failed to reveal statistically

Table 1

PDT as initial periodontal therapy in patients with ChP (data of 18 studies reported in 19 publications)

Study, Author, Year, Country, Type	Patients, Female/Male, Diagnosis Age, Smokers	Study Duration	Treatment	Photosensitizer Laser	Laser Parameters	Microbiology	Immunology	PD Reduction (mm), CAL Gain (mm), BOP Reduction (%)
Al-Zahrani & Austah,[21] 2011, Saudi Arabia, Split-mouth, RCT	ChP n = 17 0/17 41.6 ± 9.6 17 smokers	3 mo	Test: SRP + PDT (1×) Control: SRP	Methylene blue (Ondine's Periowave, Ondine Biopharma, Vancouver, BC, Canada) Diode laser	Wavelength 670 nm	Not analyzed	Not analyzed	Test: PD: from 5.60 ± 0.83 to 3.84 ± 0.85* CAL: from 6.30 ± 1.44 to 4.70 ± 1.27* BOP: from 74.50 ± 21.50 to 41.90 ± 22.30 (n.s.) Control: PD: from 5.35 ± 0.46 to 3.90 ± 0.75
Alwaeli et al,[22] 2015, Jordan, Split-mouth, RCT	ChP N = 16 11/5 40.9 ± 13.34	12 mo	Test: SRP + PDT Control: SRP	Phenothiazine chloride Diode Lasers (HELBO, Photodynamic Systems)	Wavelength 660 nm Output power 100 mW Application time: 10 s/site, 6 sites/tooth	Not analyzed	Not analyzed	Test: PD: 1.51 ± 1.54* CAL: 1.48 ± 1.89* BOP: 25%* Control: PD: 0.66 ± 1.66 CAL: 0.13 ± 1.7 BOP: 54%
Andersen et al,[23] 2007, England, Parallel, RCT	ChP N = 33 22/11 53 (18–75) Unclear	12 wk	Test 1: PDT Test 2: SRP + PDT Control: SRP	Methylene blue (Periowave) Diode laser (Periowave)	Wavelength 670 nm Energy density 10–20 J/cm² Max. power 150 mW Application time 60 s/site	Not analyzed	Not analyzed	Test 1: PD: 0.67 ± 0.44 (n.r.) CAL: 0.14 ± 0.65 (n.r.) BOP: 73% (n.r.) Test 2: PD: 1.11 ± 0.53* CAL: 0.86 ± 0.61* BOP: 59% (n.s.) Control: PD: 0.74 ± 0.43 CAL: 0.36 ± 0.35 BOP: 56%

Study	Diagnosis	Patients	Follow-up	Groups	Photosensitizer / Laser	Laser parameters			Results
Balata et al,[30] 2013, Brazil, Split-mouth, RCT	ChP	N = 22 43.18 (31–62)	6 mo	Test: SRP (ultrasonic) + PDT Control: SRP (ultrasonic)	Methylene blue 0.005% Low power laser (AsGaAl, Photon Laser III, Sao Paulo, Brazil)	Wavelength 660 nm Output power 100 mW Energy density 320 J/cm² Dose 9 J Diameter tip 600 μm Application time: 90 s/site	Not analyzed	Not analyzed	Test: PD decrease from 5.11 ± 0.56 to 2.83 ± 0.47 (n.s.) CAL change from 5.49 ± 0.76 to 3.41 ± 0.84 (n.s.) BOP: from 61.58 ± 15.64 to 36.73 ± 19.72 (n.s.) Control: PD decrease from 5.15 ± 0.46 to 2.83 ± 0.40 CAL change from 5.53 ± 0.54 to 3.39 ± 0.51 BOP: from 62.23 ± 16.91 to 38.49 ± 20.52
Berakdar et al,[24] 2012, Germany, Split-mouth, RCT	ChP	N = 22 10/12 59.3 ± 11.7 No smokers	6 mo	Test: SRP + PDT Control: SRP	Methylene blue 0.005% Diode laser (Periowave)	Wavelength 670 nm Max. power 150 mW Application time 60 s	Not analyzed	Not analyzed	Test: PD: 2.9 ± 0.8* CAL: n.s. changes n.r. BOP: from 100% to 13.6% n.s. Control: PD: 2.4 ± 0.8 BOP: from 100% to 22.7% CAL gain: n.s.

(continued on next page)

Table 1
(continued)

Study, Author, Year, Country, Type	Diagnosis	Patients, Female/Male, Age, Smokers	Study Duration	Treatment	Photosensitizer Laser	Laser Parameters	Microbiology	Immunology	PD Reduction (mm), CAL Gain (mm), BOP Reduction (%)
Betsy et al,[25] 2014, India, Parallel, RCT	ChP	N = 88 51/39 39.6 ± 8.7	6 mo	Test: SRP + PDT Control: SRP	Phenothiazine chloride trihydrate (freshly prepared, Sigma-Aldrich, St. Louis, MO, USA) Diode laser (CNI Opto-electronics Tech Co Ltd, Changchun, China)	Wavelength 655 nm, output power 1 W Power density 60 mW/cm^2 Diameter tip 0.5 mm Application time 60 s/site	Not analyzed	Not analyzed	Test: PD: from 5.7 (5.0–6.0,1.0) to 3.0 (2.0–6.0, 1.0)* CAL: from 6.5 (5.0–8.0, 1.4) to 4.0 (2.6–7.0, 2.0)* BOP: data n.r. Control: PD: from 5.5 (4.2–6.0, 1.0) to 4.0 (2.0–6.0, 1.0) CAL: from 6.0 (4.2–8.0, 1.7) to 4.5 (2.0–7.0, 2.0) BOP: data n.r.
Braun et al,[26] 2008, Germany, Split-mouth	ChP	N = 20 11/9 46.6 ± 6.1 No smokers	3 mo	Test: SRP + PDT Control: SRP	Phenothiazine chloride (HELBO Photodynamic System, Austria)	Wavelength 660 nm Power output 100 mW Application time 10 s/site	Not analyzed	Not analyzed	Test: Median (interquartile range, Max, Min) PD: 3.6 (0.6, 5.3, 3.2)* CAL: 7.04 (1.63, 9.11, 5.33)* BOP: 19 (11, 64, 2)* Control: Median (interquartile range, Max, Min) PD: 3.7 (0.6, 6.0, 3.4) CAL: 7.25 (2.02, 10.09, 5.61) BOP: 24 (21, 61, 2)

Christodoulides et al,[31] 2008, Parallel, RCT	N = 24 13/11 45 ± 8.11 3 smokers	6 mo	Test: SRP + PDT Control: SRP	Phenothiazine chloride (HELBO Blue Photosensitizer) Diode laser (HELBO TheraLite Laser)	Wavelength 670 nm Output power 75 mW Application time 60 s/tooth	No significant differences between the groups for *A.a., P.g., T.f., T.d., P.i., P.m., F.n., C.r., E.n., E.c., C.s.*	Not analyzed	Test: PD: 0.9 ± 0.3 (n.s.) CAL: 0.7 ± 0.3 (n.s.) BOP: from 54 ± 16% to 10 ± 5%* Control: PD: 0.7 ± 0.7 CAL: 0.5 ± 0.5 BOP: from 59 ± 21% to 20 ± 4%
Dilsiz et al,[27] 2013, Turkey, Split-mouth, RCT	N = 24 14/10 40.7 ± 7.3 No smokers	6 mo	Test 1: PDT + SRP Test 2: KTPL + SRP Control: SRP	Methylene blue 1% Diode laser (Doctor Smile diode, Lambda Scientifica, Vincenza, Italy)	Wavelength 808 nm Output power 100 mW Application time 60 s/site Dose 6 J Fiber tip diameter 300 µm	Not analyzed	Not analyzed	Test 1: PD: 1.54 ± 0.59* CAL: 1.54 ± 1.10* BOP: from 88 ± 0.34 to 38 ± 0.49 (n.s.) Test 2: PD: 2.08 ± 1.02* CAL: 2.42 ± 1.14* BOP: from 96 ± 0.20 to 42 ± 0.50 (n.s.) Control: PD: 1.42 ± 0.88 CAL: 1.50 ± 0.88 BOP: from 92 ± 0.28 to 46 ± 0.51

(continued on next page)

Table 1
(continued)

Study, Author, Year, Country, Type	Diagnosis	Patients, Female/Male, Age, Smokers	Study Duration	Treatment	Photosensitizer Laser	Laser Parameters	Microbiology	Immunology	PD Reduction (mm), CAL Gain (mm), BOP Reduction (%)
Ge et al,[32] 2011, China, Parallel, RCT	ChP	N = 58 28/30 43 ± 10 9 smokers	12 wk	Test 1: SRP + PDT (once) Test 2: SRP + PDT (twice) Control: SRP	Methylene blue 0.01% Diode Laser (Periowave)	Wavelength 670 nm Output power 140 mW Energy density 21 J/cm^2 Application time 60 s/site Dose 6 J	—	—	Significantly higher BOP reduction in both test groups compared with the control group
Luchesi et al,[33] 2013, Brazil, Parallel, RCT	ChP Furcation defects	N = 37 No smokers	6 mo	Test: SRP + PDT Control: SRP + nonactivated laser	Methylene blue Diode laser (Thera Lase, DMC, Sao Paulo, Brazil)	Wavelength 660 nm, power output 60 mW Energy dose 129 J/cm^2 Fiberoptics diameter 600 μm Application time 60 s/site	Significant decrease in *P.g.* and *T.f.* in PDT group; however, no significant differences between the groups	Significant reduction at 3 mo of GM-CSF, IFN-γ, IL-6, and IL-8 in favor of PDT. At 6 m, also significant reduction of IL-1β in PDT group	No significant differences between the groups Test: PD: 1.59 ± 1.11 (n.s.) CAL: 0.78 ± 1.54 (n.s.) BOP: from 100% to 37.50% (n.s.) Control: PD: 1.50 ± 1.73 CAL: 1.00 ± 1.69 BOP: from 100% to 55%

Study		N	Duration	Groups	Photosensitizer/Laser	Laser parameters	Microbiological	Immunological	Changes from baseline
Lui et al,[34] 2011, ChP China, Split-mouth, RCT		N = 24 14/10 50 No smokers	3 mo	Test: SRP + PDT Control: SRP	Methylene blue Diode laser (Ezlase, BIOLASE Tech., USA)	Wavelength 940 nm Energy 1 W Application tie 30 s/tooth Energy density 4 J/cm² Fiber tip diameter 300 μm	Not analyzed	Significant reduction of IL-1β at 1 wk in favor of PDT. Significant reduction of GCF at 1 wk and 1 min favor of PDT	Changes from baseline to 3 m: Test: PD: from 4.7 ± 0.8 to 3.1 ± 0.5 (n.s.) REC: from 0.8 ± 1.2 to 1.8 ± 1.2 (n.s.) BOP from 94 ± 6 to 39 ± 14 (n.s.) Control: PD from 4.5 ± 0.7 to 3.2 ± 0.3 REC from 1.0 ± 1.1 to 1.8 ± 1.3 BOP from 92 ± 10 to 43 ± 12
Mettraux & Hüsler,[35] 2011, Switzerland, Split-mouth, RCT	ChP	N = 19	6 mo	Test: SRP + PDT Control: SRP	Methylene blue Softlaser (Lasotronic MED-701, Orcos Medical, Switzerland)	Wavelength 670 nm, Energy output 330 mW Energy density 31 J/cm² Application: transgingival 1 min/site Fiber tip diameter 8 mm	Significant reduction of the total bacterial load in favor of PDT. Significant reduction of T.d. in both groups	Not analyzed	Test: PD: 2.1 ± 1.4 (n.s.) CAL: 1.5 ± 1.3 (n.s.) Control: PD: 1.5 ± 1.6 CAL: 0.9 ± 1.7

(continued on next page)

Table 1 (continued)

Study, Author, Year, Country, Type	Diagnosis	Patients, Female/Male, Age, Smokers	Study Duration	Treatment	Photosensitizer Laser	Laser Parameters	Microbiology	Immunology	PD Reduction (mm), CAL Gain (mm), BOP Reduction (%)
Polansky et al,[36] 2009, Austria, Parallel, RCT	ChP	N = 58 36/22 48.7 (25–67) 7 smokers	3 mo	Test: SRP + PDT Control: SRP (ultrasound)	Phenothiazine chloride (HELBO Blue Photosensitizer) Diode laser (HELBO Minilaser 2075F)	Wavelength 680 nm Output power 75 mW Application time 60 s/site	No significant difference for the reduction of *P.g.* between the groups; significant reduction of *P.g.* at 3 mo compared with baseline in both groups	Not analyzed	Test: PD: from 5.79 ± 1 to 4.55 ± 1.14 (n.s.) CAL: from 6.60 ± 1.37 to 5.25 ± 1.41 (n.s.) BOP: from 100% to 47% (n.s.) Control: PD: from 5.53 ± 1.15 to 4.50 ± 1.33 CAL: from 6.59 ± 1.23 to 5.24 ± 1.48 BOP: from 100% to 59%
Queiroz et al,[39] 2014, Brazil, Split-mouth, RCT	ChP	N = 20 11/9 46.05 ± 6.38 (35–55) Smokers only	3 mo	Test: SRP + PDT Control: SRP	Phenothiazine chloride (HELBO Blue Photosensitizer) Diode laser (HELBO Minilaser 2075F)	Wavelength 660 nm, Maximum power 60 mW/cm² Fiber tip diameter 0.6 mm Application time 10 s/site at 6 sites/tooth	40 subgingival bacteria were analyzed: no significant differences between the groups or the time points	Presented in Queiroz et al,[29] 2015	Presented in Queiroz et al,[29] 2015

Study		Sample	Duration	Groups	Photosensitizer/Laser	Laser parameters	Microbiology	Biomarkers	Clinical results
Queiroz et al,[29] 2015, Brazil, Split-mouth, RCT	ChP	N = 20, 11/9, 46.05 ± 6.38 (35–55), Smokers only	3 mo	Test: SRP + PDT, Control: SRP	Phenothiazine chloride (HELBO Blue Photosensitizer) Diode laser (HELBO Minilaser 2075F)	Wavelength 660 nm, Maximum power 60 mW/cm², Fiber tip diameter 0.6 mm, Application time 10 s/site at 6 sites/tooth	Presented in Queiroz et al,[39] 2014	Significant reduction of IL-1β at 1 wk in favor of PDT; Significant reduction of MMP 8 at 12 wk in favor of PDT	No significant differences between groups; Test: PD: 1.58 ± 1.28 (n.s.), CAL: 1.41 ± 1.58 (n.s.); Control: PD: 1.81 ± 0.52, CAL: 1.60 ± 0.92
Sigusch et al,[28] 2010, Parallel, RCT	ChP	N = 24, 17/7, 32–58, No smokers	12 wk	Test: SRP + PDT, Control: SRP	Phenothiazine chloride (HELBO Blue Photosensitizer) Diode laser (HELBO Thera Lite Laser)	Wavelength 660 nm, Power density 60 mW/cm², Application time 10 s/site	Significant reduction of F.n. in the test group compared with the control group	Not analyzed	Significant difference at 12 wk between the groups regarding mean PD* (data n.r.); Test: Median, interquartile range: CAL: 2.45, 0.68*, REC: 0.20, 0.18, BOP: from 66% to 18 %*; Control: Median, interquartile range: PD: data n.r., CAL: 0.20, 0.18, REC: 0.20, 0.10, BOP: from 68% to 72%

(continued on next page)

Table 1
(continued)

Study, Author, Year, Country, Type	Diagnosis	Patients, Female/Male, Age, Smokers	Study Duration	Treatment	Photosensitizer Laser	Laser Parameters	Microbiology	Immunology	PD Reduction (mm), CAL Gain (mm), BOP Reduction (%)
Srikanth et al,[37] 2015, India, Split-mouth, RCT	ChP	N = 39 (30–55) Nonsmokers	6 mo	Test 1: SRP + PDT Test 2: SRP + laser without photosensitizer Control: SRP	Indocyanine green (Aurogreen Aurolabs, Madurai, Tamil Nadu, India) Diode laser (firm not specified)	Wavelength 810 nm Power output 0.7 W Application time 5 s/site	Significant decrease of the % of viable bacteria in favor to PDT	Not analyzed	Test 1: PD: from 5.81 ± 0.89 to 3.07 ± 0.68 (n.s.) CAL: from 5.00 ± 0.80 to 2.53 ± 0.58 (n.s.) BOP: n.r. Test 2: PD: 5.34 ± 0.34 to 3.15 vs 0.43 (n.s.) CAL: from 4.57 ± 0.57 to 2.96 ± 0.44* BOP: n.r. Control: PD: from 5.07 ± 0.27 to 3.01 ± 0.21 CAL: from 4.50 ± 0.50 to 3.10 ± 0.01 BOP: n.r.

| Theodoro et al,[38] 2012, Brazil, Split-mouth, RCT | ChP | N = 33 21/12 43.12 ± 8.2 Nonsmokers | 6 mo | Test 1: SRP + PDT Test 2: SRP + Placebo PDT Control: SRP | Phenothiazine 100 μg/mL (Sigma Chemical, St. Louis, MO, USA) Diode Laser (BioWave) | Wavelength 660 nm Power output 30 mW Power intensity 0.4 W/cm^2 Energy density 64.28 J/cm^2 Application time 150 s/site Spot size 0.07 cm^2 | A.a., P.g., P.i., T.f., P.n. Significant differences in all investigated periodontal pathogens in favor of SRP + PDT | Not analyzed | Test 1: PD: from 5.75 ± 1.44 to 3.42 ± 1.15 (n.s.) CAL: from 6.52 ± 2.11 to 4.96 ± 2.07 (n.s.) BOP: from 93.9% to 45.5% (n.s.) Test 2: PD: from 5.88 ± 1.26 to 2.48 ± 1.0 (n.s.) CAL: from 6.37 ± 1.56 to 4.38 ± 1.82 (n.s.) BOP: from 97% to 39.4% (n.s.) Control: PD: from 5.81 ± 1.0 to 3.1 ± 0.83 CAL: from 6.23 ± 1.25 to 4.25 ± 1.73 BOP: from 97% to 27.3% |

Abbreviations: A.a., Aggregatibacter actinomycetemcomitans; C.r., Campylobacter rectus; C.s., Capnocytophaga spp; E.c., Eikenella corrodens; E.n., Eubacterium nodatum; F.n., Fusobacterium nucleatum; IFN-γ, interferon γ; *, statistical significant value; n.r., not reported; n.s., not significant; P.g., Porphyromonas gingivalis; P.i., Prevotella intermedia; P.m., Parvimonas micra; REC, recession; T.d., Treponema denticola; T.f., Tannerella forsythia.
Data from Refs.[21–39]

significant differences in these parameters.[29–38] An additional improvement for the reduction of bleeding on probing (BOP) following the use of PDT was reported in 5 of the 19 papers.[22,26,28,31,32] Changes of microbiological parameters were evaluated in 8 of 18 studies. Four studies have found a statistically significant effect of the additional use of PDT on the reduction of periodontal pathogens,[28,35,37,38] whereas 4 studies have failed to reveal any differences between the treatments groups.[31,33,36,39] Three of the 18 studies have also evaluated the changes in terms of various inflammatory markers.[29,33,34] All 3 studies have revealed statistically significantly higher reductions in the investigated inflammatory markers following the additional use of PDT (see **Table 1**).

USE OF PHOTODYNAMIC THERAPY AS ADJUNCT TO NONSURGICAL PERIODONTAL THERAPY IN PATIENTS WITH AGGRESSIVE PERIODONTITIS

Two RCTs have compared treatment with SRP + PDT to treatment with SRP alone,[40,41] and another study has compared SRP alone to PDT alone (ie, without any mechanical debridement) (**Table 2**).[42,43] Although one study found statistically significant improvements in terms of PD reduction and CAL gain in deep pockets (PD ≥7 mm) and significantly less periodontal pathogens of the red and orange complex and interleukin (IL)-1β/IL-10 ratio following treatment with PDT,[41] another study failed to reveal any statistically significant differences in the evaluated clinical and microbiological parameters between the treatments (see **Table 2**).[40]

USE OF PHOTODYNAMIC THERAPY AS AN ADJUNCT TO NONSURGICAL PERIODONTAL THERAPY IN MAINTENANCE PERIODONTITIS PATIENTS

Eight RCTs have evaluated the potential additional benefit of PDT to SRP as compared with the use of SRP alone in maintenance patients (**Table 3**). Two of the 8 studies have reported statistically significantly improvements in PD reduction and CAL gain following SRP + PDT compared with SRP alone.[44,45] An additional improvement for the reduction of BOP was reported in 5 of the 8 studies.[44–48]

Although 3 studies found a statistically significant effect of the additional use of PDT on the reduction of periodontal pathogens,[46–48] 3 other studies failed to reveal statistically significant differences between the treatment groups.[49–51] Three of the 8 studies have also evaluated the changes in terms of inflammatory markers.[47,50,52] Two studies found statistically significantly higher reductions in the investigated inflammatory markers following the use of PDT,[47,50] whereas one study detected no differences (see **Table 3**).[52]

USE OF PHOTODYNAMIC THERAPY AS AN ALTERNATIVE TO SYSTEMIC OR LOCAL ANTIBIOTICS

An extremely important aspect that must be kept in mind when considering the use of PDT is the lack of bacterial resistance to the antimicrobial mechanism, which gains even more importance in the light of the worldwide increase in bacterial resistance against conventional antibiotics.[53] Thus, its repeated application in conjunction with mechanical debridement may represent a valuable future option for treating periodontal and peri-implant infections.[11,54] At present, there is, however, limited evidence on the possibility of PDT to replace systemic or local antibiotics.

A recent RCT study evaluated the treatment of patients with aggressive periodontitis (AgP) by means of nonsurgical periodontal therapy in conjunction with either systemic administration of amoxicillin and metronidazole or 2 times topical application

Table 2
Photodynamic therapy as initial periodontal therapy in patients with aggressive periodontitis (data of 3 studies reported in 4 publications)

Study, Author, Year, Country, Type	Diagnosis	Patients, Female/Male, Age, Smokers	Study Duration	Treatment	Photo-sensitizer Laser	Laser Parameters	Microbiology	Immunology	PD Reduction (mm), CAL Gain (mm), BOP Reduction (%)
Chitsazi et al,[40] 2014, Iran, Split-mouth, RCT	AgP	N = 24 15/9 29	3 mo	Test: SRP + PDT Control: SRP	Toluidine blue photo-sensitize (Sigma Chemical Co) Diode Laser (HANDY Laser, USA)	Wavelength 670–690 nm Power 75 mW Application time 2 min/site	No significant differences for the levels of A.a. were observed between the groups	Not analyzed	Test: PD change: from 5.79 ± 1.06 to 4.29 ± 0.95 (n.s.) CAL change: from 6.58 ± 0.83 to 5.29 ± 1.26 (n.s.) BOP change: from 91.7% to 75% (n.s.) Control: PD change: from 5.45 ± 0.77 to 4.54 ± 0.88 CAL change: from 6.25 ± 1.07 to 5.50 ± 1.18 BOP change: from 100% to 37.5%

(continued on next page)

Table 2 (continued)

Study, Author, Year, Country, Type	Diagnosis	Patients, Female/Male, Age, Smokers	Study Duration	Treatment	Photo-sensitizer Laser	Laser Parameters	Microbiology	Immunology	PD Reduction (mm), CAL Gain (mm), BOP Reduction (%)
Moreira et al,[41] 2015, Brazil, Split-mouth, RCT	AgP	N = 20 30.6 ± 4.25 18/2 Nonsmokers	3 mo	Test: SRP + PDT Control: SRP	Phenothiazine chloride (HELBO Blue Photo-dynamic systems) Diode laser (HELBO Minilaser 2075F)	Wavelength 670 nm Maximum power 75 mW Fiber tip diameter 0.6 mm Energy density 2.49 J/cm^2 Application time 10 s/site	Significantly less periodontal pathogens of the red and orange complex in the test group	Significantly less IL-1β/IL-10 ratio in the test group	No differences between the groups for moderate pockets In deep pockets (PD ≥7 mm), significant PD decrease and CAL gain in favor fo PDT: Test (deep pockets): PD from 7.73 ± 0.87 to 3.77 ± 0.97* CAL: from 7.84 ± 0.89 to 5.07 ± 0.64* BOP: from 144 ± 60 to 22 ± 13.75 (n.s.) Control (deep pockets): PD: from 7.68 ± 0.92 to 5.12 ± 0.8 CAL: from 7.75 ± 1.21 to 6.00 ± 1.04. BOP: from 154 ± 64.16 to 36 ± 15

Study	Diagnosis	Sample	Follow-up	Groups	Photosensitizer/Laser	Laser parameters	Microbiological results	Clinical results	Note
Novaes et al,[43] 2012, Brazil, Split-mouth, RCT	AgP	N = 10, 8/2, 31 (18–35) Nonsmokers	3 mo	Test: PDT Control: SRP	Phenothiazine chloride (HELBO blue photosensitizer) Minilaser (HELBO)	Wavelength 660 nm, power 0.06 W/cm², fluency 212.23 J/cm² Application time 10 s/site	40 subgingival species were determined significantly, A.a. compared with SRP; SRP is more efficient for the red complex than PDT. In PDT, a recolonization of T.f. and P.g. was observed	Not analyzed	Published in Oliveira et al,[42] 2007
de Oliveira et al,[42] 2007, Brazil, Split-mouth, RCT	AgP	N = 10, 8/2, 31 (18–35) Nonsmokers	3 mo	Test: PDT Control: SRP	Phenothiazine chloride (HELBO blue photosensitizer) Minilaser (HELBO)	Wavelength 660 nm, power 60 mW/cm², fluency 212.23 J/cm² Application time 10 s/site	Not analyzed	Test: PD: from 4.92 ± 1.61 to 3.49 ± 0.98 (n.s.) CAL: from 9.93 ± 2.10 to 8.74 ± 2.12 (n.s.) BOP: from 57% to 19% (n.s.) Control: PD: from 4.92 ± 1.14 to 3.98 ± 1.76 CAL: from 10.53 ± 2.30 to 9.01 ± 3.05 BOP: from 60% to 21%	Published in Novaes et al, 2011

Abbreviations: A.a., Aggregatibacter actinomycetemcomitans; C.r., Campylobacter rectus; C.s., Capnocytophaga spp; E.c., Eikenella corrodens; E.n., Eubacterium nodatum; F.n., Fusobacterium nucleatum; *, statistical significant value; n.r., not reported; n.s., not significant; P.g., Porphyromonas gingivalis; P.i., Prevotella intermedia; P.m., Parvimonas micra; T.d., Treponema denticola; T.f., Tannerella forsythia.
Data from Refs.[40–43]

Table 3

Photodynamic therapy in supportive periodontal therapy (data of 8 studies reported in 9 publications)

Study, Author, Year, Country, Type	Diagnosis	Patients, Female/Male, Age, Smokers	Study Duration	Treatment	Photosensitizer Laser	Laser Parameters	Microbiology	Immunology	PD Reduction (mm), CAL Gain (mm), BOP Reduction (%)
Campos et al,[44] 2013, Brazil, Split-mouth, RCT	ChP	n = 13 8/5 48.15 ± 7.53 No smokers	3 mo	Test: SRP + PDT Control: SRP	Methylene blue 10 mg/mL Diode laser (Thera Lase)	Wavelength 660 nm Power output 60 mW Energy density 129 J/cm^2 Application time 60 s/site	Not analyzed	Not analyzed	Test: PD: 2.17 ± 0.91* CAL: 1.43 ± 1.61* BOP: 77.78* Control: PD: 1.14 ± 1.53 CAL: 0.51 ± 0.76* BOP: 40%
Cappuyns et al,[49] 2012, Switzerland, Split-mouth, RCT	ChP	N = 29 8/21 52 (36–74) 12 smokers	6 mo	Test 1: SRP + PDT Test 2: SRP + Diode Soft Laser (DSL) Control: SRP	Phenothiazine chloride (HELBO Blue Photosensitizer) Diode Laser (HELBO Photodynamic System)	Wavelength 660 nm Power output 40 mW Application time 60 s/site	A.a., P.g., T.f., T.d., total bacterial load No significant difference in the investigated microbiological parameters. However, P.g., T.f., and T.d. were suppressed stronger in the PDT group	Not analyzed	Test 1: PD: from 5.6 ± 1.2 to 3.8 ± 1.2 (n.s.) REC: from 0.8 ± 1.3 to 1.0 ± 1.3 (n.s.) BOP: at 6 m 15% (n.s.) Test 2: PD: from 5.5 ± 0.7 to 3.9 ± 1.0 (n.s.) REC: from 0.8 ± 1.7 to 1.3 ± 1.8 (n.s.) BOP: at 6 m 18% (n.s.) Control: PD: from 5.5 ± 1.0 to 3.6 ± 1.1 REC: from 0.7 ± 1.3 to 1.0 ± 1.3 BOP: at 6 m 12%

Study	Diagnosis	Sample	Duration	Groups	Photosensitizer/Laser	Microbiology	Laser parameters	Immunological outcomes	Clinical outcomes
Chondros et al,[46] 2009, Netherlands, Parallel, RCT	ChP	N = 24 14/10 Test: 50.6 ± 9.2 Control: 48.3 ± 7.9 7 smokers	6 mo	Test: SRP + PDT Control: SRP	Phenothiazine chloride (HELBO Blue Photosensitizer) Diode laser (HELBO minilaser 2075F)	A.a., P.g., P.i., T.f., T.d., P.m., F.n., C.r., E.n., E.c., C.s. Significant reduction of T.d., E.c., C.s. was found in favor of SRP + PDT	Wavelength 670 nm Output power 75 mW/cm² Application time 60 s/ tooth	Not analyzed	Test: PD: 0.8 ± 0.5 (n.s.) CAL: 0.7 ± 0.7 (n.s.) BOP: from 15 ± 12 to 12 ± 05* Control: PD: 0.9 ± 0.8 CAL: 0.5 ± 0.6 BOP: from 19 ± 14 to 18 ± 08
Giannopoulou et al,[52] 2012, Switzerland, Split-mouth, RCT	ChP	N = 29 8/21 52 (36–74) 12 smokers	6 mo	Test 1: SRP + PDT Test 2: SRP + diode laser (DL) Control: SRP	Phenothiazine chloride (HELBO Blue Photosensitizer) Diode Laser (HELBO Photodynamic System)	Analyzed in Cappuyns,[49] et al. 2012	Wavelength 660 nm Power output 100 mW Application time 60 s/ site	Levels of 13 cytokines and 9 acute-phase proteins were measured No significant differences were observed between the groups at any time point	See Cappuyns,[49] et al, 2012

(continued on next page)

Table 3 (continued)

Study, Author, Year, Country, Type	Diagnosis	Patients, Female/Male, Age, Smokers	Study Duration	Treatment	Photosensitizer Laser	Laser Parameters	Microbiology	Immunology	PD Reduction (mm), CAL Gain (mm), BOP Reduction (%)
Kolbe et al,[47] 2014, Brazil, Split-mouth, RCT	ChP	N = 21 12/10 48.52 (32–75) Nonsmokers	6 mo	Test 1: PDT Test 2: Photo-sensitizer Control: SRP	Methylene blue (10 mg/mL) Diode laser (Thera Lase, Brazil)	Wavelength 660 nm Power output 60 mW Energy dose 129 J/cm² Application time 60 s/ site	Lower* levels of A.a. were detected in test 1 and control groups at 3 as compared with 6 mo Lower* detection frequency of P.g. for test 1 and control groups	IL-4 increased* in Test 1. IL-10 was reduced* in Test 2. Test 1 showed significant reduction of IL-6, IL-1β IFN-γ	Test 1: PD: 1.6 ± 1.20 (n.s.) CAL: 0.95 ± 1.38 (n.s.) BOP: from 100% to 28.57% (n.s.) Test 2: PD: 1.29 ± 1.22 (n.s.) CAL: 0.69 ± 1.30 (n.s.) BOP: from 100% to 61.90%* (n.s.) Control: PD: 1.88 ± 0.97 CAL: 1.21 ± 0.96 BOP: from 100% to 28.57%

Study	Diagnosis	Duration	N	Intervention	Laser parameters	Microbiology	Immunology	Clinical outcomes
Lulic et al,[45] 2009, Parallel, RCT	ChP	12 mo	N = 10 3/7 54 (40–74) 2 smokers	Test: SRP + PDT Control: SRP + Placebo: PDT	Phenothiazine chloride (HELBO Blue Photosensitizer) Diode laser (HELBO Minilaser 2075F) Wavelength 670 nm Output power density 75 mW/cm^2 Application time 60 s/site	Not analyzed	Not analyzed	Test: PD: -0.27 ± 0.43* CAL: -0.09 ± 0.41* BOP decrease 97–77* Control: PD: -0.07 ± 0.61 CAL: -0.20 ± 0.61 BOP increase 84–87
Müller Campanile et al,[50] 2015, Switzerland, Split-mouth, RCT	ChP	6 mo	N = 27 13/14 62.8 (37–77)	Test 1: SRP + PDT (twice) Test 2: SRP + PDT (once) Control: SRP + inactivated laser	Methylene blue Diode laser (Periowave, Ondine Biomedical) Wavelength 670 nm Power output 280 mW Application time 60 s/site	No significant changes of the microorganisms from baseline to 3/6 mo in any of the group	No significant differences between the groups for IL-1β, IL-1ra, IL-8, IL-17, b-FGF, G-GSF, GM-CSF, IFN-γ, MIP-1β, VEGF, TNF-α. C-reactive protein was significantly lower in the test 1 group, compared with the others	Test 1: PD: from 5.9 ± 0.9 to 3.1 ± 1.0 (n.s.) CAL: from 7 ± 1.6 to 4.1 ± 1.6 (n.s.) BOP: from 16 to 10 sites (n.s.) Test 2: PD: from 6.3 ± 1.3 to 2.9 ± 1.8 (n.s.) CAL: from 7.9 ± 2.2 to 4.2 ± 2.8 (n.s.) BOP: from 20 to 7 sites (n.s.) Control: PD: from 6.3 ± 1.5 to 3.4 ± 1.5 CAL: from 7.6 ± 2 to 4.6 ± 2.2 BOP: from 15 to 10 sites

(continued on next page)

Table 3 (*continued*)

Study, Author, Year, Country, Type	Diagnosis	Patients, Female/ Male, Age, Smokers	Study Duration	Treatment	Photosensitizer Laser	Laser Parameters	Microbiology	Immunology	PD Reduction (mm), CAL Gain (mm), BOP Reduction (%)
Petelin et al,[48] 2014, Slovenia, Parallel, RCT	ChP	N = 27 12/15 Nonsmokers	12 mo	Test 1: ultrasonic scaling (US) + PDT Test 2: US Control: SRP	Phenothiazine chloride (HELBO Blue Photosensitizer) Diode laser (HELBO Tera Light)	Wavelength 660 nm Output power density 60 mW/cm^2 Application time 60 s/site	Assessment of *A.a., Pg., P.i., T.f., T.d.* Significant reduction of *T.d.+* sites and of *A.a., T.f., T.d* levels in favor to PDT in medium pockets (4–6 mm), and of *T.d.* in deep pockets (>6 mm)	Not analyzed	Test 1: PD: from 3.4 ± 0.2 to 2.9 ± 0.2 (n.s.) CAL: from 4.2 ± 0.3 to 3.7 ± 0.2 (n.s.) BOP from 25% to 9%* Test 2: PD: from 3.6 ± 0.2 to 3.0 ± 0.2 (n.s.) CAL: from 4.3 ± 0.3 to 3.7 ± 0.2 (n.s.) BOP: from 23% to 12% (n.s.) Control: PD: from 3.8 ± 0.2 to 3.3 ± 0.2 CAL: from 4.7 ± 0.3 to 4.0 ± 0.2 BOP: from 17% to 9%

| Rühling et al,[51] 2010, Germany, Parallel, RCT | ChP | N = 60 48 ± 8 Nonsmokers | 3 mo | Test: PDT Control: Ultrasonic debridement | 5% tolonium chloride (Asclepion Meditec, Ltd, Fife, UK) Diode laser (SaveDent Dental Laser Sydstem, Asclepion Meditec Ltd) | Wavelength 635 nm Energy dose 100 mW Application tie 60 s/site | Assessment of microbial counts were reduced after treatment but returned to baseline values after 3 mo | Not analyzed | No significant differences between the groups: Test: PD: from 3.5 ± 0.4 to 3.3 ± 0.5 (n.s.) CAL: from 11.4 ± 1.7 to 11.4 ± 1.6 (n.s.) BOP: from 5.4 ± 4.6 to 3.3 ± 4.3 (n.s.) Control: PD: from 3.3 ± 0.5 to 3.1 ± 0.4 CAL: from 10.6 ± 1.3 to 10.7 ± 1.2 BOP: from 4.7 ± 4.8 to 5.7 ± 8.7 |

Abbreviations: A.a., *Aggregatibacter actinomycetemcomitans*; b-FGF, basic fibroblast growth factor; C.r., *Campylobacter rectus*; C.s., *Capnocytophaga spp*; E.c., *Eikenella corrodens*; E.n., *Eubacterium nodatum*; F.n., *Fusobacterium nucleatum*; G-CSF, granulocyte colony stimulating factor; GM-CSF, granulocyte macrophage colony stimulating factor; IFN-γ, interferon γ; MIP-1β, macrophage inflammatory protein 1β; *, statistical significant value; n.s., not significant; n.r., not reported; P.g., *Porphyromonas gingivalis*; P.i., *Prevotella intermedia*; P.m., *Parvimonas micra*; REC, recession; T.d., *Treponema denticola*; T.f., *Tannerella forsythia*; TNF-α, tumor necrosis factor α; VEGF, vascular endothelial growth factor.
Data from Refs. 44–52

of PDT.[55,56] The results found that both treatment protocols resulted in statistically significant improvements in PD reduction, gain of CAL, and improvement in BOP compared with baseline. The systemic use of amoxicillin and metronidazole yielded, however, at both 3 and 6 months, statistically significantly higher reductions in mean PD compared with the treatment using PDT.[55,56] The most important clinical finding was the change in the total number of pockets 7 mm or greater following both treatment protocols. In the PDT group, the total number of pockets 7 mm or greater was reduced from 137 to 45 with the corresponding values of 141 and 3 in the amoxicillin and metronidazole group. Moreover, compared with the results at 3 months, at 6 months, an additional decrease in the number of pockets 7 mm or greater was measured.[55,56] On the other hand, the use of PDT also led to statistically and clinically significant improvements compared with baseline, although the number of residual pockets needing further therapy was substantially higher compared with the use of systemic antibiotics (eg, 45 vs 3). The changes in clinical parameters were also accompanied by changes in the concentration of matrix metalloproteinases 8 and 9 (MMP-8 and -9) in the gingival crevicular fluid (GCF).[57] However, although in the antibiotic group, a statistically significant decrease of MMP-8 GCF level at both 3 and 6 months after treatment was observed, these changes were not significant in the PDT group.[57] Taken together, the available data suggest a limited clinical benefit in using PDT for the treatment of patients with AgP.[40,42,43,56,57] Thus, presently, PDT cannot be recommended as a replacement for systemic antibiotics in patients with AgP. On the other hand, no studies have compared the use of PDT or systemic antibiotics in conjunction with nonsurgical treatment in patients with ChP.

The use of PDT as a potential alternative to local antibiotics has been recently evaluated in an RCT study comparing nonsurgical treatment of incipient peri-implantitis (sites with PD 4–6 mm, BOP positive, and radiographic bone loss $\geq$2 mm) by means of mechanical debridement followed by either the use of local antibiotics (eg, minocycline) or the application of PDT. The results at 6 months and at 1 year failed to reveal statistically or clinically significant differences between the 2 treatment protocols, thus suggesting that PDT may represent a valuable alternative to local antibiotics during nonsurgical treatment of incipient peri-implantitis.[58,59]

SUMMARY

Based on the available evidence from RCTs, the following conclusions can be drawn:

- In patients with ChP, the combination of SRP and PDT may result in substantially higher short-term clinical improvements evidenced by PD and BOP reductions compared with SRP alone.
- In patients with AgP, the use of PDT cannot replace the systemic administration of amoxicillin and metronidazole. Because of the lack of data, no conclusions can be made to what extent PDT may replace the use of systemic antibiotics in patients with ChP.
- Limited evidence from one study indicates that PDT may represent a possible alternative to local antibiotics in patients with incipient peri-implantitis.

CLINICAL RECOMMENDATIONS

1. In patients with ChP, clinicians may consider the use of PDT in conjunction with subgingival mechanical debridement. However, because of limitations in time and costs, the use of PDT appears to be more suitable in the maintenance phase of therapy.

2. At present, the use of PDT cannot be recommended as an alternative to systemic antibiotics in the treatment of AgP or severe cases of ChP.

REFERENCES

1. Page RC, Kornman KS. The pathogenesis of human periodontitis: an introduction. Periodontol 2000 1997;14:9–11.
2. Cobb CM. Non-surgical pocket therapy: mechanical. Ann Periodontol 1996;1(1): 443–90.
3. Lindhe J, Westfelt E, Nyman S, et al. Long-term effect of surgical/non-surgical treatment of periodontal disease. J Clin Periodontol 1984;11(7):448–58.
4. Badersten A, Nilveus R, Egelberg J. Effect of nonsurgical periodontal therapy. I. Moderately advanced periodontitis. J Clin Periodontol 1981;8(1):57–72.
5. Badersten A, Nilveus R, Egelberg J. Effect of nonsurgical periodontal therapy. II. Severely advanced periodontitis. J Clin Periodontol 1984;11(1):63–76.
6. Ramfjord SP, Caffesse RG, Morrison EC, et al. 4 modalities of periodontal treatment compared over 5 years. J Clin Periodontol 1987;14(8):445–52.
7. Adriaens PA, Adriaens LM. Effects of nonsurgical periodontal therapy on hard and soft tissues. Periodontol 2000 2004;36:121–45.
8. Umeda M, Takeuchi Y, Noguchi K, et al. Effects of nonsurgical periodontal therapy on the microbiota. Periodontol 2000 2004;36:98–120.
9. Drisko CH. Root instrumentation. Power-driven versus manual scalers, which one? Dent Clin North Am 1998;42(2):229–44.
10. Von Tappeiner HJ. On the effect of photodynamic (fluorescent) substances on protozoa and enzymes. Arch Klin Medizin 1904;39:427–87 [in German].
11. Sharman WM, Allen CM, van Lier JE. Photodynamic therapeutics: basic principles and clinical applications. Drug Discov Today 1999;4(11):507–17.
12. Wilson M, Dobson J, Harvey W. Sensitization of oral bacteria to killing by low-power laser radiation. Curr Microbiol 1992;25(2):77–81.
13. Pfitzner A, Sigusch BW, Albrecht V, et al. Killing of periodontopathogenic bacteria by photodynamic therapy. J Periodontol 2004;75(10):1343–9.
14. Dougherty TJ, Gomer CJ, Henderson BW, et al. Photodynamic therapy. J Natl Cancer Inst 1998;90(12):889–905.
15. Ochsner M. Photophysical and photobiological processes in the photodynamic therapy of tumours. J Photochem Photobiol B 1997;39(1):1–18.
16. Moan J, Berg K. The photodegradation of porphyrins in cells can be used to estimate the lifetime of singlet oxygen. Photochem Photobiol 1991;53(4):549–53.
17. Wilson M, Burns T, Pratten J, et al. Bacteria in supragingival plaque samples can be killed by low-power laser light in the presence of a photosensitizer. J Appl Bacteriol 1995;78(5):569–74.
18. Haas R, Dortbudak O, Mensdorff-Pouilly N, et al. Elimination of bacteria on different implant surfaces through photosensitization and soft laser. An in vitro study. Clin Oral Implants Res 1997;8(4):249–54.
19. Dobson J, Wilson M. Sensitization of oral bacteria in biofilms to killing by light from a low-power laser. Arch Oral Biol 1992;37(11):883–7.
20. Sigusch BW, Pfitzner A, Albrecht V, et al. Efficacy of photodynamic therapy on inflammatory signs and two selected periodontopathogenic species in a beagle dog model. J Periodontol 2005;76(7):1100–5.
21. Al-Zahrani MS, Austah ON. Photodynamic therapy as an adjunctive to scaling and root planing in treatment of chronic periodontitis in smokers. Saudi Med J 2011;32(11):1183–8.

22. Alwaeli HA, Al-Khateeb SN, Al-Sadi A. Long-term clinical effect of adjunctive anti-microbial photodynamic therapy in periodontal treatment: a randomized clinical trial. Lasers Med Sci 2015;30(2):801–7.

23. Andersen R, Loebel N, Hammond D, et al. Treatment of periodontal disease by photodisinfection compared to scaling and root planing. J Clin Dent 2007; 18(2):34–8.

24. Berakdar M, Callaway A, Eddin MF, et al. Comparison between scaling-root-planing (SRP) and SRP/photodynamic therapy: six-month study. Head Face Med 2012;8:12.

25. Betsy J, Prasanth CS, Baiju KV, et al. Efficacy of antimicrobial photodynamic therapy in the management of chronic periodontitis: a randomized controlled clinical trial. J Clin Periodontol 2014;41(6):573–81.

26. Braun A, Dehn C, Krause F, et al. Short-term clinical effects of adjunctive antimicrobial photodynamic therapy in periodontal treatment: a randomized clinical trial. J Clin Periodontol 2008;35(10):877–84.

27. Dilsiz A, Canakci V, Aydin T. Clinical effects of potassium-titanyl-phosphate laser and photodynamic therapy on outcomes of treatment of chronic periodontitis: a randomized controlled clinical trial. J Periodontol 2013;84(3):278–86.

28. Sigusch BW, Engelbrecht M, Volpel A, et al. Full-mouth antimicrobial photodynamic therapy in Fusobacterium nucleatum-infected periodontitis patients. J Periodontol 2010;81(7):975–81.

29. Queiroz AC, Suaid FA, de Andrade PF, et al. Adjunctive effect of antimicrobial photodynamic therapy to nonsurgical periodontal treatment in smokers: a randomized clinical trial. Lasers Med Sci 2015;30(2):617–25.

30. Balata ML, Andrade LP, Santos DB, et al. Photodynamic therapy associated with full-mouth ultrasonic debridement in the treatment of severe chronic periodontitis: a randomized-controlled clinical trial. J Appl Oral Sci 2013;21(2):208–14.

31. Christodoulides N, Nikolidakis D, Chondros P, et al. Photodynamic therapy as an adjunct to non-surgical periodontal treatment: a randomized, controlled clinical trial. J Periodontol 2008;79(9):1638–44.

32. Ge L, Shu R, Li Y, et al. Adjunctive effect of photodynamic therapy to scaling and root planing in the treatment of chronic periodontitis. Photomed Laser Surg 2011; 29(1):33–7.

33. Luchesi VH, Pimentel SP, Kolbe MF, et al. Photodynamic therapy in the treatment of class II furcation: a randomized controlled clinical trial. J Clin Periodontol 2013; 40(8):781–8.

34. Lui J, Corbet EF, Jin L. Combined photodynamic and low-level laser therapies as an adjunct to nonsurgical treatment of chronic periodontitis. J Periodont Res 2011;46(1):89–96.

35. Mettraux G, Hüsler J. Implementation of transgingival antibacterial photodynamic therapy (PDT) supplementary to scaling and root planing. A controlled clinical proof-of-principle study. Schweiz Monatsschr Zahnmed 2011;121(1):53–67 [in French, German].

36. Polansky R, Haas M, Heschl A, et al. Clinical effectiveness of photodynamic therapy in the treatment of periodontitis. J Clin Periodontol 2009;36(7):575–80.

37. Srikanth K, Chandra RV, Reddy AA, et al. Effect of a single session of antimicrobial photodynamic therapy using indocyanine green in the treatment of chronic periodontitis: a randomized controlled pilot trial. Quintessence Int 2015;46(5):391–400.

38. Theodoro LH, Silva SP, Pires JR, et al. Clinical and microbiological effects of photodynamic therapy associated with nonsurgical periodontal treatment. A 6-month follow-up. Lasers Med Sci 2012;27(4):687–93.

39. Queiroz AC, Suaid FA, de Andrade PF, et al. Antimicrobial photodynamic therapy associated to nonsurgical periodontal treatment in smokers: microbiological results. J Photochem Photobiol B 2014;141:170–5.
40. Chitsazi MT, Shirmohammadi A, Pourabbas R, et al. Clinical and microbiological effects of photodynamic therapy associated with non-surgical treatment in aggressive periodontitis. J Dent Res Dent Clin Dent Prospects 2014;8(3):153–9.
41. Moreira AL, Novaes AB Jr, Grisi MF, et al. Antimicrobial photodynamic therapy as an adjunct to non-surgical treatment of aggressive periodontitis: a split-mouth randomized controlled trial. J Periodontol 2015;86(3):376–86.
42. de Oliveira RR, Schwartz-Filho HO, Novaes AB Jr, et al. Antimicrobial photodynamic therapy in the non-surgical treatment of aggressive periodontitis: a preliminary randomized controlled clinical study. J Periodontol 2007;78(6):965–73.
43. Novaes AB Jr, Schwartz-Filho HO, de Oliveira RR, et al. Antimicrobial photodynamic therapy in the non-surgical treatment of aggressive periodontitis: microbiological profile. Lasers Med Sci 2012;27(2):389–95.
44. Campos GN, Pimentel SP, Ribeiro FV, et al. The adjunctive effect of photodynamic therapy for residual pockets in single-rooted teeth: a randomized controlled clinical trial. Lasers Med Sci 2013;28(1):317–24.
45. Lulic M, Leiggener Gorog I, Salvi GE, et al. One-year outcomes of repeated adjunctive photodynamic therapy during periodontal maintenance: a proof-of-principle randomized-controlled clinical trial. J Clin Periodontol 2009;36(8):661–6.
46. Chondros P, Nikolidakis D, Christodoulides N, et al. Photodynamic therapy as adjunct to non-surgical periodontal treatment in patients on periodontal maintenance: a randomized controlled clinical trial. Lasers Med Sci 2009;24(5):681–8.
47. Kolbe MF, Ribeiro FV, Luchesi VH, et al. Photodynamic therapy during supportive periodontal care: clinical, microbiologic, immunoinflammatory, and patient-centered performance in a split-mouth randomized clinical trial. J Periodontol 2014;85(8):e277–86.
48. Petelin M, Perkic K, Seme K, et al. Effect of repeated adjunctive antimicrobial photodynamic therapy on subgingival periodontal pathogens in the treatment of chronic periodontitis. Lasers Med Sci 2014. [Epub ahead of print].
49. Cappuyns I, Cionca N, Wick P, et al. Treatment of residual pockets with photodynamic therapy, diode laser, or deep scaling. A randomized, split-mouth controlled clinical trial. Lasers Med Sci 2012;27(5):979–86.
50. Muller Campanile VS, Giannopoulou C, Campanile G, et al. Single or repeated antimicrobial photodynamic therapy as adjunct to ultrasonic debridement in residual periodontal pockets: clinical, microbiological, and local biological effects. Lasers Med Sci 2015;30(1):27–34.
51. Rühling A, Fanghanel J, Houshmand M, et al. Photodynamic therapy of persistent pockets in maintenance patients—a clinical study. Clin Oral Investig 2010;14(6):637–44.
52. Giannopoulou C, Cappuyns I, Cancela J, et al. Effect of photodynamic therapy, diode laser, and deep scaling on cytokine and acute-phase protein levels in gingival crevicular fluid of residual periodontal pockets. J Periodontol 2012;83(8):1018–27.
53. van Winkelhoff AJ. Antibiotics in periodontics: are we getting somewhere? J Clin Periodontol 2005;32(10):1094–5.
54. Sgolastra F, Petrucci A, Severino M, et al. Adjunctive photodynamic therapy to non-surgical treatment of chronic periodontitis: a systematic review and meta-analysis. J Clin Periodontol 2013;40(5):514–26.

55. Arweiler NB, Pietruska M, Pietruski J, et al. Six-month results following treatment of aggressive periodontitis with antimicrobial photodynamic therapy or amoxicillin and metronidazole. Clin Oral Investig 2014;18(9):2129–35.

56. Arweiler NB, Pietruska M, Skurska A, et al. Nonsurgical treatment of aggressive periodontitis with photodynamic therapy or systemic antibiotics. Three-month results of a randomized, prospective, controlled clinical study. Schweiz Monatsschr Zahnmed 2013;123(6):532–44.

57. Anna S, Ewa D, Malgorzata P, et al. Effect of nonsurgical periodontal treatment in conjunction with either systemic administration of amoxicillin and metronidazole or additional photodynamic therapy on the concentration of matrix metalloproteinases 8 and 9 in gingival crevicular fluid in patients with aggressive periodontitis. BMC Oral Health 2015;15(1):63.

58. Bassetti M, Schar D, Wicki B, et al. Anti-infective therapy of peri-implantitis with adjunctive local drug delivery or photodynamic therapy: 12-month outcomes of a randomized controlled clinical trial. Clin Oral Implants Res 2014;25(3):279–87.

59. Schar D, Ramseier CA, Eick S, et al. Anti-infective therapy of peri-implantitis with adjunctive local drug delivery or photodynamic therapy: six-month outcomes of a prospective randomized clinical trial. Clin Oral Implants Res 2013;24(1): 104–10.

Is Radiologic Assessment of Alveolar Crest Height Useful to Monitor Periodontal Disease Activity?

CrossMark

Hattan A.M. Zaki, BDS[a,b], Kenneth R. Hoffmann, PhD[c],
Ernest Hausmann, DMD, PhD[a], Frank A. Scannapieco, DMD, PhD[a],*

KEYWORDS

- Radiologic assessment • Periodontal diagnosis • Periodontitis
- Periodontal examination • Radiographs

KEY POINTS

- Although the mainstay of periodontal assessment is clinical probing, radiographic assessment also has the potential to provide facile quantitative information on the status of tooth-supporting bone.
- Although probing measurements are viewed as more practical than radiographic measurements, radiographic assessment can be made quantitative and may prove to be more precise for routine assessment of periodontal disease activity.
- Intraoral radiographs are indispensable for assessment of periodontal disease status.
- Systems are now under development that will enable the practitioner to measure alveolar bone levels for longitudinal assessment of disease activity and could provide more objective criteria to manage patients.

INTRODUCTION

Periodontitis, which is caused by inflammatory processes initiated by bacteria that colonize as oral biofilms (dental plaque) on teeth, results in tissue destruction that manifests as gingival pockets, periodontal ligament destruction, and loss of tooth-supporting alveolar bone.[1] A variety of methods are used to evaluate the periodontium

[a] Department of Oral Biology, School of Dental Medicine, University at Buffalo, The State University of New York, 3435 Main St., Buffalo, NY 14214, USA; [b] Department of Oral Basic and Clinical Sciences, Taibah University, Madinah al Munawwarah, Kingdom of Saudi Arabia; [c] Department of Neurosurgery, School of Medicine and Biomedical Science, University at Buffalo, The State University of New York, Buffalo, NY 14214, USA
* Corresponding author. University at Buffalo, The State University of New York, 3435 Main Street, Buffalo, NY 14214.
E-mail address: fas1@buffalo.edu

Dent Clin N Am 59 (2015) 859–872
http://dx.doi.org/10.1016/j.cden.2015.06.009
0011-8532/15/$ – see front matter © 2015 Elsevier Inc. All rights reserved.

dental.theclinics.com

to assess periodontal status. These methods include visual description of the gingival tissues, periodontal probing, and radiographic assessment of underlying bone.

Tissue destruction resulting from periodontitis has been found to follow an irregular time course, and may occur as episodic "bursts."[2,3] The disease can remain stable and then progress rapidly, often at individual tooth sites. For some individuals, tissue destruction can be minimal, even in the presence of poor bacterial biofilm control, whereas for others tissue destruction can be extensive and result in tooth loss. The cause for this difference in susceptibility may be related to systemic, environmental or genetic risk factors (eg, smoking, diabetes mellitus, human immunodeficiency virus infection, and stress).[4]

Clinical examination, including periodontal probing and assessment of gingival inflammation (bleeding on probing), is the mainstay of periodontal diagnosis and disease assessment. A variety of clinical assessment indices can be used, each with its own advantages and limitations. These include the periodontal index, periodontal disease index, gingival index, and sulcus bleeding index.[1] The periodontal index is designed to give more attention to periodontal tissue destruction compared with gingival inflammatory status, and it follows a scoring system ranging from 0 to 8, where a 0 score reflects the absence of both gingival inflammation and supporting tissue destruction, and a score of 8 reflects advanced periodontal destruction with tooth mobility and/or migration. On the other hand, the periodontal disease index is designed to measure the periodontal status of 6 preselected teeth, known as the "Ramfjord teeth," which are the maxillary right first molar, maxillary left central incisor, maxillary left first premolar, mandibular left first molar, mandibular right central incisor, and mandibular right first premolar.

The gingival index system provides an overall assessment of gingival inflammatory status that can be used clinically to compare the efficiency of phase I treatment and to compare results before and after surgical therapy, as well as establishing good inter-examiner and intraexaminer calibration between dentists.[1,5] The sulcus bleeding index system is designed to give reproducible assessment of the gingival status, which is characterized by early detection of inflammatory changes at the base of the pocket or gingival crevice that are not easily detectable or visible with ordinary clinical examination. In addition, this index can be used to motivate the patient to perform better oral hygiene measures, because gingival bleeding is an early sign of disease development.[1]

Comprehensive clinical periodontal examination requires periodontal charting of all teeth. It is known, however, that probing is not precise because a good deal of variation is inherent to the procedure.[1,5] To provide periodontal care that provides timely intervention to prevent progression of disease, there is a need for a more precise method to monitor tissue destruction.

RADIOGRAPHIC ASSESSMENT OF ALVEOLAR CREST LEVEL

In most cases, clinical examination is supplemented with radiographic assessment. Radiographic examination and assessment of alveolar crest levels around individual teeth is a useful diagnostic adjunct to clinical periodontal examination. In general, radiographic examination allows for the accurate evaluation of crestal bone architecture, crown–root ratios, the presence of vertical or horizontal bone defects, furcation involvements, and the overall morphology of bone. Ideal radiographic imaging should satisfy the following criteria to achieve the most accurate diagnosis[5,6]:

1. The radiograph should record the complete area of interest, to allow assessment of alveolar crest height and the presence of furcation involvement or vertical bone defects.

2. Radiographic distortion should be minimized by use of proper x-ray projection geometry.
3. Radiographs should have the optimal contrast and density.

Periapical or bitewing radiographs are the most common types of radiographs used for the evaluation of periodontal bone loss. Periapical radiographs use 2 different types of projection techniques[6]—the parallel projection technique (or right angle-long cone technique), or the bisecting angle technique. The goal of the parallel projection technique is to position the x-ray film parallel to the tooth so that the beam hits both the tooth and the x-ray film at right angles (**Fig. 1**), resulting in minimal geometric distortion. The bisecting angle technique (**Fig. 2**) is best described by Cieszynski's rule of isometry, which states that 2 triangles are equal when they share 1 complete side and 2 equal angles. The clinical application of this is achieved by placing the film as close as possible to the lingual surface of the teeth, because the plane of the film and the long axis of the teeth will form an angle with its apex at the point where the tooth and film come in contact. An imaginary line is formed that bisects the triangle, and the x-ray beam is directed along this line and called the bisector. This results in 2 triangles with equal angles and a common side. When this technique is performed accurately, the resulting tooth image has a length equal to the tooth itself, which is an advantage compared with the parallel technique. However, the bisected angle technique has 2 limitations. The first regards multi-rooted teeth, where the central bisecting beam must be angled differently for each root. The second limitation is related to the alveolar ridge, which is usually projected more coronally than its true position when compared with the parallel projection technique. In general, periapical radiographs are preferred to bitewing radiographs when there is the need to accurately assess important anatomic structures, such as the mandibular nerve, the mental foramen, and the floor of the maxillary sinus. In addition, the periapical film can also be used to evaluate the presence or absence of periapical pathology.[7]

Bitewing radiographs differ from periapical radiographs in that they are usually limited to capturing the image of the crowns of both maxillary and mandibular posterior teeth along with the alveolar crest in the same radiographic film.[6] Bitewings are used commonly in general practice for dental caries detection as well as for evaluation of alveolar crest height around teeth. The horizontal bitewing technique uses the x-ray

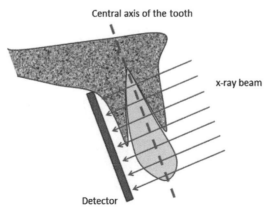

Fig. 1. The Paralleling technique. The film is placed so that its surface is parallel to the tooth axis, both of which are perpendicular to the x-ray beam.

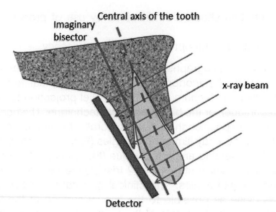

Fig. 2. The bisecting-angle technique. The film is placed as close as possible to the lingual surface of the tooth, the x-ray beam is perpendicular to the imaginary bisector plane.

beam aligned between the teeth and penetrates through the contact areas, while at the same time being parallel to the occlusal plane (**Fig. 3**A). The ideal bitewing radiograph provides a clear view of the mandibular and maxillary alveolar bone and teeth with minimal overlap between the teeth. Vertical bitewings differ from horizontal bitewings in that the radiographic film has greater vertical dimension to allow for more complete evaluation of the alveolar bone in patients expected to have moderate to severe periodontal bone loss (see **Fig. 3**B). Precise detection of proximal caries is considered an advantage of the horizontal bitewing technique, whereas the unobstructed view of the alveolar bone is the advantage of the vertical bitewing technique, which makes the latter a more valuable diagnostic tool for periodontal disease assessment.[6]

Rapid developments in computer technology have allowed for the development of digital radiographic imaging procedures, which minimize processing errors inherent to conventional (analog) radiographic techniques. Among these technological innovations is digital subtraction radiography, which is based on subtraction of 2 images of the same object, recorded at different times.[1,5,6] This technique is useful in

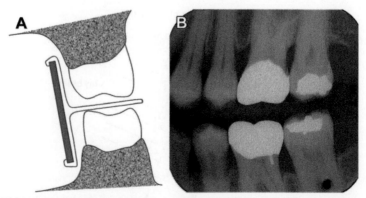

Fig. 3. (A) Horizontal bitewing geometry. Images are obtained of both the maxillar and mandibular teeth; however, less bone is imaged than in the vertical bitewing technique. (B) A bitewing radiograph.

detection of changes in tissue density between baseline and follow-up examinations. In general, the radiographic changes are either reflected as bright or dark areas. A bright area indicates gain in tissue density (mostly bone), whereas a darker area indicates tissue loss. The main disadvantage of subtraction radiography is that the geometry of the baseline image must be reproduced exactly in follow-up images or differences in geometry appropriately corrected for; otherwise, obfuscating artifacts appear in the image.[6]

Another recent advance in diagnostic imaging is the computer-assisted densitometric image analysis system (CADIA).[8] CADIA uses digitized radiographic information to measure the light transmitted through the radiograph, which is then converted into a gray-scale image that is then transferred to the computer where mathematic manipulations of the images take place that can be displayed, manipulated, and interpreted. This technique can also be used to assess alveolar bone density over time, similar to subtraction radiography. CADIA is more sensitive, accurate, and reproducible when compared with subtraction radiography. CADIA has been used in longitudinal clinical studies to follow the progression of periodontal bone loss and clinical attachment loss, and is shown to be more reliable compared with conventional radiographic techniques.[1]

As used in most clinical settings, radiographic examination of periodontal disease does not permit accurate detection of minor destruction of alveolar bone. Rather, radiographs demonstrate bone loss only after a significant amount of bone destruction has already occurred.[9] It has been reported that the difference between clinical alveolar crest height and radiographic crest height can range from 0 to 1.6 mm, with the radiographic measurements very much affected by radiographic beam angulation.[10]

Periodontal disease shows radiographic changes that usually start as a "fuzziness" or discontinuity of the lamina dura on the mesial and distal aspects of the interdental septa.[1,11] This will then transform into a wedge-shaped radiolucent area in the interdental septa. Afterward, bone destruction will seem to extend across the interdental septa and finally as a marked reduction in the height of interdental septum, resulting in a periodontal bone defect. However, there are several anatomic factors that can affect the morphology of periodontal bone defects those listed[1,11] in **Box 1**. Additional factors that can complicate interpretation of the morphology of periodontal bone include the presence of exostoses, trauma from occlusion, buttressing bone formation, and food impaction.[1,11]

Box 1
Factors affecting radiographic appearance of periodontal defects

1. The thickness, width, and angulation of the alveolar crest.

2. Thickness of lingual and facial alveolar bone plates.

3. Presence of fenestration and dehiscence.

4. Tooth alignment in the jaw.

5. Root and root trunk anatomy.

6. Root position within the alveolar process.

7. Proximity with another tooth surface.

From Manson J, Nicholson K. The distribution of bone defects in chronic periodontitis. J Periodontol 1974;45(2):88; and Newman MG, Takei HH, Klokkevold PR, et al. Carranza's clinical periodontology. 12th edition. St. Louis: Saunders Elsevier; 2015.

There are several patterns that develop regarding the distribution and classification of bone loss in periodontal disease patients.[1,11] Horizontal bone loss is the most common pattern of bone loss in chronic periodontitis.[11] Generally, the overall bone height is reduced while the margins of the alveolar crest are perpendicular to the tooth surface. Horizontal bone loss usually affects the facial and lingual plates of the interdental septa of a group of teeth or even all teeth in the mouth. In contrast, osseous defects are common in patients with periodontal disease. Osseous defects can be detected on radiographs or more precisely evaluated during surgical procedures to know their exact morphology and extent, and to plan suitable treatment approaches for each type of defect. The most common osseous defects are vertical defects, defined as bone loss occurring in a vertical or oblique direction resulting in a hollowed-out trough within the bone alongside a root surface, while the base of the defect is located apical to the surrounding bone. These types of defects usually occur as intrabony (infrabony) defects. These unique defects are often classified according to the number of the osseous walls involved in the destructive process. So, for example, 1-wall defects, 2-wall defects, and 3-wall defects can be described. However, when the number of osseous walls differs between the apical and the occlusal portion of the defect, the defect is termed a combined osseous defect. Vertical defects are more likely to occur on the mesial and distal aspects of teeth, and the molar teeth are more commonly affected (the second and third maxillary and mandibular molars), especially in the case of 3-wall defects (also referred to intrabony [infrabony] defects). One-wall defects, also termed hemiseptal defects, offer great challenge to radiographic assessment because they can be obscured by radiopaque facial, palatal, and lingual plates of bone. In some cases, the only diagnostic option is surgical exploration to appropriately assess and manage such defects.

Reverse architecture is observed more commonly in the maxilla compared with the mandible. This occurs as a result of the loss of interdental bone of the facial, lingual, and palatal plates, whereas radicular bone is preserved. Thus, bone heights seem to be reversed from the normal architecture of alveolar bone.

Osseous craters appear as continuous concavities of bone that affect multiple surfaces of teeth, for example, interdental, facial, lingual, and/or palatal bone. These defects constitute more than one-third of all defects and are most commonly found to affect the posterior teeth.[1,5,11] These types of defects tend to affect posterior teeth because bone around these teeth tends to have a flat interdental bone configuration when compared with anterior segments of teeth.

Furcation involvements are defined as the loss of bone in the bifurcation or trifurcation area of multirooted teeth. Furcation involvements are classified into four grades according to the amount of bone loss and tissue destruction (grade I, incipient bone loss; grade II, partial bone loss [or so-called CUL-DE-SAC defects]; grade III, total loss of radicular bone with a through-and-through opening of the furcation, but without gingival recession; grade IV, similar to grade III, but with gingival recession, which makes the furcation clinically visible). The radiographic assessment of furcation involvement is helpful and useful in evaluation of grade III and IV lesions. But, the angulation of the x-ray beam might result in the overlap of neighboring radiopaque structures to obscure this assessment.

Several other patterns of alveolar bone loss are encountered less commonly. A marginal gutter is defined as a shallow linear defect between the margin of a radicular cortical plate or interdental crest and along the length of 1 or more root surfaces. A dehiscence usually occurs in the form of a U-shaped or angular defect on the facial or lingual alveolar plates and also involving the marginal crest of bone of the tooth. A fenestration occurs in the form of circumscribed well-demarcated defect on the lingual or facial plate without the involvement of marginal crest of bone.

RADIOGRAPHIC MEASUREMENT OF ALVEOLAR CREST HEIGHT

A simple, inexpensive, and quantitative technique for monitoring changes in periodontal support would enable the dentist to monitor periodontal disease activity. Such a technique could be used for monitoring patients in periodontal maintenance to flag those in need of more aggressive intervention. In most cases, assessment of periodontal disease status is now performed using periodontal probing (with clinical attachment–loss measurements made in relation to a fixed anatomic landmark, usually the cementoenamel junction [CEJ]) and/or alveolar bone levels from intraoral radiographs. Both of these techniques are vulnerable to errors.[12–14] Although periodontal probing remains the gold standard for periodontal assessment, it has several limitations regarding reproducibility and sensitivity, depending on the degree of edema and probing technique (eg, probing force, angle of the probe, size of the probe and probe calibration [which can differ from 1 brand to another]), making the detection of small changes difficult.[15] Probing force is considered to be the most important factor affecting the precision, reproducibility, and consistency of the probing technique. The use of controlled force pressure probes of up to 30 g within the junctional epithelium, and of 50 g for osseous defects, is required for the accurate use of probes.[16,17] The National Institute of Dental and Craniofacial Research has proposed the development of standardized computerized physical measurement techniques for the assessment of periodontal disease with 8 criteria (**Box 2**).[1]

Examples of physical measurement techniques are the Florida Probe, the Interprobe, the Periprobe, the Foster–Miller probe, and Toronto Automated probe systems. The Florida Probe system has been modified to use the CEJ as a reference point instead of the occlusal surface.[18–21] Moreover, the Florida Probe system has been found to provide relatively reproducible measurements, with a mean standard deviation of 0.3 mm, which is superior to conventional manual probes, which show a standard deviation of 0.83 mm.[22] However, computerized automated physical measurement systems tend to underestimate deep pocket depths, which is considered to be their major drawback. Relatively few longitudinal clinical studies with long-term follow-up have been reported to evaluate these systems.[18–21]

Radiographic techniques for measuring longitudinal changes in alveolar bone levels also have several shortcomings. A review of the literature to generate guidelines to improve the reliability of radiographic measurement found that the factors affecting image formation is of prime importance to develop a clinical monitoring system

---

Box 2
Standards for computerized physical measurement techniques having a precision of 0.1 mm

1. Range of 10 mm

2. Constant and standardized probing force

3. Acceptable reach and easy access to any tooth and any location around the tooth

4. Guidance system to ensure proper angulation

5. Complete sterilization of all parts entering the mouth

6. Noninvasive, light weight, and easy to use

7. Biocompatible and safe without the risk of electrical shock to the patient

8. Direct electronic reading in a form of digital output

Data from Newman MG, Takei HH, Carranza FA. Carranza's clinical periodontology. 2006.

capable of detecting small changes in alveolar bone from serial radiographic films.[23] Two models were found to predict the length of time needed to detect marginal crestal bone loss at rate of 0.1 mm/year. The first model assumes a CEJ-crest measurement error of ±0.3 mm, whereas the second assumed ±0.9 mm. The first model estimated that it would take 7 to 13 years for the system to detect crestal bone loss of 1.0 mm caused by actual loss of 0.7 to 1.3 mm, whereas the second model estimated that 1.0 mm of crestal bone loss would take between 1 to 19 years to be detected, caused by actual bone loss between 0.1 and 1.9 mm.

The suggested guidelines for radiographic reliability and measurements include the following requirements[23]:

1. Repositionable stentless film holder to standardize the radiation geometry;
2. Very accurate reproducible measuring technique and landmarks; and
3. Automatic computer-based measuring system.

A number of studies have been published that describe computerized approaches for assessment of alveolar crest height to assess periodontal disease progression. Early on, attempts were made to standardize radiographic technique by the addition of a modified alignment system that used a reference pin in the bite block that facilitated the repositioning of the film for subsequent exposures and the preservation of geometry.[24] The measurement of alveolar bone height was then performed using a "side-by-side technique,"[25] where baseline and longitudinal radiographs are displayed on a computer monitor next to each other. The baseline radiograph is captured digitally and displayed with contrast and brightness settings chosen to optimize the visibility of structures of interest. Then the longitudinal radiograph is placed in a holder capable of translation and rotation. The longitudinal radiograph is captured and displayed. This radiograph is rotated and translated in the holder until its orientation is comparable with that of the baseline radiograph; then, its contrast and brightness are adjusted to match that of the baseline radiograph. This study showed smaller measurement differences and greater geometric accuracy than a conventional system, indicating that this approach could facilitate detection of small changes in crestal bone.[24] Later, a computerized measurement system for the analysis of nonstandardized serial radiographs was developed.[25] It was shown that a difference of 0.87 mm between the CEJ and the alveolar crest measurement is required for a significant loss in crestal bone height to be observed.[25] Thus, changes in crestal bone height of less than 1 mm can be detected using bitewing radiographs, suggesting this could be a useful diagnostic tool for monitoring periodontal disease activity.

The precision of computerized measurements of marginal alveolar bone height from bitewing radiographs has also been reported.[26] Using a digitization technique, previously shown to be useful for assessment of bone height in periapical radiographs in adults, marginal alveolar bone height on 432 sites in nonstandardized bitewing radiographs in patients with intact CEJs was assessed. The mean difference between repeated readings of the same site was 0.09 mm with a confidence limit of 99.9%. Thus, digital techniques may be reliable for measurements of alveolar bone height from nonstandardized bitewing radiographs.

Radiographic bone heights measured using the side-by-side technique for pairs of digitized images have been compared with probing attachment level measured using an electronic probing system (Florida probe).[13] Both measurements were made at baseline and after 1 year, with 13% loss found using the radiographic technique and 9.6% attachment loss measured by the Florida probe. The concordance in radiographic and attachment-level changes in 82% of the sites indicates that both techniques hold diagnostic value for assessment of disease progression. Further studies investigated the reproducibility of bone height measurement on serial radiographs using 3 different alignment systems; the results varied with the precision of each system.[27]

The correlation of histometric measurements of bone level with radiographic and probing techniques has been assessed.[28] A difference of 0.14 mm between bone probing depths and histometric bone measurements (correlation coefficient, 0.90) was reported, whereas the difference between radiographic bone level and the histometric bone measurement was 0.6 mm (correlation coefficient, 0.73). It was concluded that probing may be a more reliable measure for detecting the actual bone level after periodontal regenerative treatment. It was also suggested that changes in clinical attachment and radiographic bone level progress somewhat independently; in the short term, the different measures may not follow the same course, but in the long term the differences become minimal. However, for the purpose of longitudinal monitoring of response to therapy, or cross-sectional studies, both techniques can be used.[14]

Evaluation of radiographic assessment of periodontal endosseous defects was compared using periapical and panoramic radiographs against surgical measurements.[29,30] The results showed that the detection of periodontal bone defects from radiographs was low and that defect evaluation of periapical radiographs was affected by defect depth and buccolingual width, the number of osseous walls, and the relative location in the jaw. Furthermore, osseous defects of a small width and depth were the most difficult to detect radiographically, and detection of osseous defects was more successful in periapical radiographs than in panoramic radiographs. The difference in the accuracy of osseous defect detection between periapical and panoramic radiographs depends on the defect location and dimensions.

Two forms of radiographic analyses, linear measurements and CADIA, were compared with assess postoperative bone fill as measured by surgical reentry.[29] It was found that linear radiographic measurements significantly underestimated posttreatment bone fill compared with reentry measures, whereas the CADIA method provided the highest accuracy. Hildebolt and colleagues[31] assessed the reliability of linear alveolar bone loss measurements of mandibular posterior teeth using digitized bitewing radiographs. Linear measurements between the CEJ and the alveolar crest at 6 different sites per tooth were performed by 3 observers. It was shown that a difference in alveolar height of 0.3 mm can be detected based on digital radiograph measurements. In a subsequent study, they developed a computer-based pattern recognition system for the purpose of objective classification of periodontal disease using intraoral periapical and bitewing radiographs.[32] The system allows adjustments of the contrast and brightness level, linear measurement of bone loss and linear crown height. This pattern recognition system was able to correctly grade periodontal disease 78% to 91% of the time.

Hou and colleagues[33] evaluated the consistency and reliability of periodontal bone level measurements using a digital scanning radiographic image analysis system. Radiographic measurements were done on standardized periapical radiographs obtained using paralleling technique and were recorded by 2 examiners based on intraexaminer and interexaminer data. In assessing the consistency and reliability for each group, they found interexaminer and intraexaminer reliability coefficients ranging from 0.986 to 0.995 ($P<.001$). These results are similar to those obtained by Machtei and colleagues,[34] who compared longitudinal measurements of pocket depths, attachment level, and alveolar crest height assessment during periodontal treatment versus nontreatment. Evaluations of 108 treated and 79 nontreated patients showed change in alveolar crest height to be minimal for the treated group, whereas nontreated subjects showed greater bone loss over time. However, Eickholz and Hausmann[35] found that radiographic assessment underestimated bone loss (1.41 ± 2.58 mm) when compared with surgical measurements in a study of 22 patients. Thus, although radiographic measurements of alveolar bone loss is relatively precise, the accuracy of these measurements must be taken into account in management of periodontal disease.

Currently, standards of care in dental practice involve the use of periodontal probing for the diagnosis of periodontal disease. However, the literature has shown consistently that manual methods of measurement of alveolar crestal bone height in radiographs have a precision of approximately 0.5 mm or better.[13,23,25,26,36–42] Merchant[43] concluded that, "Periodontitis assessed as mean alveolar bone loss or the prevalence of disease based on alveolar bone loss can be accurately and reliably evaluated from non-standardized radiographs." The literature indicates that determination of accurate and precise crest heights from clinically acquired dental radiographs is possible and recommended. Until now, no one has stepped forward to provide a system which provides periodontists and general practitioners with this capability.

LOOKING TOWARD THE FUTURE OF RADIOGRAPHIC ASSESSMENT OF PERIODONTAL DISEASE

Although assessment of supporting bone can be appreciated by open flap (histometric) measurements, such an approach is not practical for routine assessment, because it is invasive and often not possible in most cases. Although probing measurements continue to be viewed as more accurate than radiographic measurements, radiographic assessment can be made quantitative and likely made easier and more precise than probing. Unfortunately, appropriate image analysis requires more manipulation of the images than is currently available from most digital imaging systems.

Over the past several years, digital acquisition devices (photostimulable phosphor plates) or direct digital capture are being used more frequently in dental imaging. Although digital detectors do not have the physical flexibility of film in terms of positioning the detector in the mouth and thus tend to reduce patient comfort, they do provide the ability for digital archiving of images, for adjusting the brightness and contrast to correct for incorrect exposures allowing better visualization of anatomic features, and for some measurements, including alveolar crest height. However, the potential for the use of digital imaging to contribute to periodontal assessment has yet to be realized, even though digital analysis of intraoral radiographs is not new, as discussed. Indeed, the vast majority of radiographic analysis by dentists remains qualitative, for example, simply "eyeballing" radiographs. Vendors are providing measurement tools with their image presentation software (**Fig. 4**). Currently, manual indications or measurements are time consuming and can introduce some level of error arising primarily from projection geometry differences.[13,44]

However, a number of digital analysis systems have been proposed that have been shown to provide improved precision and accuracy. Hausmann and colleagues[25] have shown, using the side-by-side technique, that adjustment of orientation, contrast, and brightness improves the accuracy and precision of radiographic change measurements. Subtraction techniques[1,5,6] after image registration[45,46] may not only facilitate change measurement, but perhaps more importantly subtle change detection.

In general, longitudinal assessment of alveolar crest height by radiographic analysis may require use of standardized geometry to minimize angulation differences that

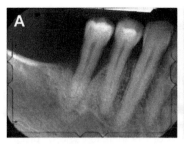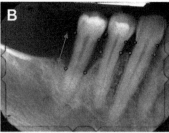

Fig. 4. Radiograph with landmarks. (*A*) Radiograph of the right posterior jaw with the cementoenamel junction (CEJ) and the base of defect (BD) indicated by the red and yellow markers (*B*), respectively. The CEJ can be identified as the interface of the higher contrast enamel and the lower contrast dentin. The BD can be identified as the interface between the lower density of the bone-free or bone-reduced regions and the alveolar bone. Bone height or crest height (*green double arrow*) is taken as the distance between the CEJ and BD.

introduce errors in the measurements.[36,44] Rotations about the jaw axis introduce foreshortening of the tooth and the measurements of bone height as well as introducing false contours that can be take as horizontal defects. Rotations about the vertical axis can introduce double lateral edges and reduce the contrast of the CEJ. Foreshortening can be overcome using alignment and rescaling techniques based on concepts used in the Schei ruler method.[47] The false contouring can be identified if the foreshortening is first recognized via the alignment results. Identification of double lateral edges can also be identified by aligning images of the same tooth taken at different angles and/or times. With the image having higher contrast CEJ providing "guidance" on the location of the CEJ in the angulated image, the effects of the double lateral edge or reduced contrast can be minimized.

Such effects can be reduced substantially (and the results of the analyses described can be improved) if a film positioning device is used, as has been shown using the Rinn positioning device, which improves not only the quality of the images but also the reproducibility of the geometry of the acquisition.[27] In addition, as has been discussed by Jeffcoat[36] and Byrd,[44] the issues that arise from the placement of the imaging plate in the mouth can also be addressed using similar approaches. More automated, accurate, geometry correcting analyses of digital dental radiographs should facilitate monitoring of alveolar bone levels around teeth and implants.

However, there are 2 additional issues that may limit progress and use of more complete digital analysis in periodontics. The first is the acceptance and use of digital imaging technology itself. Here, patient comfort remains an issue because film is more pliable than the photostimulable phosphor plate devices and the direct capture devices. We expect that the technology will continue to advance to improve patient comfort. The second issue is the impact of these analyses on clinical work flow. Ultimately, artificial intelligence principles will allow application of algorithms that will require minimal user input. Ideally, fully automated techniques would be developed where teeth, surrounding bone levels, and background are identified automatically, adjustments are made, and the results are available for quantitative inspection within seconds. However, before that some user input will be required; full automation is daunting. Indication of the tooth or teeth of interest, perhaps some points along the tooth or in the bone to guide the subsequent analyses, will be required initially (see **Fig. 4**). But the user interface will need to facilitate these indications while minimizing the number of mouse clicks (our experience is that none is ideal, 1–5 is tolerable, whereas >10 is unacceptable). An additional consideration is the use of hygienists to provide the necessary input, with the dentist interpreting the results.

SUMMARY

Intraoral radiographs are indispensable for the assessment of periodontal disease status. Systems are now under development that will enable the practitioner to easily and conveniently measure alveolar bone levels of individual patients for longitudinal assessment of disease activity. Such systems will provide more objective criteria to properly manage patients for the prevention of the initiation and/or progression of inflammatory periodontal diseases.

ACKNOWLEDGMENTS

Funding for portions of the work described in the article was provided from grant R44DE019593 from the National Institute of Dental and Craniofacial Research.

REFERENCES

1. Newman MG, Takei H, Klokkevold PR, et al. Carranza's Clinical Periodontology. 12th edition. St. Louis: Saunders Elsevier; 2015.
2. Haffajee AD, Socransky SS. Microbial etiological agents of destructive periodontal diseases. Periodontol 2000 1994;5(1):78–111.
3. Socransky SS, Haffajee AD. The bacterial etiology of destructive periodontal disease: current concepts. J Periodontol 1992;63(4 Suppl):322–31.
4. Khocht A, Albandar JM. Aggressive forms of periodontitis secondary to systemic disorders. Periodontol 2000 2014;65(1):134–48.
5. Rose LF. Periodontics: medicine, surgery, and implants. St. Louis (MO): Mosby; 2004.
6. White SC, Pharoah MJ. Oral radiology: principles and interpretation. St. Louis (MO): Mosby-Elsevier; 2013.
7. Lang NP, Lindhe J. Clinical Periodontology and Implant Dentistry. 6th edition. Chichester (England): Wiley-Blackwell; 2015.
8. Brägger U, Pasquali L, Rylander H, et al. Computer-assisted densitometric image analysis in periodontal radiography. A methodological study. J Clin Periodontol 1988;15(1):27–37.
9. Ramadan A-BE, Mitchell DF. A roentgenographic study of experimental bone destruction. Oral Surg Oral Med Oral Pathol 1962;15(8):934–43.
10. Regan J, Mitchell D. Roentgenographic and dissection measurements of alveolar crest height. J Am Dent Assoc 1963;66:356–9.
11. Manson J, Nicholson K. The distribution of bone defects in chronic periodontitis. J Periodontol 1974;45(2):88.
12. Jeffcoat MK, Reddy MS. Advances in measurements of periodontal bone and attachment loss. Monogr Oral Sci 2000;17:56–72.
13. Hausmann E, Allen K, Norderyd J, et al. Studies on the relationship between changes in radiographic bone height and probing attachment. J Clin Periodontol 1994;21(2):128–32.
14. Machtei EE, Hausmann E, Grossi SG, et al. The relationship between radiographic and clinical changes in the periodontium. J Periodontal Res 1997; 32(8):661–6.
15. Listgarten M, Mao R, Robinson P. Periodontal probing and the relationship of the probe tip to periodontal tissues. J Periodontol 1976;47(9):511–3.

16. Armitage GC, Svanberc GK, Löe H. Microscopic evaluation of clinical measurements of connective tissue attachment levels. J Clin Periodontol 1977;4(3): 173–90.
17. Kalkwarf KL, Kaldahl WB, Patil KD. Comparison of manual and pressure-controlled periodontal probing. J Periodontol 1986;57(8):467–71.
18. Alves Rde V, Machion L, Andia DC, et al. Reproducibility of clinical attachment level and probing depth of a manual probe and a computerized electronic probe. J Int Acad Periodontol 2005;7(1):27–30.
19. Christensen MM, Joss A, Lang NP. Reproducibility of automated periodontal probing around teeth and osseointegrated oral implants. Clin Oral Implants Res 1997;8(6):455–64.
20. Wang SF, Leknes KN, Zimmerman GJ, et al. Intra - and inter-examiner reproducibility in constant force probing. J Clin Periodontol 1995;22(12):918–22.
21. Wang SF, Leknes KN, Zimmerman GJ, et al. Reproducibility of periodontal probing using a conventional manual and an automated force-controlled electronic probe. J Periodontol 1995;66(1):38–46.
22. Haffajee A, Socransky S, Goodson J. Comparison of different data analyses for detecting changes in attachment level. J Clin Periodontol 1983;10(3): 298–310.
23. Benn DK. A review of the reliability of radiographic measurements in estimating alveolar bone changes. J Clin Periodontol 1990;17(1):14–21.
24. Carpio LC, Hausmann E, Dunford RG, et al. Evaluation of a simple modified radiographic alignment system for routine use. J Periodontol 1994;65(1):62–7.
25. Hausmann E, Allen K, Carpio L, et al. Computerized methodology for detection of alveolar crestal bone loss from serial intraoral radiographs. J Periodontol 1992; 63(8):657–62.
26. Fredriksson M, Zimmerman M, Martinsson T. Precision of computerized measurement of marginal alveolar bone height from bite-wing radiographs. Swed Dent J 1988;13(4):163–7.
27. Hausmann E, Allen K. Reproducibility of bone height measurements made on serial radiographs. J Periodontol 1997;68(9):839–41.
28. Yun JH, Hwang SJ, Kim CS, et al. The correlation between the bone probing, radiographic and histometric measurements of bone level after regenerative surgery. J Periodontal Res 2005;40(6):453–60.
29. Pepelassi EA, Tsiklakis K, Diamanti-Kipioti A. Radiographic detection and assessment of the periodontal endosseous defects. J Clin Periodontol 2000; 27(4):224–30.
30. Toback GA, Brunsvold MA, Nummikoski PV, et al. The accuracy of radiographic methods in assessing the outcome of periodontal regenerative therapy. J Periodontol 1999;70(12):1479–89.
31. Hildebolt C, Pilgram TK, Yokoyama-Crothers N, et al. Reliability of linear alveolar bone loss measurements of mandibular posterior teeth from digitized bitewing radiographs. J Clin Periodontol 1998;25(11):850–6.
32. Hildebolt C, Vannier M. Automated classification of periodontal disease using bitewing radiographs. J Periodontol 1988;59(2):87–94.
33. Hou GL, Lin CH, Hung CC, et al. The consistency and reliability of periodontal bone level measurements using digital scanning radiographic image analysis– a pilot study. Kaohsiung J Med Sci 2000;16(11):566–73.
34. Machtei EE, Schmidt M, Hausmann E, et al. Outcome variables in periodontal research: means and threshold-based site changes. J Periodontol 2000;71(4): 555–61.

35. Eickholz P, Hausmann E. Accuracy of radiographic assessment of interproximal bone loss in intrabony defects using linear measurements. Eur J Oral Sci 2000; 108(1):70–3.

36. Jeffcoat MK, Jeffcoat RL, Williams RC. A new method for the comparison of bone loss measurements on non-standardized radiographs. J Periodont Res 1984; 19(4):434–40.

37. Hausmann E, Allen K, Dunford R, et al. A reliable computerized method to determine the level of the radiographic alveolar crest. J Periodontal Res 1989;24(6): 368–9.

38. Hausmann E, Allen K, Christersson L, et al. Effect of x-ray beam vertical angulation on radiographic alveolar crest level measurement. J Periodontal Res 1989; 24(1):8–19.

39. Hildebolt CF, Vannier MW, Shrout MK, et al. Periodontal disease morbidity quantification. II. Validation of alveolar bone loss measurements and vertical defect diagnosis from digital bite-wing images. J Periodontol 1990;61(10):623–32.

40. Verdonschot EH, Sanders AJ, Plasschaert AJ. Applicability of an image analysis system in alveolar bone loss measurement. J Clin Periodontol 1991;18(1):30–6.

41. Wyatt CC, Bryant SR, Avivi-Arber L, et al. A computer-assisted measurement technique to assess bone proximal to oral implants on intraoral radiographs. Clin Oral Implants Res 2001;12(3):225–9.

42. Hildebolt CF, Couture R, Garcia NM, et al. Alveolar bone measurement precision for phosphor-plate images. Oral Surg Oral Med Oral Pathol Oral Radiol Endod 2009;108(3):e96–107.

43. Merchant AT, Pitiphat W, Parker J, et al. Can nonstandardized bitewing radiographs be used to assess the presence of alveolar bone loss in epidemiologic studies? Community Dent Oral Epidemiol 2004;32(4):271–6.

44. Byrd V, Mayfield-Donahoo T, Reddy MS, et al. Semiautomated image registration for digital subtraction radiography. Oral Surg Oral Med Oral Pathol Oral Radiol Endod 1998;85(4):473–8.

45. Zitová B, Flusser J. Image registration methods: a survey. Image Vis Comput 2003;21(11):977–1000.

46. Fitzpatrick JM, Hill DLG, Maurer CR. Image registration. In: Sonka M, Fitzpatrick JM, editors. Medical Image Processing and Analysis. Bellingham WA: SPIE Press; 2000. p. 447–513.

47. Bassiouny MA, Grant AA. The accuracy of the Schei ruler: a laboratory investigation. J Periodontol 1975;46(12):748–52.

Do Mobility and Occlusal Trauma Impact Periodontal Longevity?

Richard A. Reinhardt, DDS, PhD*, Amy C. Killeen, DDS, MS

KEYWORDS

- Tooth mobility • Occlusal trauma • Periodontal bone loss • Periodontitis
- Periodontal inflammation • Periodontal maintenance therapy

KEY POINTS

- Occlusal trauma and tooth mobility are associated with periodontal bone and attachment loss. It follows that over many years, this association may lead to enough destruction of periodontal support to threaten periodontal longevity. However, strong evidence of cause and effect is lacking.
- Tooth mobility may enhance the probability for further attachment loss during periodontal maintenance therapy, but most mobile teeth can be maintained in function and comfort for many years.
- Increasing mobility during periodontal maintenance therapy is a concern, because it may indicate increased deterioration of the periodontium. This may be a result of increasing size of the lesion of occlusal trauma (periodontal ligament space) from increased forces, or from loss of periodontal attachment. Accurate initial measurement of mobility, and monitoring for change over time, is often overlooked in clinical practice. Systematic methods for recording mobility changes need to be integrated into recall protocols.
- Control of periodontal inflammation is a key element in minimizing the progression of periodontal attachment loss associated with excessive occlusal forces. Reduction of inflammation should precede definitive occlusal therapy, and occlusal therapy usually should precede periodontal regenerative surgery when significant mobility exists in the teeth targeted for regenerative therapy.
- Occlusal therapy is also important in improving the function and comfort of the dentition, which may also enhance the desire by the patient to retain teeth, thereby increasing tooth longevity.

Department of Surgical Specialties, University of Nebraska Medical Center College of Dentistry, 4000 East Campus Loop South, Lincoln, NE 68583-0740, USA
* Corresponding author.
E-mail address: rareinha@unmc.edu

Dent Clin N Am 59 (2015) 873–883
http://dx.doi.org/10.1016/j.cden.2015.06.003
0011-8532/15/$ – see front matter © 2015 Elsevier Inc. All rights reserved.

HISTORICAL EVIDENCE

Several articles in *Dental Clinics of North America* in the late 1990s reviewed the state of knowledge as to the impact of trauma from occlusion and mobility on periodontitis.[1–3] Occlusal trauma was defined as an injury (usually a histologically demonstrable lesion) to the attachment apparatus or tooth as a result of excessive occlusal forces.[3] Common symptoms of occlusal trauma were described to include pain or discomfort, dental hypersensitivity, tooth mobility (fremitus), or pathologic migration of teeth.[1] Classic animal studies by Lindhe and colleagues[4] using a dog model suggested that experimental occlusal trauma alone does not initiate periodontal pockets or periodontal attachment loss, but requires concomitant inflammatory periodontal disease.[5,6] Treatment of periodontitis and control of inflammation in the presence of experimental occlusal trauma reversed periodontal disease activity.[7] However, monkey studies by Polson and colleagues[8,9] found minimal changes in the rate of periodontal attachment loss when experimental occlusal trauma was combined with inflammatory periodontal disease, but no regeneration of bone took place when experimental occlusal trauma was removed in the presence of active inflammation. Osseous regeneration occurred only when both occlusal trauma and periodontal inflammation were eliminated, but with reduced level of periodontal attachment resulting from the previous loss.[10]

Although most tooth mobility is not the result of occlusal trauma, mobility is one of the primary clinical signs of occlusal trauma. However, Ericsson and Lindhe[11] concluded that increased tooth mobility did not exacerbate clinical attachment loss caused by plaque-induced periodontitis.

Human clinical studies reviewed in *Dental Clinics of North America* were sparse, mostly because of the difficulty in performing such investigations. Cross-sectional evaluations or investigations where mobility was noted included the finding that teeth with mobility may have a detrimental effect on postsurgical healing (following curettage, modified Widman, or pocket elimination surgery) and do not gain as much attachment.[12] More recent evidence that mobility impacts surgical outcomes was reported by Cortellini and colleagues[13] showing that baseline tooth mobility was significantly associated with reduced clinical attachment gains following procedures to regenerate deep intrabony defects.

Occlusal contacts, even if abnormal, do not necessarily lead to occlusal trauma, but excessive occlusal forces by definition are a needed initiator of the injury of occlusal trauma.[3] Early work indicated that abnormal occlusal contacts were associated with increased periodontal bone loss and mobility,[14,15] yet later studies were contradictory.[16] Pihlstrom and coworkers[17] found that occlusal contacts (centric relation, working, nonworking, or protrusive) did not lead to more severe periodontitis than in teeth without these contacts. Ismail and colleagues[18] reported on a group of 165 subjects who were re-examined for clinical attachment loss following a 28-year evaluation period, and determined that increased age, smoking, and tooth mobility were the factors most closely related to attachment loss. Wang and colleagues[19] reported that mobile teeth had significantly more attachment loss during the maintenance years than the nonmobile teeth. Jin and Cao[20] found no significant difference in probing depth, clinical attachment level, or bone height loss in teeth with or without abnormal occlusal contact, but teeth with mobility or widened periodontal ligaments had greater probing depths, more attachment loss, and increased alveolar bone loss. McGuire and Nunn[21,22] found that parafunctional habits and mobility were correlated with worsening prognosis and tooth loss over 5 to 8 years of periodontal maintenance.

In a rare interventional trial, Burgett and colleagues[23] found that occlusal adjustment designed to reduce occlusal trauma resulted in a 0.4-mm improvement in mean probing attachment compared with patients with no occlusal adjustment over a 6-year period. However, there was no significant difference in mobility between those receiving occlusal adjustment and those who did not.

The evidence reported in these manuscripts, written near the turn of the century, is summarized in **Box 1**. It is the purpose of this current review to analyze subsequent literature to cast new light on the question "Do mobility and occlusal trauma impact periodontal longevity?"

RECENT EVIDENCE: OCCLUSAL TRAUMA AND MOBILITY IMPACT ON PERIODONTITIS PROGRESSION

Support for abnormal occlusal contacts, which may lead to occlusal trauma, as a risk factor in periodontitis progression and eventually tooth longevity was found in a series of retrospective studies by Harrel and Nunn. These authors reported that teeth with occlusal discrepancies had significantly deeper probing depths and worse prognoses and mobility.[24] Occlusal discrepancies were defined as differences between retruded position (centric relation) and maximum intercuspation (centric occlusion), and working and balancing contacts in lateral and protrusive movements. After adjusting for other risk factors, such as smoking and poor oral hygiene, occlusal discrepancy continued as an independent contributor to increased probing depths.

Furthermore, teeth with untreated occlusal discrepancies had a significantly greater increase in probing depth per year than teeth without initial occlusal discrepancies or with occlusal treatment designed to correct occlusal discrepancies.[25] In fact, only teeth with untreated occlusal discrepancies showed a significant increase in probing depth during periodontal maintenance (0.066 mm/year over an undefined period, at least 1 year). The authors concluded that occlusal treatment reduces the progression of periodontitis.

Finally, characterization of the occlusal discrepancies revealed that deeper probing depths were associated with premature contacts in centric relation (0.89 mm), posterior protrusive contact (0.51 mm), balancing contacts (1.01 mm), and combined working and balancing contacts (1.13 mm, all $P<.0001$).[26] Although this series of studies had several major shortcomings, including a small sample size (<100), lack of standardized treatment and appropriate longitudinal evaluation protocols, and not being randomized or blinded, they do suggest that discrepancies potentially leading to occlusal trauma could impact progressive periodontal breakdown, even during periodontal maintenance.

The importance of nonworking (balancing) side contacts was extended in a large cross-sectional epidemiologic study,[27] wherein it was reported that nonworking side contacts only were related to probing depth ($P<.0001$) and attachment loss

---

Box 1
State of evidence in 2000: role of occlusal trauma and mobility in periodontitis progression

- Occlusal trauma is a risk factor in the progression of periodontitis, but routine occlusal treatment may not be necessary for successful periodontal maintenance outcomes.

- Tooth mobility may result from a variety of factors in addition to occlusal trauma, but there does seem to be a relationship between tooth mobility and progressing periodontitis.

- Occlusal trauma and mobility may threaten periodontal longevity and impede successful therapy, thereby prompting consideration of occlusal therapy along with inflammation control.

(P = .001), although it was weak in terms of magnitude and specificity. In another cross-sectional investigation,[28] the number of premature and balancing contacts increased with the severity of periodontitis (loss of clinical attachment, $P<.001$). The authors concluded that secondary trauma from occlusion, which was erroneously defined as premature and balancing contacts, is positively correlated with the severity of attachment loss. The lack of longitudinal data limits determination of the role of occlusal trauma in periodontal longevity.

A recent systematic review of occlusal adjustment in periodontal therapy[29] found no new evidence to encourage the use of routine occlusal adjustment to maintain periodontal health. However, it was concluded that it is not detrimental, and occlusal adjustment in conjunction with periodontal therapy may improve patient comfort and function. A similar conclusion was reached in a review article on the biologic effects of occlusal trauma, based on evidence primarily from animal studies.[30]

POTENTIAL INDICATIONS AND SCIENTIFIC RATIONALE FOR REDUCING OCCLUSAL TRAUMA IN PERIODONTITIS

Although reduction of occlusal trauma by occlusal therapy has not been proved to be a mandatory part of routine periodontal therapy, are there certain comorbidities that accelerate the damage caused by occlusal trauma? Kawamoto and Nagaoka[31] found that ovariectomized rats subjected to experimental occlusal trauma demonstrated significantly more bone resorption around the periodontal ligament than sham-treated animals. Nicotine also enhanced bone loss in rats with combined occlusal trauma and ligature-induced periodontitis compared with animals without either nicotine or both nicotine and occlusal trauma.[32] de Oliveira Diniz and colleagues[33] confirmed that occlusal trauma augmented the bone loss seen with ligature-induced periodontitis in rats, and this effect was further enhanced by diabetes mellitus. These rat studies suggest that attempts to reduce occlusal trauma in certain vulnerable cohorts, such as those with estrogen deficiency, diabetes, or smoking habits, may have merit, or at least deserves further investigation.

The scientific rationale for how occlusal trauma may contribute to increased periodontal bone loss has received some attention over the past decade. Central to occlusal trauma-induced (and periodontitis-induced) bone resorption seems to be stimulation of receptor activator of nuclear factor kappa B ligand (RANKL), the primary driver of osteoclast activation. RANKL interacts with RANK receptor on osteoclasts to initiate bone resorption. In a rat model where occlusal trauma was initiated by raising the occlusal surface, immunohistochemistry demonstrated RANKL associated with osteoclasts and osteoblasts.[34] A similar occlusal trauma protocol combined with lipopolysaccharide-induced periodontitis extended the length of time that osteoclasts were present on the interproximal bone surface, and the increased expression of RANKL in osteoclasts, endothelial cells, inflammatory cells, and periodontal ligament cells.[35] Human periodontal ligament cells exposed to mechanical stress also increased interleukin-6 production, a potent stimulator of RANKL, periodontal inflammation, and bone resorption.[36]

The recent evidence for occlusal trauma and mobility impacting tooth longevity is summarized in **Box 2**.

IMPACT OF OCCLUSAL TRAUMA ON PERI-IMPLANT BONE LOSS

With the surge of dental implant placements over the last 15 years, the role of occlusal trauma or overload in peri-implant bone resorption has been investigated. It was proposed that excessive occlusal force may contribute to bone loss around implants.[37]

Box 2
Recent evidence of the role of occlusal trauma and mobility in periodontitis progression

- Occlusal discrepancies, especially balancing interferences, are associated with accelerated periodontal breakdown during periodontal maintenance.
- Systemic comorbidities, such as estrogen deficiency, diabetes, and smoking, seem to enhance the impact of occlusal trauma on periodontal bone loss.

Monkey studies[38,39] found that, as with natural teeth, occlusal overload did not induce peri-implant inflammation but did cause bone resorption around implants. However, when inflammation was added to the occlusal overload by withholding tooth brushing, no acceleration of bone resorption was noted. A subsequent review paper of cellular biomechanics, engineering principles, bone mechanical properties, animal studies, clinical reports, bone physiology, and implant design biomechanics reported that occlusal overload on implants may increase the incidence of marginal bone loss.[40] A systematic review of animal studies on the effects of occlusal overload on peri-implant tissue[41] revealed only two appropriate controlled trials (in dogs),[42,43] which concluded that overload alone is not associated with peri-implant tissue breakdown, but when combined with plaque accumulation is key to increased pocket depths and loss of bone-to-implant contact. A more recent review came to the same conclusion,[44] whereas another pointed to the poor level of evidence and conflicting results.[45]

In a retrospective analysis of 3578 patient records, occlusal trauma was identified as one of several iatrogenic conditions, together responsible for 17.5% of causes for implant loss.[46] Sakka and colleagues[47] also found that occlusal overload is an important factor in late implant failure. Despite these pronouncements, well-designed clinical trials are lacking.

CLINICAL CONSIDERATIONS

Radiographic changes, such as widened periodontal ligament spaces and alveolar crest density changes, support the clinical evidence of mobility.[48] Increased mobility may be an adaptation to short roots, poor crown-to-root ratios, or increased forces in the absence of inflammation, whereas mobility associated with periodontal inflammation or occlusal trauma may contribute to the pathogenesis of disease and require treatment. It could be argued that parafunctional habits or increased occlusal forces in nonperiodontitis patients will eventually result in adaptive mobility and not lead to pathologic consequences.

The source of the occlusal force becomes much less important than the interaction of the resultant tooth movement and periodontal inflammation, which may lead to accelerated loss of bone and periodontal attachment. This may be analogous to orthodontic tooth movement through inflamed tissue in a periodontitis-susceptible individual. Careful inflammation reduction and management is important for successful active orthodontic therapy, and similar inflammation control is important when mobility from excessive occlusal forces is superimposed on periodontitis. Pathogenic mobility becomes more problematic when it increases over time, suggesting that widening of the periodontal ligament space or possible attachment loss is occurring.

The degree of tooth mobility can be difficult to determine because of varying systems that have been proposed, and operator subjectivity. The most common manual measure of tooth mobility is the Miller Index (**Box 3**)[49] based on the amount of tooth movement. Other mobility classification schemes have much more subjective criteria,

---

Box 3
Miller Index for measuring tooth mobility

- Class I: First distinguishable sign of movement greater than "normal."
- Class II: Movement of the crown up to 1 mm in any direction.
- Class III: Movement of the crown more than 1 mm in any direction and/or vertical depression or rotation of the crown in its socket.

Data from Miller SC. Textbook of periodontia. 3rd edition. Philadelphia: The Blakeston Co; 1950.

---

such as grade II as moderately more than normal and grade III as severe mobility facio-lingually and mesiodistally, combined with vertical displacement.[50]

Even though the Miller system uses definitive distances of movement, the ability of the clinician to judge 1 mm of horizontal movement is questionable.[51] Subjectivity and lack of reliability in using the Miller technique for the measurement of mobility have been demonstrated.[52] Various instruments have been developed to rule out "operator subjectivity" in determining tooth mobility. Historically, the most prominent and objective of these instruments is the Periotest (**Fig. 1**). The Periotest (Medizintechnik Gulden, Modautal, Germany) instrument uses an electromagnetically retracting tapping head that automatically makes contact with the tooth or implant 16 times (four times per second). The contact time on impact with the tooth is less in teeth with greater periodontal support and, therefore, less mobility. It has been shown[53] that a strong association exists between Periotest values and bone loss, but adaptation of the instrument to posterior teeth is difficult and use of the instrument in clinical practice has not become common. Modification of standard mirror handles to allow calibration of horizontal movement may be simpler and more helpful (**Fig. 2**). This would allow easier measurement of mobility during routine periodontal examinations, which then should be recorded and evaluated against previous findings to reveal increasing mobility.

Determining the prognosis of a tooth based on mobility is questionable.[48] However, mobility can affect prognosis and, therefore, subsequent treatment options. Patients considered "high risk" (those with aggressive periodontitis, smoking habit, estrogen deficiency, diabetes) are especially vulnerable to generalized periodontal breakdown

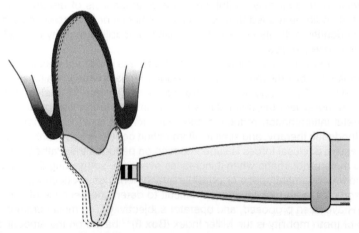

Fig. 1. The Periotest tooth mobility measurement device.

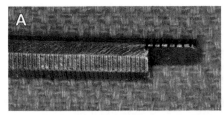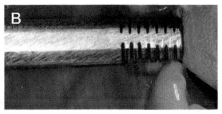

Fig. 2. (*A*) Standard mouth mirror handle that has been notched to allow the notched edge (inferior) to be placed on the lateral aspect of the tooth. The remaining superior surface has been calibrated in millimeters. (*B*) Notched inferior edge placed on the facial aspect of mandibular first premolar allowing the 1-mm calibrated superior surface to measure movement against the canine landmark. Handle and gloved finger (*blue*) are used to move the tooth.

and mobile teeth may have an even worse prognosis. Miller class II+ mobile teeth should be assigned "questionable prognosis" according to McGuire.[54] Teeth in fremitus during centric or excursive contacts may be removed from occlusion early in treatment. However, it is prudent to perform definitive occlusal therapy following completion of the inflammation control stage of therapy, specifically scaling and root planing. It is not uncommon for periodontally mobile teeth to tighten or shift position following scaling and root planing (**Fig. 3**), and adjusting occlusion at a subsequent visit will likely yield more appropriate results. However, occlusal therapy before surgical pocket reduction or regenerative treatment may enhance healing and clinical outcomes.[12,13]

The positive effect of routine, quality supportive periodontal maintenance therapy has been established many times, but the impact of mobility on outcomes remains unclear. However, it is reasonable that special attention should be directed toward patients with increasing mobility and sustained inflammation, and then focusing on inflammation reduction and controlling forces in these mobile teeth.

As was emphasized in the point-counterpoint discussion in 2006,[55,56] the clinician should recognize that occlusal discrepancies are not the pathology, but rather the pathology is the potential resulting lesion of occlusal trauma, the symptom of which is mobility. Not all occlusal discrepancies cause mobility.

Overall, the periodontal literature has weak evidence that mobility and occlusal trauma impact periodontal longevity. However, a prudent approach may dictate that focused occlusal therapy (following inflammation reduction) be directed toward teeth with mobility associated with parafunctional habits or increasing severity. Furthermore, occlusal therapy should be considered if it could result in improved patient comfort and function. A suggested algorithm is presented in **Fig. 4**.

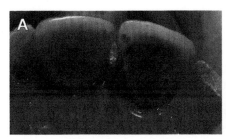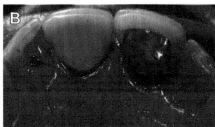

Fig. 3. (*A*) Diastema between central maxillary incisors before scaling and root planing or occlusal adjustment. (*B*) Diastema closed because of tooth movement following scaling and root planing, but before any occlusal adjustment.

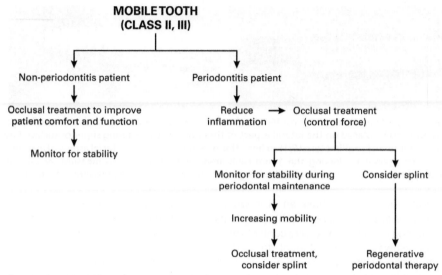

Fig. 4. Algorithm for occlusal adjustment for mobile teeth during periodontal therapy.

ACKNOWLEDGMENTS

The authors thank Bobby Simetich for fabrication of the calibrated mirror handles for measuring mobility, Kim Theesen for graphic designs, and Susan McCoy for preparation of the article. They also thank Dr Wayne Kaldahl for his critical review of this article.

REFERENCES

1. Burgett FG. Trauma from occlusion. Periodontal concerns. Dent Clin North Am 1995;39:301–11.
2. Gher ME. Changing concepts. The effects of occlusion on periodontitis. Dent Clin North Am 1998;42:285–99.
3. Serio FG, Hawley CE. Periodontal trauma and mobility. Diagnosis and treatment planning. Dent Clin North Am 1999;43:37–44.
4. Svanberg G. Influence of trauma from occlusion on the periodontium of dogs with normal or inflamed gingiva. Odontol Revy 1974;25:165–78.
5. Lindhe J, Svanberg G. Influence of trauma from occlusion on progression of experimental periodontitis in the beagle dog. J Clin Periodontol 1974;1:3–14.
6. Ericsson I, Lindhe J. Effect of longstanding jiggling on experimental marginal periodontitis in the beagle dog. J Clin Periodontol 1982;9:497–503.
7. Lindhe J, Ericsson I. The influence of trauma from occlusion on reduced but healthy periodontal tissues in dogs. J Clin Periodontol 1976;3:110–22.
8. Polson AM, Meitner SW, Zander HA. Trauma and progression of marginal periodontitis in squirrel monkeys. III. Adaptation of inter-proximal alveolar bone to repetitive injury. J Periodontal Res 1976;11:279–89.
9. Polson AM, Meitner SW, Zander HA. Trauma and progression of marginal periodontitis in squirrel monkeys. IV. Reversibility of bone loss due to trauma alone and trauma superimposed upon periodontitis. J Periodontal Res 1976;11:290–8.
10. Kantor M, Polson AM, Zander HA. Alveolar bone regeneration after removal of inflammatory and traumatic factors. J Periodontol 1976;47:687–95.

11. Ericsson I, Lindhe J. Lack of significance of increased tooth mobility in experimental periodontitis. J Periodontol 1984;55:447–52.
12. Fleszar TJ, Knowles JW, Morrison EC, et al. Tooth mobility and periodontal therapy. J Clin Periodontol 1980;7:495–505.
13. Cortellini P, Tonetti MS, Lang NP, et al. The simplified papilla preservation flap in the regenerative treatment of deep intrabony defects: clinical outcomes and postoperative morbidity. J Periodontol 2001;72:1702–12.
14. Youdelis RA, Mann WV Jr. The prevalence of a possible role of nonworking contacts in periodontal disease. Periodontics 1965;3:219–23.
15. Glickman I, Smulow JB. Effect of excessive occlusal forces upon the pathway of gingival inflammation in humans. J Periodontol 1965;36:141–9.
16. Shefler GJ, McFall WT Jr. Occlusal relations and periodontal status in human adults. J Periodontol 1984;55:368–74.
17. Pihlstrom BL, Anderson KA, Aeppli D, et al. Association between signs of trauma from occlusion and periodontitis. J Periodontol 1986;57:1–6.
18. Ismail AI, Morrison EC, Burt BA, et al. Natural history of periodontal disease in adults: findings from the Tecumseh Periodontal Disease Study, 1959–87. J Dent Res 1990;69:430–5.
19. Wang HL, Burgett FG, Shyr Y, et al. The influence of molar furcation involvement and mobility on future clinical periodontal attachment loss. J Periodontol 1994;65:25–9.
20. Jin LJ, Cao CF. Clinical diagnosis of trauma from occlusion and its relation with severity of periodontitis. J Clin Periodontol 1992;19:92–7.
21. McGuire MK, Nunn ME. Prognosis versus actual outcome. II. The effectiveness of clinical parameters in developing an accurate prognosis. J Periodontol 1996;67:658–65.
22. McGuire MK, Nunn ME. Prognosis versus actual outcome. III. The effectiveness of clinical parameters in accurately predicting tooth survival. J Periodontol 1996;67:666–74.
23. Burgett FG, Ramfjord SP, Nissle RR, et al. A randomized trial of occlusal adjustment in the treatment of periodontitis patients. J Clin Periodontol 1992;19:381–7.
24. Nunn ME, Harrel SK. The effect of occlusal discrepancies on periodontitis. I. Relationship of initial occlusal discrepancies to initial clinical parameters. J Periodontol 2001;72:485–94.
25. Harrel SK, Nunn ME. The effect of occlusal discrepancies on periodontitis. II. Relationship of occlusal treatment to the progression of periodontal disease. J Periodontol 2001;72:495–505.
26. Harrel SK, Nunn ME. The association of occlusal contacts with the presence of increased periodontal probing depth. J Clin Periodontol 2009;36:1035–42.
27. Bernhardt O, Gesch D, Look JO, et al. The influence of dynamic occlusal interferences on probing depth and attachment level: results of the Study of Health in Pomerania (SHIP). J Periodontol 2006;77:506–16.
28. Branschofsky M, Beikler T, Schäfer R, et al. Secondary trauma from occlusion and periodontitis. Quintessence Int 2011;42:515–22.
29. Foz AM, Artese HP, Horliana AC, et al. Occlusal adjustment associated with periodontal therapy—a systematic review. J Dent 2012;40:1025–35.
30. Liu H, Jiang H, Wang Y. The biological effects of occlusal trauma on the stomatognathic system—a focus on animal studies. J Oral Rehabil 2013;40:130–8.
31. Kawamoto S, Nagaoka E. The effect of oestrogen deficiency on the alveolar bone resorption caused by traumatic occlusion. J Oral Rehabil 2000;27:587–94.

32. Nogueira-Filho GR, Fróes Neto EB, Casati MZ, et al. Nicotine effects on alveolar bone changes induced by occlusal trauma: a histometric study in rats. J Periodontol 2004;75:348–52.

33. de Oliveira Diniz CK, Correa MG, Casati MZ. Diabetes mellitus may increase bone loss after occlusal trauma and experimental periodontitis. J Periodontol 2012;83:1297–303.

34. Kaku M, Uoshima K, Yamashita Y, et al. Investigation of periodontal ligament reaction upon excessive occlusal load—osteopontin induction among periodontal ligament cells. J Periodontal Res 2005;40:59–66.

35. Yoshinaga Y, Ukai T, Abe Y, et al. Expression of receptor activator of nuclear factor kappa B ligand relates to inflammatory bone resorption, with or without occlusal trauma, in rats. J Periodontal Res 2007;42:402–9.

36. Yamamoto T, Kita M, Yamamoto K, et al. Mechanical stress enhances production of cytokines in human periodontal ligament cells induced by Porphyromonas gingivalis. Arch Oral Biol 2011;56:251–7.

37. Goldberg PV, Higginbottom FL, Wilson TG. Periodontal considerations in restorative and implant therapy. Periodontol 2000 2001;25:100–9.

38. Miyata T, Kobayashi Y, Araki H, et al. The influence of controlled occlusal overload on peri-implant tissue. Part 3. A histologic study in monkeys. Int J Oral Maxillofac Implants 2000;15:425–31.

39. Miyata T, Kobayashi Y, Araki H, et al. The influence of controlled occlusal overload on peri-implant tissue. Part 4. A histologic study in monkeys. Int J Oral Maxillofac Implants 2002;17:384–90.

40. Misch CE, Suzuki JB, Misch-Dietsh FM, et al. A positive correlation between occlusal trauma and peri-implant bone loss: literature support. Implant Dent 2005;14:108–16.

41. Chambrone L, Chambrone LA, Lima LA. Effects of occlusal overload on peri-implant tissue health: a systematic review of animal-model studies. J Periodontol 2010;81:1367–78.

42. Heitz-Mayfield LJ, Schmid B, Weigel C, et al. Does excessive occlusal load affect osseointegration? an experimental study in the dog. Clin Oral Implants Res 2004; 15:259–68.

43. Kozlovsky A, Tal H, Laufer BZ, et al. Impact of implant overloading on the peri-implant bone in inflamed and non-inflamed peri-implant mucosa. Clin Oral Implants Res 2007;18:601–10.

44. Naert I, Duyck J, Vandamme K. Occlusal overload and bone/implant loss. Clin Oral Implants Res 2012;23(Suppl 6):95–107.

45. Chang M, Chronopoulos V, Mattheos N. Impact of excessive occlusal load on successfully-osseointegrated dental implants: a literature review. J Investig Clin Dent 2013;4:142–50.

46. Montes CC, Pereira FA, Thomé G, et al. Failing factors associated with osseointegrated dental implant loss. Implant Dent 2007;16:404–12.

47. Sakka S, Baroudi K, Nassani MZ. Factors associated with early and late failure of dental implants. J Investig Clin Dent 2012;3:258–61.

48. Anderegg CR, Metzler DG. Tooth mobility revisited. J Periodontol 2001;72:963–7.

49. Miller SC. Textbook of periodontia. 3rd edition. Philadelphia: The Blakeston Co; 1950.

50. Glickman I. Clinical periodontology. 4th edition. Philadelphia: W.B. Saunders; 1972.

51. Laster L, Laudenbach KW, Stoller NH. An evaluation of clinical tooth mobility measurements. J Periodontol 1975;46:603–7.

52. Pameijer CH, Stallard RE. A method for quantitative measurement of tooth mobility. J Periodontol 1973;44:339–46.

53. Schulte W, d-Hoedt B, Lukas D, et al. Periotest for measuring periodontal characteristics—correlation with periodontal bone loss. J Periodont Res 1992;27:184–90.

54. McGuire MK. Prognosis versus actual outcome: a long-term survey of 100 treated periodontal patients under maintenance care. J Periodontol 1991;62:51–8.

55. Harrel SK, Nunn ME. Yes – occlusal forces can contribute to periodontal destruction. J Am Dent Assoc 2006;137:1380–92.

56. Deas DE, Mealey BL. Only in limited circumstances does occlusal force contribute to periodontal disease progression. J Am Dent Assoc 2006;137:1381–9.

Does Treatment of Periodontal Disease Influence Systemic Disease?

Wenche S. Borgnakke, DDS, MPH, PhD

KEYWORDS

- Arthritis, rheumatoid • Atherosclerosis • Bacteremia • Cardiovascular diseases
- Inflammation • Intervention studies • Oral – general health • Pneumonia, aspiration

KEY POINTS

- Infection of the periodontal tissues causes inflammatory responses, both locally and systemically.
- Routine activities, such as chewing hard food items or tooth brushing or flossing, and periodontal treatment cause bacteremia in persons with periodontal infection.
- Periodontal treatment can lower levels of oral bacteria, several systemic disease endpoints, and markers of inflammation, and hence does influence systemic diseases.
- There is insufficient scientific evidence to claim that periodontal treatment should be performed solely to prevent or treat systemic diseases.

INTRODUCTION

Much attention is drawn to the notion that oral health is an important and indispensable element of general health. The lay press has widely touted the links between oral and systemic health, but not always with attention to the quality of the source information and with close scrutiny of the underlying scientific evidence. Indeed, an entire industry based on the oral-systemic relationship has developed and gained foothold in the conscience of professional colleagues and the public alike. However, claims are often loosely based on scientific evidence and are the result of overinterpretation of the available data (recall "Floss or Die"). With patients accumulating widely available (mis)information, it is increasingly important for the dental practitioner to be knowledgeable about the actual current scientific evidence regarding the effects of periodontal disease and its treatment on systemic health.

Disclosure Statement: The author has not received any support for this work and have no conflict of interest.
Department of Periodontics and Oral Medicine, University of Michigan School of Dentistry, 1011 North University Avenue, Room# G049, Ann Arbor, MI 48109-1078, USA
E-mail address: wsb@umich.edu

From public health and economic viewpoints, this is an important issue. Given that the estimated diabetes-related costs in the United States amount to $245 billion, with $176 billion in direct medical and $69 billion indirect (disability, work loss, premature death),[1] the possibility that dental professionals could improve the quality of life of patients and diminish the economic burden for individuals affected and for society is an intriguing notion.

The overarching goal of this article is to summarize the existing evidence for the effects of periodontal treatment on general health. The specific goals are to provide an update on the state of the science regarding mechanisms that may explain the connections between periodontal disease and systemic diseases and effects of periodontal treatment on general health.

This goal will enable the reader to

- Understand that the underlying mechanisms are similar for most all of the diseases described
- Understand the systemic effects of periodontal treatment
- Be able to critically interpret future scientific reports
- Explain to their patients what is known and what is not known
- Avoid the pitfalls of the current trends to overinterpret the evidence
- Practice evidence-based dentistry.

Scannapieco and colleagues[2] described in a comprehensive review published in January 2010 the then existing evidence for the effects of periodontal treatment on various general diseases. Therefore, this review focuses on the evidence published since 2010 and preferentially cites systematic reviews and meta-analyses in the relevant areas because they pool several studies to gain more weight and statistical power for their conclusions.

Periodontitis—What Is It?

Everyone knows what periodontal disease is—or do they? Dental clinicians know the condition when they see it, but their diagnosis and successful treatment will depend on their knowledge of each individual patient. Research teams have historically created their own periodontitis case definitions, based on a multitude of periodontal parameters. This lack of a global, generally accepted and applied case definition for periodontitis is often overlooked, but is one of the most important factors in periodontal research that prevents direct comparison of results generated by different study teams.[3] For example, Manau and collaborators[4] examined 1296 individuals while using more than 50 different measures of periodontitis used in 23 different published studies. Then they applied 14 periodontitis published case definitions to their data and found the prevalence of periodontitis in their study group ranged from 2.2% to 70.8%, with a mean of 35.9% and a median of 29.7%, depending on how periodontitis was defined. So whether an association is statistically significant can depend on which measures were made and on the definition of the disease. This disparity in definitions is one of the main reasons it is so difficult to compare the results of different studies—and so challenging to come to firm conclusions about the strength of the association between periodontal disease and treatment and any systemic disease or condition.

SYSTEMIC EFFECTS OF PERIODONTAL INFECTION
How Does Periodontal Infection Affect Systemic Health?

Fig. 1 depicts the 3 major mechanisms by which periodontal infection is thought to affect the rest of the body. Because these 3 mechanistic pathways also present the

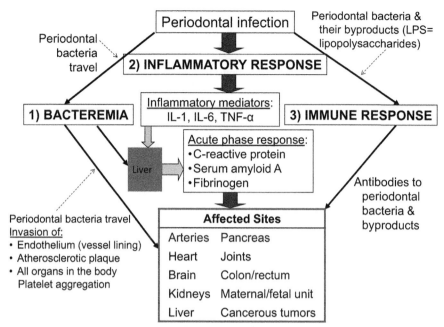

Fig. 1. Conceptual model illustrating the ways in which periodontal infection affects the human body: (1) bacteremia (direct effect): periodontal bacteria travel in the blood through the entire body; (2) inflammatory responses (indirect effect): pro-inflammatory mediators (cytokines) cause the liver to produce acute phase reactants (CRP, and others); and (3) immune response (indirect effect): production of antibodies to the bacterial antigens, including their lipopolysaccharides (LPS) and various cross-reactive agents. (*Data from* Refs.[2,5,6])

options for periodontal treatment to interrupt the deleterious effects, the evidence will be presented based on these pathways, with an emphasis on inflammation as the predominant mechanism.

Bacteremia

The bacteria in deep periodontal pockets can easily penetrate through ulcerations of the inflamed epithelium into the bloodstream. Once in the blood, the bacteria can travel everywhere in the body, and many of the species have developed sophisticated ways to survive the host defense system.[7] Not only can they survive; when they reach an inviting location, they make a landing and multiply in that remote location, for instance, an atherosclerotic plaque. The frequent, but consistent, dissemination of oral microbes via the bloodstream causes a chronic inflammatory response and can occur on daily activities, as reviewed by Tomas and colleagues[8]: chewing of hard food items[9] or chewing gum,[10] tooth brushing,[10–12] and flossing.[13]

Invasive dental procedures also can cause bacteremia,[14–16] for instance: tooth extraction,[11] endodontic procedures,[17,18] oral surgical treatment,[19] nonsurgical soft tissue treatment,[20] nonsurgical periodontal therapy,[10,19] and periodontal probing.[19,21] Even though bacteremia can be identified within 1 to 5 minutes after a procedure or activity, it is typically transient, with the bacteria usually undectable in the blood within 15 to 30 minutes, although bacteremia on chewing, tooth brushing, and scaling can last longer in persons with periodontitis.[10]

The oral bacterial burden The tooth is the only tissue that does not shed its surface cells and constantly undergoes renewal; this is the reason that bacterial biofilm can be established on teeth and over time grow and organize itself. This biofilm consists of a complicated system of bacteria and "glue" (extracellular polymers) that binds the members of this community together and makes it difficult for antibiotics to penetrate and reach bacteria that otherwise would be sensitive to their effects.

Novel laboratory techniques and development of powerful computers and software have enabled an exponentially growing understanding of the composition and function of oral microbiomes (the collective pool of microbes consisting of bacteria, virus, fungi, and archea) in various locations in the oral cavity.

It is important for periodontal treatment to target this pathway of bacteremia with the goal of reducing the quantity and changing the composition of the dental plaque in order to reduce the presence of particularly virulent bacteria that would cause bacteremia.

Inflammation

Only recently has the pivotal role of inflammation as the mechanistic basis for many chronic diseases come to the attention of health care professionals and medical researchers.[22] For instance, in 1997, Ridker and colleagues[23] suggested that inflammation, manifested by the general acute phase inflammatory biomarker C-reactive protein (CRP), is an important risk factor for a first thrombotic event (myocardial infarction or ischemic stroke). Ten years later, Ridker and Silvertown[24] argued that CRP, which has been shown to be elevated in patients with periodontitis, might be more important than low-density cholesterol levels as a cause of atherosclerosis. It was therefore suggested that periodontal disease may indirectly influence"risk, manifestation and progression of vascular events."[24]

What is inflammation? Inflammation is a biological process that describes the host's response against any attack on its integrity, including exogenous infections; bacterial overgrowth of commensal periodontal bacteria that flourish due to environmental changes; injuries, with or without breakage of the skin or any other visible surface; sunburn; chronic autoimmune disease; physical, chemical, thermal, or hormone-induced irritation; and exercise. Inflammation is a response for the host's protection and consists of

- Vascular reactions: vasodilation, increased permeability
- Plasma cascade systems producing molecular mediators: coagulation system (thrombin); fibrinolysis system (plasmin)
- Immune cell-derived mediators: enzymes; vasoactive amine (histamine); cytokines (tumor necrosis factor-α [TNF-α], interleukin-1 [IL-1], interferon-γ [IFN-γ]); chemokines (IL-8); soluble gas (nitric oxide)
- Leukocyte extravasation (the process of movement of the leukocytes from the blood through the vessel wall to the site of injury)
- Phagocytosis (engulfing and ingestion of bacteria, cell debris, and so on by phagocytes [eg, macrophages, neutrophils, and monocytes]).

The purposes of inflammation are to eliminate the initial cause of cell injury; remove necrotic cells and tissues damaged both from the original insult and from the subsequent inflammatory process; and to initiate tissue repair. The classic cardinal signs of inflammation are heat, pain, redness, swelling, and loss of function. Inflammation can be local or systemic; acute or chronic; and of various morphologic patterns (granulomatous, fibrinous, purulent, serous, or ulcerative). Resolution of inflammation occurs via several mechanisms, for example:

- Production and release of anti-inflammatory substances
- Apoptosis (normal, programmed cell death) of pro-inflammatory cells
- Production of resolvins that promote healing, especially in the presence of aspirin.

If the inflammation does not resolve by complete healing, an abscess can form. Otherwise, the inflammation becomes chronic. Tissue affected by chronic inflammation will be dominated by macrophages whose toxins eventually will cause destruction of both foreign and host soft and hard tissue, as seen in chronic periodontitis that, if left untreated, may result in tooth loss.

Inflammation originating in the periodontal microbiome It is now gaining acceptance that a microbial imbalance (dysbiosis) in the oral microbiome mediates inflammation not only locally in the periodontal tissues but also systemically, via the host response to the bacteremia and via the inflammatory biomarkers from the periodontium spreading in the body. Inflammation is thought to be the common mechanism underlying the links between periodontitis and most of the systemic diseases that periodontitis affects.[25]

Oral biofilm on the teeth and in the periodontal pocket induces inflammation that will continue as long as biofilm is present. Periodontitis is the polymicrobial inflammatory disease that emerges because of disruption of the ecologic equilibrium (homeostasis) between the periodontal microbiome and its host that then can enter a vicious cycle of increasing imbalance and loss of alveolar bone.[26] The inflammatory mediators that are produced in the periodontium will cause local inflammatory effects, but also spill into the bloodstream and travel to all parts of the body. However, the intensity of the inflammatory response will depend more on the individual host's immune system than simply the amount and microbial composition of the dental plaque.

Therefore, the inflammatory pathway is the most important target for periodontal therapy.

Immune response
The immune system will be stimulated to form antibodies to the bacteria and their toxins that are found both in the periodontium and in distant sites due to bacteremia. This pathway seems to be protective and to not have deleterious effects on the development of diseases, although cross-reactive antibodies to heat shock proteins from bacteria in the oral biofilm may be formed and could contribute to atherogenesis.[27]

SYSTEMIC EFFECTS OF PERIODONTAL TREATMENT

The often overlooked, overarching goal for periodontal therapy is to improve or maintain the patient's quality of life, via the preservation of functional teeth surrounded by a healthy periodontium. A multitude of studies have demonstrated that nonsurgical periodontal treatment is effective in improving the periodontal health status, also in persons who suffer from various other medical conditions, such as diabetes, kidney disease, and pregnancy. Moreover, successful periodontal intervention may not only reduce periodontal disease and extend tooth survival but also prevent the initiation or progression of, as well as ameliorate, several chronic systemic diseases.

Effects on Bacterial Load, Inflammation, and Immune Response

It has been demonstrated that periodontal treatment can reduce the

- Bacterial load on the teeth
- General inflammatory response to the microbes usually associated with periodontal breakdown and their toxins
- Specific immune response to these microbes and toxins.[28]

Therefore, it intuitively follows that such reduction of bacteria and inflammatory biomarkers that cause or aggravate the systemic consequences of their circulation by periodontal treatment should have significant and clinically relevant effects on the systemic diseases that are wholly or partially caused by these bacteria and substances.

However, it is not straightforward to measure the end effects of reduction of oral bacteria directly on disease outcomes for a variety of reasons, including

- Chronic, multicausal, and complex nature of the diseases
- Changing composition of the microbiomes in the oral cavity
- Variability in methods used to detect the microbes
- Inability to identify many of the microbes involved
- Variability of case definitions for periodontitis and many chronic diseases.

Effects of Periodontal Treatment on Local and Systemic Inflammation

The 3 main systemic disease pathways for periodontal infection to influence the body and that periodontal treatment may therefore target are depicted in **Fig. 1**, namely, (1) bacteremia, (2) inflammatory response, and (3) immune response.

Bacteremia

- Sudden, transient increase in blood levels of periodontal bacteria immediately following tooth brushing or periodontal treatment
- Decreased blood levels of periodontal bacteria on resolution of the immediate bacteremia in saliva, supragingival and subgingival plaque[29]
  - Total periodontal bacterial load
  - *Aggregatibacter actinomycetemcomitans*
  - *Fusobacterium nucleatum*
  - *Porphyromonas gingivalis*
  - *Prevotella intermedia*
  - Several other periodontal bacteria

Inflammatory response

- Sudden, transient increase in blood levels of inflammatory markers immediately on periodontal treatment[30,31]

Followed after 1 week by

- Decreased levels of pro-inflammatory mediators
  - Cytokines (cell signaling proteins)
    - Interleukins (IL-1, IL-6,[32] IL-8, IL-18)[30,33]
    - Tumor necrosis factors (TNF-α,[32] TNF-β)
    - IFN-γ
- Decreased levels of other acute phase reactants
  - CRP[32] with a significant reduction of 0.50 mg/mL[32,34]
  - Serum amyloid A

- ○ Fibrinogen[32,35]
- ○ Plasminogen-activator inhibitor 1
- Decreased levels of blood glucose
  - ○ Fasting
  - ○ Random
  - ○ Glycated hemoglobin (Hb_{A1c}, A_{1c})

Immune response

- Only a modest or temporary decrease in levels of antibodies to periodontal bacteria and their toxins
  - ○ Immunoglobulins (IgG, IgA)

A Special Note on Antibodies (Immune Response) to Periodontal Bacteria

Antibodies to periodontal bacteria persist in the human body long after periodontal treatment, for instance, after full-mouth extraction. Lakio and colleagues[36] showed that serum and salivary immunoglobulin to *P gingivalis* and *A actinomycetemcomitans* remained remarkably stable over a period of 15 years in all individuals who at the end were periodontally examined and found to have slight to moderate periodontitis.

Despite successful periodontal therapy, antibodies to 16 of 19 periodontal bacteria declined only modestly after 30 months and remained much higher than in the control group with periodontal health.[37] Therefore, Papapanou and colleagues[37] suggest that such antibodies may reflect a history of periodontal infection, not only current periodontal status.

Serum antibody titers against bacteria associated with periodontitis are linked to several systemic diseases, such as diabetes[38] and metabolic syndrome.[39] Although no treatment studies have been published, several interesting observations supporting links to other diseases also are reported, such as impaired cognitive function:

- High-serum IgG levels to an oral bacterium, *Actinomyces naeslundii,* doubles the hazard risk for development of new Alzheimer disease over a period of 5 years, whereas high anti-*Eubacterium nodatum* IgG was associated with half the risk of developing Alzheimer disease over a period of 5 years.[40]
- In an analysis of the US population-based NHANES III data, high levels of antibodies to *P gingivalis* were associated with poorer performance in three cognitive tests (cognitive impairment).[41]

Gingivitis Treatment Alone Also Has a Positive Effect on Bacterial Load and Inflammation

Even in otherwise healthy persons with gingivitis only (no periodontitis), ultrasonic debridement supplemented with rinsing with mouthwash containing essential oils is shown to lead to a decrease in levels of overall bacterial load, *Tannerella forsythia, A actinomycetemcomitans,* gingival crevicular fluid (GCF) volume, and IL-1β.[16] Rinsing with essential oil mouthwash alone also reduced the levels of selected bacteria individually and the total bacterial load by half, on average, with 21% to 52% in saliva, on average 53% in supragingival plaque, and by 21% to 38% in subgingival plaque.[29] However, these reductions by oral rinse were less pronounced than after scaling and root planing in the same study (52%–63% in saliva, 68%–81% in supragingival plaque, and 68%–93% in subgingival plaque).

Effects on Systemic Diseases

Diabetes
Diabetes is a growing public health problem in the United States and in many other countries. Almost half of the roughly 240 million adults living in the United States have hyperglycemia (**Box 1**). Prediabetes is defined in **Table 1**.

Table 1 illustrates how to translate HbA_{1c} into mean plasma glucose levels (Panel A) and to categorize diabetes status by HbA_{1c} or fasting or 1-hour postoral glucose tolerance test (OGTT) plasma glucose levels (Panel B).

The epidemic of obesity parallels the increasing prevalence of type 2 diabetes (**Fig. 2**).

Periodontitis: associations with diabetes and prediabetes
There is a widespread belief that all persons with diabetes are at much higher risk for developing or having periodontitis and that the extent and severity of periodontitis are greatly increased. However, this is true mostly when the long-term blood sugar known as glycated hemoglobin (HbA_{1c} or A_{1c}) exceeds about 7%, the threshold above which diabetes complications mostly occur and below which glucose levels generally are considered to be under control. Hyperglycemia negatively impacts the structure and function of many tissues.[44] A large German population study illustrates this: the association between clinical attachment loss was stronger in poorly controlled diabetes than in well-controlled diabetes, and absent in prediabetes.[44]

Nevertheless, a large study of mostly Hispanics in Northern Manhattan reported that periodontitis severity and extent was associated with both newly diagnosed prediabetes and diabetes.[45] The periodontal breakdown in prediabetes ranged between that in persons with normal blood sugar levels and those with overt diabetes, suggesting hyperglycemia as potentially causing the periodontal damage even before the diagnosis of prediabetes. Persons with prediabetes had worse clinical periodontal health, radiographic bone loss, and self-reported oral health (gingival bleeding, chewing pain, dry mouth, and burning mouth) than individuals with normal glycemic levels.[46]

Interestingly, even among persons with prediabetes, periodontal health assessed clinically, radiographically, and subjectively was better in those with better controlled prediabetes.[47] Furthermore, hyperglycemia in smokers actually seemed to have a stronger effect on poor periodontal health than smoking.[48] A systematic review and meta-analysis estimate that type 2 diabetes is 5 to 6 times more likely to develop in a person with prediabetes than in one with normal glucose levels.[49]

Periodontal infection: effects on blood glucose levels The first systematic review of the effect of periodontal infection on blood glucose levels included studies in which directionality could be determined, that is, periodontitis occurred before the outcome

---

Box 1
Estimated US population with diagnosed and undiagnosed prediabetes and manifest diabetes[1]

It is estimated that among the US adults, there are:[1]

21.0 million diagnosed with manifest diabetes

8.1 million with undiagnosed manifest diabetes

28.9 million with manifest diabetes

86.0 million with prediabetes (up to 90% being unaware)

114.9 million adults with diabetes or prediabetes (see **Table 1**)

Table 1
Glycated hemoglobin, plasma glucose levels, and classification of diabetes: Panel A: HbA1c and corresponding average plasma glucose levels; Panel B: American Diabetes Association criteria for diabetes status using HbA1c, fasting plasma glucose, and OGTT levels

Panel A[42]

HbA1c (%)	Average Plasma Glucose (mg/dL) (CI)
4	~68
5	97 (76–120)
5.6	~114
5.7	~117
6	126 (100–152)
6.4	~137
6.5	~140
7	154 (123–185)
8	183 (147–217)
9	212 (170–249)
10	240 (193–282)
11	269 (217–314)
12	298 (240–347)

Panel B[43]

HbA1c (%)	Fasting Plasma Glucose (mg/dL)	2-h OGTT (75 g Glucose) (mg/dL)	Diabetes Status
≤5.6	<100	—	No diabetes
		n/a	
5.7–6.4	100–125	—	Prediabetes
		n/a	
≥6.5	≥126	—	Diabetes
		≥200	

Panel A: Translating HbA1c into estimated average blood glucose concentration. *Note:* Each percentage point HbA1c is equivalent to a mean glucose level of ~29 mg/dL; numbers in italics are estimates.
Panel B: Diabetes status classification. Fasting: no caloric intake for 8+ hours.
Abbreviation: CI, confidence interval.
Data from Nathan DM, Kuenen J, Borg R, et al. Translating the A1c assay into estimated average glucose values. Diabetes Care 2008;31(8):1473–8; and American Diabetes Association. Classification and diagnosis of diabetes. Diabetes Care 2015;38(Suppl 1):S8–16.

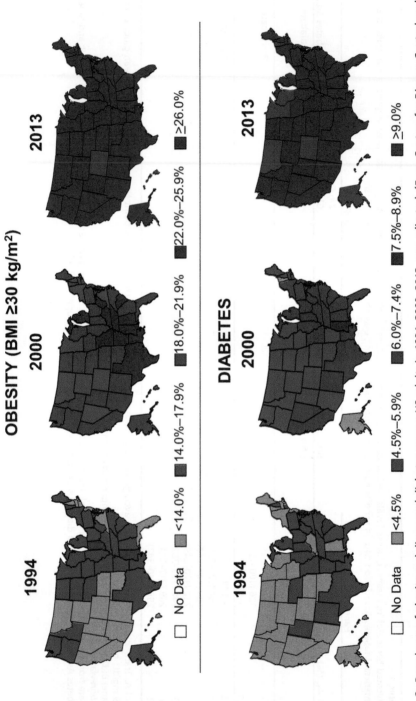

Fig. 2. Prevalence of obesity and diagnosed diabetes among US adults in 1994, 2000, 2013, age-adjusted. (*From* Centers for Disease Control and Prevention, Division of Diabetes Translation, National Diabetes Surveillance System. Maps of diagnosed diabetes and obesity in 1994, 2000, and 2013. 2015. Available at: http://www.cdc.gov/diabetes/data/center/slides.html. Accessed June 1, 2015.)

Table 2
Effect of nonsurgical periodontal treatment on glycemic control in type 2 diabetes: meta-analyses published as of June 1, 2015

Author, Year	No. of Studies	No. of RCT	Pooled No. of Subjects	HbA$_{1c}$ Change (Percentage Point)	95% CI	P Value
Janket et al,[57] 2005	4	1	268	−0.66[f]	−2.2; 0.9	n/s
Darré et al,[58] 2008	9	5	485	−0.46[e]	−0.82; −0.11	.01
Teeuw et al,[59] 2010	5	3	180	−0.40[f]	−0.77; −0.04	.03
Simpson et al,[60] 2010 (Cochrane Review)	3	3	244	−0.40	−0.78; −0.01	.04
Sgolastra et al,[61] 2013	5	5	315	−0.65[f]	−0.88; −0.43	<.05
Engebretson & Kocher,[62] 2013	9	9	775	−0.36	−0.54; −0.19	<.0001
Liew et al,[63] 2013	6	6	422	−0.41	−0.73; −0.09	.013
Wang et al,[64] 2014[a]	3	3	143	−0.24[e]	−0.62; 0.14	.217
Sun et al,[65] 2014	8	8	515	1.03%(3 mo)[d]	−0.31%; −1.70%[d]	.003
Sun et al,[65] 2014 (6 mos)	3	3	150	−1.18%(6 mo)[d]	−1.64%[d]; −0.72	<.001
Additional reviews that each includes one study on type 1 diabetes						
Corbella et al,[66] 2013 (3 mo)[b]	8	8	678	−0.38	−0.53; −0.23	<.001
Corbella et al,[66] 2013 (6 mo)[b]	3	3	235	−0.31	−0.74; 0.11	.15
Wang et al,[67] 2014[c]	10	10	1135	−0.36	−0.52; −0.19	<.0001

Abbreviations: CI, confidence interval; HbA1c, glycated hemoglobin; n/s, nonsignificant; RCT, randomized controlled trial.
[a] Includes only studies using adjunct doxycycline.
[b] Includes one study with type 1 + type 2 diabetes subjects; 1 study with only type 1 diabetes subject.
[c] Includes one study with 39 type 1 + 66 type 2 diabetes subjects and 9 studies with type 2 diabetes subjects, including DPTT study.
[d] Percent of initial HbA$_{1c}$ value; 3 mo/6 mo, 3/6 months after treatment.
[e] Standardized mean difference.
[f] Weighted Mean Difference.
Data from Refs.[57–67]

diabetes. Such meta-analyses combine data from sufficiently similar studies to obtain more robust results.

Even though many individual nonsurgical periodontal treatment studies are conducted among small numbers of participants and use different exposure and outcome measures and case definitions of periodontitis, and even though the different meta-analyses do not include the same studies, the conclusions of the meta-analyses are remarkably similar:

- None show a posttreatment increase in HbA_{1c}
- All show a (short-term) posttreatment reduction in HbA_{1c}
- The mean HbA_{1c} reduction hovers around 0.4 percentage points.

Of special note is the *Cochrane Collaboration* systematic review from 2010 that, based on 3 studies, reported a decrease of 0.40 percentage points, but calls for "larger, carefully conducted and reported studies."[60] As well, it should be noted that the DPTT study is included in the 2014 meta-analysis by Wang and colleagues,[67] but the HbA_{1c} decrease is still 0.36 (or 0.4) percentage points.

Is a reduction of 0.4 percentage points HbA₁c clinically meaningful?

When a person is diagnosed with type 2 diabetes, the first mode of action to bring the blood sugar under control is to try to improve eating and drinking habits and to do more physical exercise. If that is not sufficient, the first-line medication of choice is metformin taken by mouth, the actions of which are to suppress hepatic glucose production (gluconeogenesis), increase insulin sensitivity, and enhance peripheral glucose uptake while decreasing glucose absorption from the intestinal tract.[68] The expected effect of metformin on HbA_{1c} is a reduction of about 1 percentage point,[69] which is about twice that of which nonsurgical periodontal treatment is shown to lead to. Therefore, the effect of successful nonsurgical periodontal treatment may be clinically significant in diabetes management.

This improvement in glycemic control can help reduce the risk of potentially serious and even fatal complications of poorly controlled diabetes

- Retinopathy (blindness)
- Nephropathy (chronic kidney disease/renal failure/end-stage renal disease)
- Neuropathy (numbness or pain in feet or fingers, burning mouth syndrome, dry mouth/hyposalivation)
- Hypertension
- Heightened susceptibility to infections, delayed wound healing
- Amputation
- Cardiovascular disease (CVD)/myocardial infarction (premature death)
- Stroke (premature death)

Periodontal Treatment in Prediabetes: Effects on Blood Glucose Levels

Recent attention to the importance of prediabetes has resulted in the emergence of intervention studies among that population group. For instance, in 35 to 65 years old individuals with prediabetes, the HbA_{1c} level decreased significantly 3 months after nonsurgical periodontal treatment, namely from 6.08($\pm$0.23)% to 5.67($\pm$0.33)%.[70] Another small study of persons between 35 and 75 years old with prediabetes reported a clinically and statistically significant decrease in HbA_{1c} level 3 months after nonsurgical periodontal treatment, namely, from 6.08($\pm$0.51)% to 5.89($\pm$0.45)%.[71] Finally, among 66 persons with prediabetes, the HbA_{1c} level improved from an average of 6.0% (5.7%–6.3%) to 5.1% (4.9%–5.3%) in the 33 who received nonsurgical periodontal therapy only and from

6.2% (5.7%–6.4%) to 5% (4.8%–5.3%) in participants who additionally received oral doxycycline.[46] Notably, the antibiotic made no difference in the clinical or glycemic outcomes.

In all 3 studies, nonsurgical periodontal treatment was sufficient to reverse prediabetes to healthy in a large proportion of the participants, with an HbA_{1c} level of 5.7% being the lower cut point for the diagnosis of prediabetes (see **Table 1**).

Gingivitis Treatment Only: Effect on Inflammation in Diabetes

Even in persons with type 2 diabetes and only gingivitis (not periodontitis), ultrasonic debridement (prophylaxis) leads to decreased gingival inflammation.[16,72] Such 3-month routine prophylaxes also prevent progression of chronic periodontitis in both poorly controlled and well-controlled patients with type 2 diabetes mellitus.[72] After professional prophylaxis, daily use of essential oils mouth rinse for 90 days is shown to lead to a decrease in levels of overall bacterial load, *T forsythia, A actinomycetemcomitans,* GCF volume, and IL-1β.[16]

In summary

It makes intuitive sense that treatment of periodontal infection would diminish the inflammatory response and elevated blood glucose levels. This is because periodontal treatment is shown to reduce the levels of inflammatory mediators caused by periodontal infections, such as IL-β and TNF-α, which in turn reduce the blood glucose level that was elevated due to the inflammatory response to periodontal infection. Taking this chain of events further back, it could be speculated that effective daily oral hygiene measures, possibly supplemented with professional intervention, would contribute to a decrease in the bacterial burden from the biofilm, thereby help prevent or reduce the subsequent inflammation, and consequently that cleaning the teeth would function as both a preventive and a therapeutic measure.

There is evidence that nonsurgical periodontal treatment in persons with type 2 diabetes can

- Reduce systemic inflammation
- Improve periodontal health both in gingivitis only and in periodontitis
- Improve periodontal health both in poorly and in well-controlled diabetes
- Decrease levels of HbA_{1c} and thereby improve glycemic control in the short term (3 months)

What can be said to patients

- Periodontal disease can increase the amount of sugar in the blood
- Treatment of periodontal disease may lower the amount of sugar in the blood
- Treatment of periodontal disease may help control type 2 diabetes
- It is important to keep the mouth as clean as possible in people with diabetes.

Metabolic Syndrome

Metabolic syndrome is a cluster of metabolic and physiologic abnormalities that are risk factors for both diabetes and atherosclerotic CVD. A person is diagnosed with metabolic syndrome if 3 or more of the following conditions are present:

- Hyperglycemia (fasting glucose ≥100 mg/dL or receiving drug therapy for reduction)
- Hypertension (blood pressure ≥130/85 mm Hg or receiving drug therapy for reduction)

- Hyperlipidemia (triglycerides ≥150 mg/dL or receiving drug therapy for reduction)
- Low HDL cholesterol level (HDL-C <40 mg/dL in men or <50 mg/dL in women or receiving drug therapy for increase)
- Large waistline (abdominal or central obesity: waist circumference ≥102 cm [40 in] in men or ≥88 cm [35 in] in women; if Asian American, ≥90 cm [35 in] in men or ≥80 cm [32 in] in women).

Nonalcoholic Fatty Liver Disease

Nonalcoholic fatty liver disease (NAFLD) is a hepatic manifestation of metabolic syndrome. The highly virulent type of the periodontal bacterium *P gingivalis* is shown to be present with high frequency in oral samples from NAFLD sufferers.[73] Importantly, nonsurgical periodontal treatment over a period of 3 months in such patients improved their liver function parameters, as measured by serum levels of aspartate aminotransferase and alanine aminotransaminase.[73] The effects of periodontal treatment are mentioned under diabetes and cerebrovascular diseases, respectively.

In summary
There is evidence that

- Periodontitis is associated with metabolic syndrome[74] (also in hemodialysis patients),[75] diabetes, and gestational diabetes[76]
- Serum antibody against specific periodontal bacteria is associated with metabolic syndrome[77]
- Periodontitis is significantly associated with development of one or more components of metabolic syndrome over a period of 4 years[78]
- Tooth loss is associated with metabolic syndrome[77,79]
- Periodontal therapy improves total leukocyte count and levels of CRP, triglycerides, and HDL[80]
- Tooth brushing at least once a day leads to
  - Lower levels of triglycerides[81]
  - Lower prevalence and incidence (new cases) of metabolic syndrome[81]

What can be said to patients

- Maintaining good periodontal health may control fat or blood sugar levels and help prevent metabolic syndrome.

Cerebrocardiovascular Disease

Bacteremia
Several reports have found periodontal bacteria in atheromatous plaque.[82–84] *T forsythia* has been identified in the same location as hemoglobin and is therefore regarded as a potential trigger for intraplaque hemorrhage, which may increase the risk for plaque rupture.[85] The periodontal bacterium, *A actinomycetemcomitans*, has been identified in the same person's subgingival plaque, blood, and blood vessels, demonstrating the spread via bacteremia.[86] Dorn and colleagues[87] showed for the first time in 1999 that periodontal bacteria are able to invade both human coronary artery endothelial cells and coronary artery smooth muscle cells, so persons with periodontal infection have greater risk of myocardial infarction.[88] Even though periodontal intervention studies with clinically important outcomes such as myocardial infarction and ischemic stroke are lacking, evidence exists that

- Viable bacteria originating from the periodontium are found in atherosclerotic plaque[89]
- Periodontal bacteria can contribute to atherogenesis[89,90]
- Periodontal bacteria most likely can contribute to destabilization of atherosclerotic plaque[85]
- *P gingivalis* infection is associated with aortic aneurysms and with proliferation of smooth muscle cell tissue in developing aneurysms.[91]

Inflammation

Cardiovascular and cerebral diseases and events considered in this review are those caused by atherosclerosis, which is related to inflammation. Atherosclerosis is the thickening and subsequent calcification of the inner artery wall with deposition of a waxy substance (plaque) that consists of fat, cholesterol, calcium, and other substances from the blood. Atherosclerosis may affect arteries anywhere in the body.

Previous notions of the cause of atherosclerosis centered on the role of lipids, but recent research has indicated that inflammation plays a crucial role. For example, as recently as in 2013, Abdelbaky and colleagues[92] demonstrated for the first time in humans that inflammation actually precedes calcification of the arterial wall in atherogenesis.

Periodontal disease that is inflammatory in nature is recognized as an independent risk factor for atherosclerosis, regardless of other risk factors.[93,94] For example, periodontitis was shown to predict recurrent cardiovascular events in a study that followed 668 survivors of a myocardial infarction for 3 years. Never-smokers with periodontal disease were found to have a 43% higher risk of experiencing another fatal or nonfatal cardiovascular event than such individuals without periodontal disease.[95] In Japanese and US participants with clinical echocardiograms, 77% had cardiac calcifications and 51% had moderate to severe periodontitis.[96] Calcification of structures of the heart is viewed as a marker of subclinical atherosclerosis. Not only were periodontitis and cardiac calcification significantly associated up on adjustment for confounders, their relationship was also dose dependent regarding severity of both conditions.

Periodontal treatment: effect on cardiovascular diseases and events

A systematic *Cochrane Review* from 2014 concluded that there were no studies that assessed periodontal therapy for primary prevention of CVD in persons with periodontitis.[97] Although another 2014 systematic review also agreed that no trials used hard clinical endpoints of CVD, it concluded that periodontal treatment significantly reduces several risk factors for atherosclerotic CVD.[33]

Periodontal treatment: effects on risk factors for cardiovascular events

Instead of exploring the direct effect of periodontal treatment on the actual end points, such as heart attacks, the effect on factors that are known to be risk factors for such events has been investigated. There is evidence that periodontal therapy improves

- Levels of several pro-inflammatory cytokines[33,98]
- Concentrations of CRP in patients without and with coronary heart disease[33,98–100]
- Levels of fibrinogen and white blood cells[100]
- Levels of total cholesterol[33,101]
- Levels of low-density ("bad") cholesterol[32,101]

- Levels of high-density ("good") cholesterol[101]
- Triglyceride levels[33]
- Blood glucose levels (hyperglycemia is a risk factor for CVD)
- Endothelial function,[31] especially in persons with diabetes and CVD[33]
- Systolic and diastolic blood pressure[35]
- Left ventricular mass (improvement is a reduction)[35]
- Pulse-wave velocity (measure of arterial function).[35]

Of particular interest is that the concentrations of the cytokines IL-18 and IFN-γ are shown to be decreased by 90% at 12 months postperiodontal therapy.[102] This finding is of special interest because levels of IL-18 are reported to significantly predict acute myocardial infarction in people with coronary artery disease and major cardiovascular events 6 months after hospitalization for acute coronary syndrome.[103] IL-18 independently predicts congestive heart failure, myocardial infarction, cardiovascular death, and all-cause non-CVD death.[104]

Periodontal treatment: effect on intima media thickness and endothelial dysfunction
Increased intima media thickness (IMT) assessed by ultrasound is a marker for atherosclerosis and is demonstrated to be associated with future cardiovascular events.[105] Endothelial dysfunction is an impairment of the arteries to dilate and contract properly to adjust blood pressure and is a sign of atherosclerotic changes in vessels. It is most often measured on the brachial artery on the inside of the upper arm or on the carotid artery on the side of the neck.

A 2014 meta-analysis concluded that the presence of periodontitis is associated with an increased IMT and a decreased flow-mediated dilation (a measure of endothelial dysfunction),[106] with both differences being clinically significant. Importantly, the authors also concluded that periodontal treatment leads to improvement in endothelial function. Later, it was demonstrated that periodontal therapy can lead to decreased IMT of the carotid artery.[107]

Rheumatoid Arthritis

Rheumatoid arthritis (RA) is an autoimmune, systemic inflammatory chronic disorder that leads to pain and deformity of the joints. Inflammatory mediators, such as TNF-α, and levels of P gingivalis are known to aggravate or partially cause the disease.[108–110] The presence of periodontitis is also shown to hamper RA treatment with TNF-α blockers.[111]

The periodontal bacterium P gingivalis is unique among the oral flora because it possesses an enzyme needed for protein citrullination, a major hallmark of RA.[109] Therefore, it would follow logically that reduction of the P gingivalis level and inflammation levels via periodontal treatment should decrease the severity of RA.

The following is a brief summary of the most recent relevant evidence for periodontal therapy affecting RA:

- Based on 3 treatment studies,[112–114] a 2013 systematic review concluded that evidence is emerging for periodontal treatment leading to improvement in *biochemical markers* in persons suffering from RA.[115]
- A 2014 systematic review concluded, based on 5 eligible intervention studies,[112–114,116,117] that nonsurgical periodontal treatment leads to significant improvement in both *biomarkers* and *clinical arthritis manifestations*, citing reductions in erythrocyte sedimentation rate (ESR) and a trend toward decreasing levels of TNF-α and the 28-joint count disease activity score (DAS28)[118] assessed by CRP or ESR scores.[110]

- More recent treatment studies confirm these findings, with a significant decrease in TNF-α levels.[119–121]
- Improvement in signs and symptoms of RA occurred, regardless of whether the RA patients were under anti-TNF-α treatment.[117]
- Anti-TNF-α RA treatment had no effect on the periodontal health without periodontal therapy.[117]

Interestingly, a case report reported that periodontal treatment resulted in resolution of the RA disease, suggesting that in this case, RA was actually caused by the periodontal infection, specifically by *P gingivalis*.[122]

Gingivitis treatment alone: effect on rheumatoid arthritis manifestation
Among persons suffering from RA, even plaque control consisting of supragingival scaling and oral hygiene instruction decreased the DAS28 as well as serum levels of IgG to *P gingivalis* hemin binding protein 35 and citrulline.[116]

In summary There is evidence to suggest

- A 2-way relationship exists between periodontitis and RA
- Periodontal treatment leads to improved biochemical markers of RA
- Periodontal treatment may ameliorate the clinical manifestations of RA.

What can be said to patients:

- Periodontal treatment and home oral hygiene can help lessen the swelling and pain of arthritic joints (symptoms of RA) and may help prevent RA.

Respiratory Tract Diseases

Aspiration pneumonia
Aspiration pneumonia is an infection of the lungs that is caused by aspiration of oral contents into the larynx and continuing via trachea and the primary bronchi to the lungs. Aspiration pneumonia is common among frail elderly and persons with swallowing disorders. Individuals who for any reason are not able to maintain good oral hygiene are also at risk.

The term nosocomial pneumonia describes a lung infection that is caused by microbes, typically in the hospital or other health care institution, at least 48 to 72 hours after being admitted and is therefore also known as hospital-acquired pneumonia (HAP). Bacteria from dental plaque are associated with pneumonia.[123] Patients with periodontitis have more than a 3-fold higher risk of having lower respiratory tract infection than those without periodontitis among hospital patients.[124] Among nursing home residents, those without oral health care have 3.6 times higher mortality from pneumonia than those who were assigned oral hygiene care by nursing assistants.[125]

Systematic reviews published in 2003,[126] 2006,[127] 2008,[128] and 2013[129] explored whether oral health care interventions in frail older persons in nursing homes or at hospitals could prevent aspiration pneumonia, and concluded that

- Mechanical oral hygiene and local chemical disinfection with antiseptics or antibiotics prevent aspiration pneumonia.[127,128]
- About 40% of pneumonia cases are preventable by improved oral hygiene.[126]
- Oral health care lowers not only the risk for both development and progression of aspiration pneumonia[127] but also the risk of death from the disease.[128,129]
- About 10% of deaths caused by pneumonia might be prevented by oral interventions.[128]

Ventilator-assisted pneumonia

Mechanical ventilation contributes to the risk for HAP, but a 2013 *Cochrane Systematic Review* concluded that effective oral health care is important for adult patients in intensive care, and the use of either mouth rinse or gel that contains chlorhexidine is associated with a 40% decrease in the risk of developing ventilator-assisted pneumonia.[130] However, there is no evidence for a decrease in risk for death from pneumonia, duration of mechanical ventilation, or duration of intensive care. Furthermore, the review found no difference regarding prevention of ventilator-assisted pneumonia in adults whether using (a) chlorhexidine together with tooth brushing versus chlorhexidine alone or (b) povidone iodine mouthwash versus saline, although weak evidence favors the former. Finally, the *Cochrane Review* did not find sufficient evidence to determine if other mouth rinses like saline, triclosan, or water can decrease the development of ventilator-related pneumonia.[130]

Chronic obstructive pulmonary disease

Chronic obstructive pulmonary disease (COPD) is strongly associated with poor periodontal status,[131] frequency of professional dental care, and knowledge about oral health.[132] In COPD, periodontal treatment is reported to improve lung capacity function[133] and lessen the frequency of exacerbations.[133,134] However, a small study with 30 participants did not find any effect of periodontal therapy on quality of life 4 weeks after treatment, nor was there any effect on the COPD. The study did demonstrate that power brushes could be used without any adverse events.[135]

Chronic Kidney Disease

Individuals undergoing dialysis typically have very poor oral health,[136–142] and for those with long-term hemodialysis, periodontitis is associated with an increased mortality.[137,140,143] One study reported a higher periodontitis risk for older Japanese women with lower cystatin C-based estimated glomerular filtration rate (eGFR).[144]

Periodontal treatment: effect on chronic kidney disease

Some evidence indicates that periodontal treatment can reduce chronic systemic inflammation (measured as CRP level) and improve nutritional status in patients who receive both hemodialysis[145] and peritoneal dialysis.[145]

Periodontal treatment reduces the concentration of IL-18, a pro-inflammatory cytokine that is shown to be significantly elevated in persons with type 2 diabetes in whom IL-18 also may be a predictor for both development and progression of diabetic nephropathy.[146,147]

A systematic review concluded that "There is quite consistent evidence to support the positive association between periodontitis and CKD [chronic kidney disease], as well as the positive effect of PT [periodontal treatment] on eGFR."[138] However, a critical review of this paper concluded that "periodontitis may be associated with chronic kidney disease, but current evidence is insufficient."[148] Specifically, the reviewer considered the inclusion of only 3, nonrandomized treatment studies with ambiguous results inadequate to support the last part of the authors' statement.

In summary There is some evidence to suggest that periodontal treatment

- Can reduce systemic inflammation in persons receiving hemodialysis or peritoneal hemodialysis
- Can decrease systemic inflammation (importantly, IL-18 levels) that may predict incidence and progression of nephropathy in people with type 2 diabetes

- Can improve nutritional status in persons receiving hemodialysis or peritoneal hemodialysis

What can be said to patients:

- Periodontal disease treatment and home oral hygiene might help people with kidney disease, but there is not enough proof for that yet.
- It is important to keep the mouth as clean as possible also in persons with long-term kidney disease who typically have poorer oral health habits than persons without kidney disease.

Cancer

The notion that infection/inflammation plays a potentially pivotal role in development of cancer has recently gained support, as it is realized that cancer is not only due to genes and their mutations, obesity, or pollution. For instance, a 24-year follow-up study of 1390 Swedes showed that a history of chronic dental infections due to caries or periodontitis that had caused tooth loss was strongly linked to the development of cancer.[149]

Specifically related to periodontitis is the role that lately has been demonstrated by *F nucleatum*, a commensal member of the periodontal microbiome that is predominant in chronic periodontitis[150] and which can turn into a pathogen that travels to locations outside the oral cavity.[151] *F nucleatum* is not only found to invade colorectal cancerous lesions, but a causal role is established. Other members of the periodontal microbiome also invade oral and pharyngeal cancers and may contribute to their development.[152,153]

In summary

There is evidence for

- Various periodontal bacteria and virus as known risk factors for cancers of the digestive tract, including the oral cavity
- *F. nucleatum* contributing to the development of colorectal cancer
- Oral human papilloma virus infection or a history of periodontitis being associated with squamous cell carcinomas of the head and neck, with a stronger link in oropharyngeal cancer than in cancers of the mouth and larynx.

What can be said to patients:

- Normal bacteria in the dental plaque (biofilm) may contribute to the cause of cancer of the gut (colon/rectum), even more so when there also is periodontal disease.
- There is no proof that treatment of periodontal disease can prevent cancer from developing.

Other Diseases

Evidence is emerging that illuminates the understanding of the systemic effects of members of the "traveling oral microbiome."[7,154] There is also evidence for the association between periodontal disease and systemic diseases thought to be caused by the general inflammatory responses. There is emerging evidence for links between periodontal infection with its subsequent inflammation and systemic disease, such as

- Alzheimer disease/cognitive function decline[40,155]
- Appendicitis[151]
- Benign prostatic hyperplasia[156]

- Erectile dysfunction[157–159] even in large population-based studies[160,161]
- Human T-lymphotropic virus type I associated myelopathy/tropical spastic paraparesis and adult T-cell leukemia[162]
- Inflammatory bowel disease[163,164]
- Lemierre syndrome[165,166]
- Ruptured intracranial aneurysms, abdominal aortic aneurysms[167]
- Spondyloarthritis.[164]

However, no findings from intervention studies to support these reported associations are available at this time.

Obesity

Obesity has recently been declared a disease, but will not be described in any detail because studies have not attempted to show whether periodontal treatment has any direct effect on this condition. However, it should be borne in mind that the excess fat cells in all body organs and tissues cause a chronic, low-grade inflammation (see **Fig. 1**) that has been called metainflammation.[168] It has the same negative consequences as any other inflammation and hence contributes to the total load of systemic inflammatory responses, which in turn affects all the inflammation-related diseases. Obesity, metabolic syndrome, type 2 diabetes, and CVD are part of a cardiovascular-metabolic dysfunction continuum that without sharp borders develop together. Finally, obesity is shown to be a predictor for poorer outcome of periodontal treatment.[169–171]

Pregnancy

Even though pregnancy is not a disease, but a temporary condition, it should be mentioned that there is some evidence for associations between periodontal infection and adverse pregnancy outcomes, especially pre-eclampsia (hypertension and protein in the urine or organ damage), as demonstrated by 3 meta-analyses in 2013 and 2014.[172–174] Although cautioning against the studies' heterogeneity, they all conclude that mothers with periodontitis have about 2 to 4 times higher risk for pre-eclampsia than those with healthy periodontal tissues and suggest that periodontitis may be regarded as a possible, independent risk factor for pre-eclampsia. Moreover, identical bacteria have been identified in the mother's subgingival plaque and in the stillborn fetus and were declared the cause of such negative outcome.

A multitude of smaller studies report that periodontal treatment leads to a lower incidence of various adverse pregnancy outcomes, most often preterm birth and babies born too small for their gestational age. However, there is no evidence from large, well-designed and well-executed RCTs that nonsurgical periodontal treatment can prevent adverse pregnancy outcomes. Importantly, all studies concur that periodontal treatment during pregnancy is safe for both mother and child.

Why It Is so Difficult to Determine Whether Periodontal Treatment Has Systemic Effects

Clinical research findings of high quality are trickling in, but here follow some reasons it is difficult to unambiguously determine whether periodontal therapy improves general health:

- The systemic diseases are typically chronic and require many years to develop.
- Periodontal disease and many chronic systemic diseases are multifactorial with a multitude of causes and modifying internal and external factors.
- Some individuals seem to cope well (exhibit resistance) with the frequent, recurrent, or constant microbial offense, whereas others are more susceptible to

periodontal breakdown. That is, the amount of damage caused seems to depend more on the host than on the amount and composition of the offending plaque.

- There has never been one globally accepted case definition for periodontitis, which prevents direct comparison of results from different studies.
- A therapeutic effect could be caused by something other than the periodontal treatment provided—or be overshadowed by other factors.
- Most people with a given disease suffer from more than one disease or condition, complicating both study participant enrollment and statistical analyses of the data collected.
- Human studies are inherently costly to conduct.
- The current systems to determine whether a relationship between 2 factors is one of cause and effect (causal, so one leads to the other) versus association ("vary together" without knowing whether one factor causes the other) were developed for infectious diseases that had mostly one major cause.
- As yet unknown genetic and environmental factors cannot be controlled, but may impact the end results.

SUMMARY

Associations between periodontal disease and chronic systemic diseases exist. The main underlying mechanisms are thought to include (1) the direct effect of bacterial invasion on bacteremia; and (2) the indirect effect of inflammatory responses.

Furthermore, there is evidence that periodontal treatment leads to decreased blood concentrations of periodontal bacteria and inflammatory markers, up on any transient increases immediately on such treatment. Therefore, it would follow intuitively to expect that incidence and severity of such systemic diseases would be ameliorated by periodontal treatment. The current scientific evidence suggests that periodontal treatment can have positive effects on glycemic control in type 2 diabetes, aspiration pneumonia, and RA. There is emerging evidence for periodontal therapy having significant, clinical effects on other systemic diseases and conditions.

What can be said to patients regarding the effect of periodontal treatment, based on the current evidence:

- Dental plaque (biofilm) should be removed often because it is starts inflammation that in some persons leads to periodontal disease (periodontitis).
- Persons with the most severe periodontal breakdown likely have a compromised defense (immune) system and therefore should be extra careful to have good oral hygiene and regular dental checkups.
- Treating periodontal disease can help decrease the amount of sugar in the blood and improves control in type 2 diabetes in the short run (3 months).
- Treating periodontal disease seems to lower the sugar level in persons with prediabetes.
- Cleaning the mouth can help keep frail or very ill persons on ventilators from getting pneumonia.
- Treating periodontal disease may help lessen the swelling and pain in joint disease (RA).
- Keeping the teeth as clean as possible may help lower the risk for heart attacks, stroke, some cancers, and other diseases.
- Cleaning the teeth is necessary for having a healthy body, because the mouth is part of the body.
- Cleaning the teeth is necessary to have a healthy mouth, and a healthy mouth increases the quality of life.

REFERENCES

1. Centers for Disease Control and Prevention. National diabetes statistics report: estimates of diabetes and its burden in the United States, 2014. Atlanta (GA): U.S. Department of Health and Human Services. Available at: http://www.Cdc.Gov/diabetes/pubs/statsreport14/national-diabetes-report-web.Pdf. Accessed June 1, 2015.
2. Scannapieco FA, Dasanayake AP, Chhun N. Does periodontal therapy reduce the risk for systemic diseases? Dent Clin North Am 2010;54(1):163–81.
3. Eke PI, Page RC, Wei L, et al. Update of the case definitions for population-based surveillance of periodontitis. J Periodontol 2012;83(12):1449–54.
4. Manau C, Echeverria A, Agueda A, et al. Periodontal disease definition may determine the association between periodontitis and pregnancy outcomes. J Clin Periodontol 2008;35(5):385–97.
5. Donahue RP, Wu T. Insulin resistance and periodontal disease: an epidemiologic overview of research needs and future directions. Ann Periodontol 2001; 6(1):119–24.
6. Taylor GW, Borgnakke WS, Graves DT. Association between periodontal diseases and diabetes mellitus. Chapter 6. In: Genco RJ, Williams RC, editors. Periodontal disease and overall health; a clinician's guide. Yardley (PA): Professional Audience Communication; 2010. p. 83–104. Available at: http://www.colgateprofessional.com/professionaleducation/Periodontal-Disease-and-Overall-Health-A-Clinicians-Guide/article. Accessed June 1, 2015.
7. Borgnakke WS. The traveling oral microbiome. Chapter 4. In: Glick M, editor. The oral-systemic health connection: a guide to patient care. Chicago: Quintessence; 2014. p. 61–102.
8. Tomas I, Diz P, Tobias A, et al. Periodontal health status and bacteraemia from daily oral activities: systematic review/meta-analysis. J Clin Periodontol 2012; 39(3):213–28 [Systematic review/meta-analysis].
9. Cobe HM. Transitory bacteremia. Oral Surg Oral Med Oral Pathol 1954;7(6): 609–15.
10. Forner L, Larsen T, Kilian M, et al. Incidence of bacteremia after chewing, tooth brushing and scaling in individuals with periodontal inflammation. J Clin Periodontol 2006;33(6):401–7.
11. Bahrani-Mougeot FK, Paster BJ, Coleman S, et al. Diverse and novel oral bacterial species in blood following dental procedures. J Clin Microbiol 2008;46(6): 2129–32.
12. Lockhart PB, Brennan MT, Sasser HC, et al. Bacteremia associated with toothbrushing and dental extraction. Circulation 2008;117(24):3118–25.
13. Carroll GC, Sebor RJ. Dental flossing and its relationship to transient bacteremia. J Periodontol 1980;51(12):691–2.
14. Olsen I. Update on bacteraemia related to dental procedures. Transfus Apher Sci 2008;39(2):173–8.
15. Graziani F, Cei S, Tonetti M, et al. Systemic inflammation following non-surgical and surgical periodontal therapy. J Clin Periodontol 2010;37(9): 848–54.
16. Raslan SA, Cortelli JR, Costa FO, et al. Clinical, microbial, and immune responses observed in patients with diabetes after treatment for gingivitis: a three-month randomized clinical trial. J Periodontol 2015;86(4):516–26.
17. Bender IB, Bender AB. Diabetes mellitus and the dental pulp. J Endod 2003; 29(6):383–9.

18. Debelian GJ, Olsen I, Tronstad L. Anaerobic bacteremia and fungemia in patients undergoing endodontic therapy: an overview. Ann Periodontol 1998;3(1):281–7.
19. Horliana AC, Chambrone L, Foz AM, et al. Dissemination of periodontal pathogens in the bloodstream after periodontal procedures: a systematic review. PLoS One 2014;9(5):e98271 [Systematic review/meta-analysis].
20. Zhang W, Daly CG, Mitchell D, et al. Incidence and magnitude of bacteraemia caused by flossing and by scaling and root planing. J Clin Periodontol 2013; 40(1):41–52.
21. Daly CG, Mitchell DH, Highfield JE, et al. Bacteremia due to periodontal probing: a clinical and microbiological investigation. J Periodontol 2001;72(2):210–4.
22. Ross R. Cell biology of atherosclerosis. Annu Rev Physiol 1995;57:791–804.
23. Ridker PM, Cushman M, Stampfer MJ, et al. Inflammation, aspirin, and the risk of cardiovascular disease in apparently healthy men. N Engl J Med 1997;336(14): 973–9.
24. Ridker PM, Silvertown JD. Inflammation, C-reactive protein, and atherothrombosis. J Periodontol 2008;79(8 Suppl):1544–51.
25. Hajishengallis G. Periodontitis: from microbial immune subversion to systemic inflammation. Nat Rev Immunol 2015;15(1):30–44.
26. Hajishengallis G. Immunomicrobial pathogenesis of periodontitis: keystones, pathobionts, and host response. Trends Immunol 2014;35(1):3–11.
27. Bartova J, Sommerova P, Lyuya-Mi Y, et al. Periodontitis as a risk factor of atherosclerosis. J Immunol Res 2014;2014:636893.
28. Darby IB, Mooney J, Kinane DF. Changes in subgingival microflora and humoral immune response following periodontal therapy. J Clin Periodontol 2001;28(8): 796–805.
29. He JY, Qi GG, Huang WJ, et al. Short-term microbiological effects of scaling and root planing and essential-oils mouthwash in Chinese adults. J Zhejiang Univ Sci B 2013;14(5):416–25.
30. D'Aiuto F, Nibali L, Mohamed-Ali V, et al. Periodontal therapy: a novel non-drug-induced experimental model to study human inflammation. J Periodontal Res 2004;39(5):294–9.
31. Tonetti MS, D'Aiuto F, Nibali L, et al. Treatment of periodontitis and endothelial function. N Engl J Med 2007;356(9):911–20.
32. Teeuw WJ, Slot DE, Susanto H, et al. Treatment of periodontitis improves the atherosclerotic profile: a systematic review and meta-analysis. J Clin Periodontol 2014;41(1):70–9 [Systematic review/meta-analysis].
33. D'Aiuto F, Nibali L, Parkar M, et al. Short-term effects of intensive periodontal therapy on serum inflammatory markers and cholesterol. J Dent Res 2005; 84(3):269–73.
34. Moura Foz A, Alexandre Romito G, Manoel Bispo C, et al. Periodontal therapy and biomarkers related to cardiovascular risk. Minerva Stomatol 2010;59(5): 271–83.
35. Vidal F, Cordovil I, Figueredo CM, et al. Non-surgical periodontal treatment reduces cardiovascular risk in refractory hypertensive patients: a pilot study. J Clin Periodontol 2013;40(7):681–7.
36. Lakio L, Antinheimo J, Paju S, et al. Tracking of plasma antibodies against *Aggregatibacter actinomycetemcomitans* and *Porphyromonas gingivalis* during 15 years. J Oral Microbiol 2009;1.
37. Papapanou PN, Neiderud AM, Disick E, et al. Longitudinal stability of serum immunoglobulin G responses to periodontal bacteria. J Clin Periodontol 2004; 31(11):985–90.

38. Choi YH, Mckeown RE, Mayer-Davis EJ, et al. Serum C-reactive protein and immunoglobulin G antibodies to periodontal pathogens may be effect modifiers of periodontitis and hyperglycemia. J Periodontol 2014;85(9):1172–81.
39. Iwasaki M, Minagawa K, Sato M, et al. Serum antibody to Porphyromonas gingivalis in metabolic syndrome among an older Japanese population. Gerodontology 2014. Accessed July 13, 2015.
40. Noble JM, Scarmeas N, Celenti RS, et al. Serum IgG antibody levels to periodontal microbiota are associated with incident Alzheimer disease. PLoS One 2014;9(12):e114959.
41. Noble JM, Borrell LN, Papapanou PN, et al. Periodontitis is associated with cognitive impairment among older adults: analysis of NHANES-III. J Neurol Neurosurg Psychiatry 2009;80(11):1206–11.
42. Nathan DM, Kuenen J, Borg R, et al. Translating the A1c assay into estimated average glucose values. Diabetes Care 2008;31(8):1473–8.
43. American Diabetes Association. Classification and diagnosis of diabetes. Diabetes Care 2015;38(Supplement 1):S8–16.
44. Kowall B, Holtfreter B, Völzke H, et al. Prediabetes and well-controlled diabetes are not associated with periodontal disease: the SHIP Trend Study. J Clin Periodontol 2015;42(5):422–30.
45. Lamster IB, Cheng B, Burkett S, et al. Periodontal findings in individuals with newly identified prediabetes or diabetes mellitus. J Clin Periodontol 2014; 41(11):1055–60.
46. Javed F, Ahmed HB, Mehmood A, et al. Effect of nonsurgical periodontal therapy (with or without oral doxycycline delivery) on glycemic status and clinical periodontal parameters in patients with prediabetes: a short-term longitudinal randomized case-control study. Clin Oral Investig 2014;18(8):1963–8.
47. Javed F, Thafeed Alghamdi AS, Mikami T, et al. Effect of glycemic control on self-perceived oral health, periodontal parameters, and alveolar bone loss among patients with prediabetes. J Periodontol 2014;85(2):234–41.
48. Javed F, Al-Askar M, Samaranayake LP, et al. Periodontal disease in habitual cigarette smokers and nonsmokers with and without prediabetes. Am J Med Sci 2013;345(2):94–8.
49. Santaguida PL, Balion C, Hunt D, et al. Diagnosis, prognosis, and treatment of impaired glucose tolerance and impaired fasting glucose. Evidence Report/Technology Assessment No. 128. AHRQ publication no. 05-e026-2. Rockville (MD): Agency for Healthcare Research and Quality; 2005. p. 312. Available at: http://archive.ahrq.gov/downloads/pub/evidence/pdf/impglucose/impglucose.pdf. Accessed June 1, 2015.
50. Borgnakke WS, Ylöstalo PV, Taylor GW, et al. Effect of periodontal disease on diabetes: systematic review of epidemiologic observational evidence. J Clin Periodontol 2013;40(Suppl 14):S135–52 [Systematic review/meta-analysis]. Available at: http://onlinelibrary.wiley.com/doi/10.1111/jcpe.2013.40.issue-s14/issuetoc. Accessed June 1, 2015.
51. Sooray KV, Suchetha A, Lakshmi P, et al. The effect of scaling and root planing on glycaemic control, periodontal status and gingival crevicular fluid TNF-α levels in an Indian population—to reveal the ambivalent link. J Clin Diagn Res 2014;8(11):ZC22–6.
52. Engebretson SP, Hyman LG, Michalowicz BS, et al. The effect of nonsurgical periodontal therapy on hemoglobin A1c levels in persons with type 2 diabetes and chronic periodontitis: a randomized clinical trial. JAMA 2013;310(23): 2523–32.

53. Borgnakke WS, Chapple IL, Genco RJ, et al. The multi-center randomized controlled trial (RCT) published by the Journal of The American Medical Association (JAMA) on the effect of periodontal therapy on glycated hemoglobin (HbA1c) has fundamental problems. J Evid Based Dent Pract 2014;14(3):127–32.
54. Chapple IL, Borgnakke WS, Genco RJ. Hemoglobin A1c levels among patients with diabetes receiving nonsurgical periodontal treatment. JAMA 2014;311(18): 1919–20.
55. Pihlstrom BL. Selections from the current literature. J Am Dent Assoc 2014; 145(5):479–81.
56. Pihlstrom BL, Buse JB. Diabetes and periodontal therapy. J Am Dent Assoc 2014;145(12):1208–10.
57. Janket SJ, Wightman A, Baird AE, et al. Does periodontal treatment improve glycemic control in diabetic patients? a meta-analysis of intervention studies. J Dent Res 2005;84(12):1154–9 [Systematic review/meta-analysis].
58. Darré L, Vergnes JN, Gourdy P, et al. Efficacy of periodontal treatment on glycaemic control in diabetic patients: a meta-analysis of interventional studies. Diabetes Metab 2008;34(5):497–506 [Systematic review/meta-analysis].
59. Teeuw WJ, Gerdes VE, Loos BG. Effect of periodontal treatment on glycemic control of diabetic patients: a systematic review and meta-analysis. Diabetes Care 2010;33(2):421–7 [Systematic review/meta-analysis].
60. Simpson TC, Needleman I, Wild SH, et al. Treatment of periodontal disease for glycaemic control in people with diabetes. Cochrane Database Syst Rev 2010;(5):CD004714. [Systematic review/meta-analysis].
61. Sgolastra F, Severino M, Pietropaoli D, et al. Effectiveness of periodontal treatment to improve metabolic control in patients with chronic periodontitis and type 2 diabetes: a meta-analysis of randomized clinical trials. J Periodontol 2013;84(7):958–73 [Systematic review/meta-analysis].
62. Engebretson S, Kocher T. Evidence that periodontal treatment improves diabetes outcomes: a systematic review and meta-analysis. J Clin Periodontol 2013;40(Suppl 14):S153–63 [Systematic review/meta-analysis].
63. Liew AK, Punnanithinont N, Lee YC, et al. Effect of non-surgical periodontal treatment on HbA1c: a meta-analysis of randomized controlled trials. Aust Dent J 2013;58(3):350–7 [Systematic review/meta-analysis].
64. Wang TF, Jen IA, Chou C, et al. Effects of periodontal therapy on metabolic control in patients with type 2 diabetes mellitus and periodontal disease: a meta-analysis. Medicine (Baltimore) 2014;93(28):e292 [Systematic review/meta-analysis].
65. Sun QY, Feng M, Zhang MZ, et al. Effects of periodontal treatment on glycemic control in type 2 diabetic patients: a meta-analysis of randomized controlled trials. Chin J Physiol 2014;57(6):305–14 [Systematic review/meta-analysis].
66. Corbella S, Francetti L, Taschieri S, et al. Effect of periodontal treatment on glycemic control of patients with diabetes: a systematic review and meta-analysis. J Diabetes Investig 2013;4(5):502–9 [Systematic review/meta-analysis].
67. Wang X, Han X, Guo X, et al. The effect of periodontal treatment on hemoglobin A1c levels of diabetic patients: a systematic review and meta-analysis. PLoS One 2014;9(9):e108412 [Systematic review/meta-analysis].
68. Bailey CJ, Turner RC. Metformin. N Engl J Med 1996;334(9):574–9.
69. Agency for Healthcare Research and Quality (AHRQ). Effective health care program. Comparing medications for adults with type 2 diabetes. pub. No. 11-ehc038-3. Rockville, MD: AHRQ; 2011. p. 8. Available at: http://www.Effectivehealthcare. Ahrq.Gov/ehc/products/155/720/ecbcm_oral%20meds%20t2%20diab_clinician 06282011.Pdf. Accessed June 1, 2015.

70. Perayil J, Suresh N, Fenol A, et al. Comparison of glycated hemoglobin levels in individuals without diabetes and with and without periodontitis before and after non-surgical periodontal therapy. J Periodontol 2014;85(12):1658–66.
71. Giblin LJ, Boyd LD, Rainchuso L, et al. Short-term effects of non-surgical periodontal therapy on clinical measures of impaired glucose tolerance in people with prediabetes and chronic periodontitis. J Dent Hyg 2014;88(Suppl 1):23–30.
72. Lopez NJ, Quintero A, Casanova PA, et al. Routine prophylaxes every 3 months improves chronic periodontitis status in type 2 diabetes. J Periodontol 2014; 85(7):e232–40.
73. Yoneda M, Naka S, Nakano K, et al. Involvement of a periodontal pathogen, *Porphyromonas gingivalis* on the pathogenesis of non-alcoholic fatty liver disease. BMC Gastroenterol 2012;12:16.
74. Watanabe K, Cho YD. Periodontal disease and metabolic syndrome: a qualitative critical review of their association. Arch Oral Biol 2014;59(8):855–70.
75. Chen LP, Hsu SP, Peng YS, et al. Periodontal disease is associated with metabolic syndrome in hemodialysis patients. Nephrol Dial Transplant 2011;26(12):4068–73.
76. Bullon P, Jaramillo R, Santos-Garcia R, et al. Relation of periodontitis and metabolic syndrome with gestational glucose metabolism disorder. J Periodontol 2014;85(2):e1–8.
77. Hyvärinen K, Salminen A, Salomaa V, et al. Systemic exposure to a common periodontal pathogen and missing teeth are associated with metabolic syndrome. Acta Diabetol 2014;52:179–82.
78. Morita T, Yamazaki Y, Mita A, et al. A cohort study on the association between periodontal disease and the development of metabolic syndrome. J Periodontol 2010; 81(4):512–9.
79. Zhu Y, Hollis JH. Associations between the number of natural teeth and metabolic syndrome in adults. J Clin Periodontol 2015;42(2):113–20.
80. Acharya A, Bhavsar N, Jadav B, et al. Cardioprotective effect of periodontal therapy in metabolic syndrome: a pilot study in Indian subjects. Metab Syndr Relat Disord 2010;8(4):335–41.
81. Kobayashi Y, Niu K, Guan L, et al. Oral health behavior and metabolic syndrome and its components in adults. J Dent Res 2012;91(5):479–84.
82. Figuero E, Sanchez-Beltran M, Cuesta-Frechoso S, et al. Detection of periodontal bacteria in atheromatous plaque by nested polymerase chain reaction. J Periodontol 2011;82(10):1469–77.
83. Haraszthy VI, Zambon JJ, Trevisan M, et al. Identification of periodontal pathogens in atheromatous plaques. J Periodontol 2000;71(10):1554–60.
84. Kozarov EV, Dorn BR, Shelburne CE, et al. Human atherosclerotic plaque contains viable invasive *Actinobacillus actinomycetemcomitans* and *Porphyromonas gingivalis*. Arterioscler Thromb Vasc Biol 2005;25(3):e17–8.
85. Range H, Labreuche J, Louedec L, et al. Periodontal bacteria in human carotid atherothrombosis as a potential trigger for neutrophil activation. Atherosclerosis 2014;236(2):448–55.
86. Figuero E, Lindahl C, Marin MJ, et al. Quantification of periodontal pathogens in vascular, blood, and subgingival samples from patients with peripheral arterial disease or abdominal aortic aneurysms. J Periodontol 2014;85(9):1182–93.
87. Dorn BR, Dunn WA Jr, Progulske-Fox A. Invasion of human coronary artery cells by periodontal pathogens. Infect Immun 1999;67(11):5792–8.
88. Andriankaja O, Trevisan M, Falkner K, et al. Association between periodontal pathogens and risk of nonfatal myocardial infarction. Community Dent Oral Epidemiol 2011;39(2):177–85.

89. Kozarov E. Bacterial invasion of vascular cell types: vascular infectology and atherogenesis. Future Cardiol 2012;8(1):123–38.

90. Reyes L, Herrera D, Kozarov E, et al. Periodontal bacterial invasion and infection: contribution to atherosclerotic pathology. J Clin Periodontol 2013;40(Suppl 14): S30–50.

91. Wada K, Kamisaki Y. Roles of oral bacteria in cardiovascular diseases – from molecular mechanisms to clinical cases: involvement of *Porphyromonas gingivalis* in the development of human aortic aneurysm. J Pharmacol Sci 2010;113(2):115–9.

92. Abdelbaky A, Corsini E, Figueroa AL, et al. Focal arterial inflammation precedes subsequent calcification in the same location: a longitudinal FDG-PET/CT study. Circ Cardiovasc Imaging 2013;6(5):747–54.

93. Kebschull M, Haupt M, Jepsen S, et al. Mobilization of endothelial progenitors by recurrent bacteremias with a periodontal pathogen. PLoS One 2013;8(1): e54860.

94. Katsiki N, Athyros VG, Karagiannis A, et al. Should we expand the concept of coronary heart disease equivalents? Curr Opin Cardiol 2014;29(4):389–95.

95. Dorn JM, Genco RJ, Grossi SG, et al. Periodontal disease and recurrent cardiovascular events in survivors of myocardial infarction (MI): the Western New York Acute MI study. J Periodontol 2010;81(4):502–11.

96. Pressman GS, Qasim A, Verma N, et al. Periodontal disease is an independent predictor of intracardiac calcification. Biomed Res Int 2013;2013:854340.

97. Li C, Lv Z, Shi Z, et al. Periodontal therapy for the management of cardiovascular disease in patients with chronic periodontitis. Cochrane Database Syst Rev 2014;(8):CD009197. [Systematic review/meta-analysis].

98. Zhou SY, Duan XQ, Hu R, et al. Effect of non-surgical periodontal therapy on serum levels of TNF-a, Il-6 and C-reactive protein in periodontitis subjects with stable coronary heart disease. Chin J Dent Res 2013;16(2):145–51.

99. Offenbacher S, Beck JD, Moss K, et al. Results from the Periodontitis and Vascular Events (PAVE) Study: a pilot multicentered, randomized, controlled trial to study effects of periodontal therapy in a secondary prevention model of cardiovascular disease. J Periodontol 2009;80(2):190–201.

100. Bokhari SA, Khan AA, Butt AK, et al. Non-surgical periodontal therapy reduces coronary heart disease risk markers: a randomized controlled trial. J Clin Periodontol 2012;39(11):1065–74.

101. Buhlin K, Hultin M, Norderyd O, et al. Periodontal treatment influences risk markers for atherosclerosis in patients with severe periodontitis. Atherosclerosis 2009;206(2):518–22.

102. Li ZG, Li JJ, Sun CA, et al. Interleukin-18 promoter polymorphisms and plasma levels are associated with increased risk of periodontitis: a meta-analysis. Inflamm Res 2014;63(1):45–52.

103. Furtado MV, Rossini AP, Campani RB, et al. Interleukin-18: an independent predictor of cardiovascular events in patients with acute coronary syndrome after 6 months of follow-up. Coron Artery Dis 2009;20(5):327–31.

104. Hartford M, Wiklund O, Hulten LM, et al. Interleukin-18 as a predictor of future events in patients with acute coronary syndromes. Arterioscler Thromb Vasc Biol 2010;30(10):2039–46.

105. van den Oord SC, Sijbrands EJ, ten Kate GL, et al. Carotid intima-media thickness for cardiovascular risk assessment: systematic review and meta-analysis. Atherosclerosis 2013;228(1):1–11 [Systematic review/meta-analysis].

106. Orlandi M, Suvan J, Petrie A, et al. Association between periodontal disease and its treatment, flow-mediated dilatation and carotid intima-media thickness: a

systematic review and meta-analysis. Atherosclerosis 2014;236(1):39–46 [Systematic review/meta-analysis].

107. Kapellas K, Maple-Brown LJ, Jamieson LM, et al. Effect of periodontal therapy on arterial structure and function among Aboriginal Australians: a randomized, controlled trial. Hypertension 2014;64(4):702–8.

108. Arvikar SL, Collier DS, Fisher MC, et al. Clinical correlations with *Porphyromonas gingivalis* antibody responses in patients with early rheumatoid arthritis. Arthritis Res Ther 2013;15(5):R109.

109. El-Shinnawi U, Soory M. Associations between periodontitis and systemic inflammatory diseases: response to treatment. Recent Pat Endocr Metab Immune Drug Discov 2013;7(3):169–88.

110. Kaur S, Bright R, Proudman SM, et al. Does periodontal treatment influence clinical and biochemical measures for rheumatoid arthritis? A systematic review and meta-analysis. Semin Arthritis Rheum 2014;44(2):113–22 [Systematic review/meta-analysis].

111. Savioli C, Ribeiro AC, Fabri GM, et al. Persistent periodontal disease hampers anti-tumor necrosis factor treatment response in rheumatoid arthritis. J Clin Rheumatol 2012;18(4):180–4.

112. Al-Katma MK, Bissada NF, Bordeaux JM, et al. Control of periodontal infection reduces the severity of active rheumatoid arthritis. J Clin Rheumatol 2007; 13(3):134–7.

113. Pinho Mde N, Oliveira RD, Novaes AB Jr, et al. Relationship between periodontitis and rheumatoid arthritis and the effect of non-surgical periodontal treatment. Braz Dent J 2009;20(5):355–64.

114. Ribeiro J, Leao A, Novaes AB. Periodontal infection as a possible severity factor for rheumatoid arthritis. J Clin Periodontol 2005;32(4):412–6.

115. Kaur S, White S, Bartold PM. Periodontal disease and rheumatoid arthritis: a systematic review. J Dent Res 2013;92(5):399–408 [Systematic review/meta-analysis].

116. Okada M, Kobayashi T, Ito S, et al. Periodontal treatment decreases levels of antibodies to *Porphyromonas gingivalis* and citrulline in patients with rheumatoid arthritis and periodontitis. J Periodontol 2013;84(12):e74–84.

117. Ortiz P, Bissada NF, Palomo L, et al. Periodontal therapy reduces the severity of active rheumatoid arthritis in patients treated with or without tumor necrosis factor inhibitors. J Periodontol 2009;80(4):535–40.

118. Prevoo ML, van 't Hof MA, Kuper HH, et al. Modified disease activity scores that include twenty-eight-joint counts. Development and validation in a prospective longitudinal study of patients with rheumatoid arthritis. Arthritis Rheum 1995; 38(1):44–8.

119. Biyikoglu B, Buduneli N, Aksu K, et al. Periodontal therapy in chronic periodontitis lowers gingival crevicular fluid interleukin-1 beta and DAS28 in rheumatoid arthritis patients. Rheumatol Int 2013;33(10):2607–16.

120. Erciyas K, Sezer U, Ustun K, et al. Effects of periodontal therapy on disease activity and systemic inflammation in rheumatoid arthritis patients. Oral Dis 2013; 19(4):394–400.

121. Monsarrat P, Vergnes JN, Cantagrel A, et al. Effect of periodontal treatment on the clinical parameters of patients with rheumatoid arthritis: study protocol of the randomized, controlled ESPERA trial. Trials 2013;14:253.

122. Salemi S, Biondo MI, Fiorentino C, et al. Could early rheumatoid arthritis resolve after periodontitis treatment only?: Case report and review of the literature. Medicine (Baltimore) 2014;93(27):e195.

123. Heo SM, Haase EM, Lesse AJ, et al. Genetic relationships between respiratory pathogens isolated from dental plaque and bronchoalveolar lavage fluid from patients in the intensive care unit undergoing mechanical ventilation. Clin Infect Dis 2008;47(12):1562–70.

124. Gomes-Filho IS, Santos CM, Cruz SS, et al. Periodontitis and nosocomial lower respiratory tract infection: preliminary findings. J Clin Periodontol 2009;36(5): 380–7.

125. Bassim CW, Gibson G, Ward T, et al. Modification of the risk of mortality from pneumonia with oral hygiene care. J Am Geriatr Soc 2008;56(9):1601–7.

126. Scannapieco FA, Bush RB, Paju S. Associations between periodontal disease and risk for nosocomial bacterial pneumonia and chronic obstructive pulmonary disease; a systematic review. Ann Periodontol 2003;8(1):54–69 [Systematic review/meta-analysis].

127. Azarpazhooh A, Leake JL. Systematic review of the association between respiratory diseases and oral health. J Periodontol 2006;77(9):1465–82 [Systematic review/meta-analysis].

128. Sjogren P, Nilsson E, Forsell M, et al. A systematic review of the preventive effect of oral hygiene on pneumonia and respiratory tract infection in elderly people in hospitals and nursing homes: effect estimates and methodological quality of randomized controlled trials. J Am Geriatr Soc 2008;56(11):2124–30 [Systematic review/meta-analysis].

129. van der Maarel-Wierink CD, Vanobbergen JN, Bronkhorst EM, et al. Oral health care and aspiration pneumonia in frail older people: a systematic literature review. Gerodontology 2013;30(1):3–9 [Systematic review/meta-analysis].

130. Shi Z, Xie H, Wang P, et al. Oral hygiene care for critically ill patients to prevent ventilator-associated pneumonia. Cochrane Database Syst Rev 2013;(8):CD008367. [Systematic review/meta-analysis].

131. Liu Z, Zhang W, Zhang J, et al. Oral hygiene, periodontal health and chronic obstructive pulmonary disease exacerbations. J Clin Periodontol 2012;39(1): 45–52.

132. Wang Z, Zhou X, Zhang J, et al. Periodontal health, oral health behaviours, and chronic obstructive pulmonary disease. J Clin Periodontol 2009;36(9): 750–5.

133. Zhou X, Han J, Liu Z, et al. Effects of periodontal treatment on lung function and exacerbation frequency in patients with chronic obstructive pulmonary disease and chronic periodontitis: a 2-year pilot randomized controlled trial. J Clin Periodontol 2014;41:564–72.

134. Kucukcoskun M, Baser U, Oztekin G, et al. Initial periodontal treatment for prevention of chronic obstructive pulmonary disease exacerbations. J Periodontol 2013;84(7):863–70.

135. Agado BE, Crawford B, Delarosa J, et al. Effects of periodontal instrumentation on quality of life and illness in patients with chronic obstructive pulmonary disease: a pilot study. J Dent Hyg 2012;86(3):204–14.

136. Wilczynska-Borawska M, Baginska J, Malyszko J. Dental problems in a potential kidney transplant recipient: case report and literature review. Ann Acad Med Stetin 2010;56(2):51–4.

137. Chen LP, Chiang CK, Peng YS, et al. Relationship between periodontal disease and mortality in patients treated with maintenance hemodialysis. Am J Kidney Dis 2011;57(2):276–82.

138. Chambrone L, Foz AM, Guglielmetti MR, et al. Periodontitis and chronic kidney disease: a systematic review of the association of diseases and the effect of

periodontal treatment on estimated glomerular filtration rate. J Clin Periodontol 2013;40(5):443–56 [Systematic review/meta-analysis].

139. Strippoli GF, Palmer SC, Ruospo M, et al. Oral disease in adults treated with hemodialysis: prevalence, predictors, and association with mortality and adverse cardiovascular events: the rationale and design of the oral diseases in hemodialysis (ORAL-D) study, a prospective, multinational, longitudinal, observational, cohort study. BMC Nephrol 2013;14:90 [Systematic review/meta-analysis].

140. De Souza CM, Braosi AP, Luczyszyn SM, et al. Association among oral health parameters, periodontitis, and its treatment and mortality in patients undergoing hemodialysis. J Periodontol 2014;85(6):e169–78.

141. Palmer SC, Ruospo M, Wong G, et al. Dental health and mortality in people with end-stage kidney disease treated with hemodialysis: A multinational cohort study. Am J Kidney Dis 2015. http://dx.doi.org/10.1053/j.ajkd.2015.04.051.

142. Sharma P, Dietrich T, Sidhu A, et al. The periodontal health component of The Renal Impairment In Secondary Care (RIISC) cohort study: a description of the rationale, methodology and initial baseline results. J Clin Periodontol 2014; 41(7):653–61.

143. Ruospo M, Palmer SC, Craig JC, et al. Prevalence and severity of oral disease in adults with chronic kidney disease: a systematic review of observational studies. Nephrol Dial Transplant 2014;29(2):364–75 [Systematic review/meta-analysis].

144. Iwasaki M, Taylor GW, Sato M, et al. Cystatin C-based estimated glomerular filtration rate and periodontitis. Gerodontology 2014. http://dx.doi.org/10.1111/ger.12159.

145. Siribamrungwong M, Yothasamutr K, Puangpanngam K. Periodontal treatment reduces chronic systemic inflammation in peritoneal dialysis patients. Ther Apher Dial 2013;18(3):305–8.

146. Nakamura A, Shikata K, Hiramatsu M, et al. Serum interleukin-18 levels are associated with nephropathy and atherosclerosis in Japanese patients with type 2 diabetes. Diabetes Care 2005;28(12):2890–5.

147. Shimizu C, Matsumoto K, Fujita T, et al. Imbalance of interleukin-18 and interleukin-18 binding protein in patients with IgA nephropathy implicating renal vasculopathy. Clin Lab 2015;61(1–2):23–30.

148. Borgnakke WS. Periodontitis may be associated with chronic kidney disease, but current evidence is insufficient. J Evid Based Dent Pract 2013;13(3): 88–90.

149. Virtanen E, Söder B, Andersson LC, et al. History of dental infections associates with cancer in periodontally healthy subjects: a 24-year follow-up study from Sweden. J Cancer 2014;5(2):79–85.

150. Han YW. Oral bacteria as drivers for colorectal cancer. J Periodontol 2014;85(9): 1155–7.

151. Han YW. Fusobacterium nucleatum: a commensal-turned pathogen. Curr Opin Microbiol 2015;23:141–7.

152. Tezal M, Scannapieco FA, Wactawski-Wende J, et al. Local inflammation and human papillomavirus status of head and neck cancers. Arch Otolaryngol Head Neck Surg 2012;138(7):669–75.

153. Tezal M. Interaction between chronic inflammation and oral HPV infection in the etiology of head and neck cancers. Int J Otolaryngol 2012;2012:575242.

154. Han YW, Wang X. Mobile microbiome: oral bacteria in extra-oral infections and inflammation. J Dent Res 2013;92(6):485–91.

155. Gil-Montoya JA, Sanchez-Lara I, Carnero-Pardo C, et al. Is periodontitis a risk factor for cognitive impairment and dementia? a case-control study. J Periodontol 2014;86:1–14.

156. Boland MR, Hripcsak G, Albers DJ, et al. Discovering medical conditions associated with periodontitis using linked electronic health records. J Clin Periodontol 2013;40(5):474–82.
157. Oguz F, Eltas A, Beytur A, et al. Is there a relationship between chronic periodontitis and erectile dysfunction? J Sex Med 2013;10(3):838–43.
158. Sharma A, Pradeep AR, Raju PA. Association between chronic periodontitis and vasculogenic erectile dysfunction. J Periodontol 2011;82(12):1665–9.
159. Zadik Y, Bechor R, Galor S, et al. Erectile dysfunction might be associated with chronic periodontal disease: two ends of the cardiovascular spectrum. J Sex Med 2009;6(4):1111–6.
160. Tsao CW, Liu CY, Cha TL, et al. Exploration of the association between chronic periodontal disease and erectile dysfunction from a population-based view point. Andrologia 2015;47(5):513–8.
161. Keller JJ, Chung SD, Lin HC. A nationwide population-based study on the association between chronic periodontitis and erectile dysfunction. J Clin Periodontol 2012;39(6):507–12.
162. Caskey MF, Morgan DJ, Porto AF, et al. Clinical manifestations associated with HTLV type I infection: a cross-sectional study. AIDS Res Hum Retroviruses 2007;23(3):365–71.
163. Brito F, Zaltman C, Carvalho AT, et al. Subgingival microflora in inflammatory bowel disease patients with untreated periodontitis. Eur J Gastroenterol Hepatol 2013;25(2):239–45.
164. Yeoh N, Burton JP, Suppiah P, et al. The role of the microbiome in rheumatic diseases. Curr Rheumatol Rep 2013;15(3):314.
165. Karkos PD, Asrani S, Karkos CD, et al. Lemierre's syndrome: a systematic review. Laryngoscope 2009;119(8):1552–9 [Systematic review/meta-analysis].
166. Wu AY, Tseng HK, Su J, et al. Lemierre's syndrome in a patient with habitual toothpick usage. J Microbiol Immunol Infect 2013;46(3):237–40.
167. Pyysalo MJ, Pyysalo LM, Pessi T, et al. The connection between ruptured cerebral aneurysms and odontogenic bacteria. J Neurol Neurosurg Psychiatry 2013;84(11):1214–8.
168. Janket SJ, Javaheri H, Ackerson LK, et al. Oral infections, metabolic inflammation, genetics, and cardiometabolic diseases. J Dent Res 2015. http://dx.doi.org/10.1177/0022034515580795.
169. Suvan J, Petrie A, Moles DR, et al. Body mass index as a predictive factor of periodontal therapy outcomes. J Dent Res 2014;93(1):49–54.
170. Palomo L. BMI is a predictor of periodontal therapy outcomes. J Evid Based Dent Pract 2014;14(2):82–4.
171. Goncalves TE, Feres M, Zimmermann GS, et al. Effects of scaling and root planing on clinical response and serum levels of adipocytokines in obese patients with chronic periodontitis. J Periodontol 2015;86(1):53–61.
172. Huang X, Wang J, Liu J, et al. Maternal periodontal disease and risk of preeclampsia: a meta-analysis. J Huazhong Univ Sci Technolog Med Sci 2014;34(5):729–35 [Systematic review/meta-analysis].
173. Sgolastra F, Petrucci A, Severino M, et al. Relationship between periodontitis and pre-eclampsia: a meta-analysis. PLoS One 2013;8(8):e71387 [Systematic review/meta-analysis].
174. Wei BJ, Chen YJ, Yu L, et al. Periodontal disease and risk of preeclampsia: a meta-analysis of observational studies. PLoS One 2013;8(8):e70901 [Systematic review/meta-analysis].

Should Antibiotics Be Prescribed to Treat Chronic Periodontitis?

John Walters, DDS, MMSc[a],*, Pin-Chuang Lai, DDS[a,b]

KEYWORDS

- Antimicrobials-systemic • Periodontitis microbiology • Oral biofilm
- Periodontitis therapy • Scaling and root planing • Clinical trials

KEY POINTS

- Although chronic periodontitis often responds to mechanical debridement alone, patients with progressive attachment loss, invasive subgingival pathogens, or multiple deep pockets may benefit from combining systemic antibiotics with mechanical therapy.
- Bacteria in subgingival biofilm are resistant to antibiotics. Antibiotics should only be prescribed after biofilm has been mechanically disrupted, not as the sole approach to treatment.
- Meta-analyses suggest that metronidazole (in combination with amoxicillin or alone) or azithromycin produce statistically significant adjunctive benefits in combination with mechanical therapy.
- When used to treat chronic periodontitis, the combination of mechanical therapy and antibiotics yields its greatest benefit at sites with deep initial probing depths.
- Systemic antibiotics have the potential to produce adverse reactions that must be considered in balance with their expected benefits.

INTRODUCTION

Periodontitis is a chronic inflammatory disease that leads to destruction of the supporting tissues of teeth and, if left untreated, tooth loss. Severe periodontitis was the world's sixth-most prevalent condition in 2010; its age-standardized prevalence

Conflict of interest disclosure: The authors have nothing to disclose.
Financial support disclosure: The authors received support from US Public Health Service research grant R21 DE018804 from the National Institutes of Health, Bethesda, MD.
[a] Division of Periodontology, College of Dentistry, The Ohio State University, 3015 Postle Hall, 305 West 12th Avenue, Columbus, OH 43210, USA; [b] Division of Biosciences, College of Dentistry, The Ohio State University, 3015 Postle Hall, 305 West 12th Avenue, Columbus, OH 43210, USA
* Corresponding author.
E-mail address: walters.2@osu.edu

between 1990 and 2010 among all countries was 11.2%.[1] Consistent with this estimate, a study based on data from the 2009 and 2010 National Health and Nutrition Examination Survey cycle reported prevalence rates of 8.7%, 30.0%, and 8.5% for mild, moderate, and severe periodontitis, respectively, in the United States.[2]

Studies from the past 3 decades have revealed that only a small subset of microorganisms from among the hundreds of species found in the oral cavity is highly associated with periodontitis.[3] Although specific biofilm-producing bacterial pathogens and other cooperative species are required, bacteria alone are not sufficient to induce periodontitis. The host immune-inflammatory response is a determinant of susceptibility to periodontitis and is responsible for most of the periodontal tissue destruction.[4] During persistent bacterial infection and prolonged homeostatic imbalance, cytokines and enzymes released by host leukocytes mediate destruction of periodontal connective tissue and bone. Systemic diseases (eg, diabetes), immune dysfunction, and environmental factors (eg, smoking) can also contribute to disruption of the homeostatic balance.[5] The goal of periodontal therapy is to preserve the natural dentition in stability, comfort, and function by eliminating pathologic biofilm and resolving inflammation.

Microbial complexes in subgingival biofilm have been recently characterized using molecular techniques. Individual species in these complexes have been assigned using a color-coded system that reflects community ordination and cluster analysis.[6] The red complex, consisting of *Tannerella forsythia*, *Porphyromonas gingivalis*, and *Treponema denticola*, is strongly associated with severe chronic periodontitis. The orange complex, which includes *Prevotella intermedia*, *Fusobacterium nucleatum*, *Campylobacter rectus*, and *Peptostreptococcus micros*, is closely associated with the red complex. The green complex includes *Aggregatibacter actinomycetemcomitans*, which has a strong association with aggressive periodontitis and a less frequent association with chronic periodontitis.[7] *Porphyromonas gingivalis*, *A actinomycetemcomitans* and other pathogens possess virulence factors that can overcome the host response and damage periodontal tissues.[8,9]

Porphyromonas gingivalis, *A actinomycetemcomitans*, and *Prevotella intermedia* are capable of invading the epithelium of periodontal pockets, which protects them from elimination by the host response, making them exceptionally difficult to eliminate by conventional periodontal scaling and root planing (SRP). Persistent infections by these bacteria are frequently associated with progressive chronic periodontitis.[10] Another limitation of SRP is that it is not effective in removing bacteria from deep pockets, furcations, dentinal tubules, and other subgingival sites where access is poor. The difficulties associated with eliminating bacteria that have colonized the soft tissue wall of the pocket and other inaccessible areas provide a rationale for incorporating systemic antibiotics into the treatment of periodontitis.

A broad range of systemic antibiotics has been used to treat chronic periodontitis. The pharmacokinetic and antimicrobial properties of the agents used most commonly are presented in **Table 1** and information on dosage is detailed in **Table 2**. In general, amoxicillin, metronidazole, azithromycin, tetracycline, and doxycycline are capable of attaining levels that can effectively inhibit periodontal pathogens when they are growing as single (planktonic) cells in a periodontal pocket or the soft tissue wall of a pocket. The exception is metronidazole, which exhibits relatively poor activity against *A actinomycetemcomitans* at typical in vivo concentrations. However, it is important to remember that subgingival bacteria live in a biofilm, not as single cells. Bacteria growing in a biofilm are substantially more difficult to inhibit with antibiotics. For this reason, antibiotics should only be used to treat periodontitis in patients who have already had their subgingival biofilm disrupted by SRP.

Table 1
Characteristics of antibiotics used to treat chronic periodontitis

Agent	Half-Life in Serum (h)	Action	GCF Level (μg/mL)	MIC₉₀ (μg/mL) for *Porphyromonas gingivalis*	MIC₉₀ (μg/mL) for *T forsythia*	MIC₉₀ (μg/mL) for *Prevotella intermedia*	MIC₉₀ (μg/mL) for *A actinomycetemcomitans*
Amoxicillin	1–2	Bactericidal	3–4	<0.016	0.38	0.25–1.5	0.4–1
Metronidazole	6–12	Bactericidal	8–10	<0.016	0.005	0.032–0.25	64–96
Azithromycin	40–68	Bacteriostatic or bactericidal	3–10	0.094–0.5	0.5–1	0.25–0.4	0.875–4
Tetracycline	6–8	Bacteriostatic	5–10	0.023–0.25	0.19	2–4	0.2–1.5
Doxycycline	12–22	Bacteriostatic	2–8	0.047	0.38	0.05	1

Abbreviations: GCF, gingival crevicular fluid; MIC₉₀, minimal inhibitory concentration of an antibiotic at which 90% of bacterial isolates are inhibited.
Data from Refs.[11–19]

Table 2
Representative antibiotic regimens for adjunctive use in treatment of chronic periodontitis

Antibiotic	Prescription	Potential Adverse Reactions
Amoxicillin + Metronidazole	500 mg tid for 8 d 250 mg tid for 8 d	Hypersensitivity to amoxicillin, nausea, diarrhea, vomiting, altered taste sensations, Antabuse effect
Metronidazole	500 mg tid for 7 d	Nausea, vomiting, altered taste sensations, Antabuse effect
Azithromycin	500 mg qd for 3 d	Diarrhea, nausea, vomiting, abdominal pain, cholestatic jaundice, increased risk of serious cardiac arrhythmia (prolonged Q-T interval) Inhibition of bactericidal agents if used in combination
Doxycycline	200 mg initial dose, then 100 mg qd for 21 d	Photosensitivity, nausea, diarrhea, vomiting, and abdominal pain Inhibition of bactericidal agents if used in combination

Unlike the other agents in **Table 1**, azithromycin and doxycycline have relatively long half-lives and are normally administered in a single daily dose. Azithromycin and tetracycline compounds are actively taken up and concentrated inside oral epithelial cells,[20,21] whereas amoxicillin and metronidazole enter cells by passive diffusion.[22,23] This property may be useful for targeting periodontal pathogens that have invaded the pocket epithelium. When cultured gingival epithelial cells infected with *A actinomycetemcomitans* are incubated with physiologic concentrations of azithromycin (8 μg/mL), azithromycin accumulates inside the epithelial cells at levels that kill more than 80% of the intracellular *A actinomycetemcomitans* within 2 hours. In the same experimental conditions, treatment with amoxicillin at its peak therapeutic concentration (4 μg/mL) kills only 14% of the intracellular bacteria.[21]

PATIENT EVALUATION FOR POTENTIAL USE OF AN ANTIBIOTIC: OVERVIEW

Although it is difficult to completely remove subgingival biofilm and root deposits with SRP, most patients with chronic periodontitis respond favorably to treatment with conventional SRP without antibiotics. However, some cases can derive an additional increment of clinical attachment gain or probing depth reduction from combining systemic antibiotics with SRP. The literature provides guidance for predicting which patients could potentially benefit.

Characteristics of chronic periodontitis patients who may benefit from use of antibiotics

- Patients who exhibit a poor response to adequate SRP, with continuing loss of clinical attachment
- Patients who test positive for *Porphyromonas gingivalis* or *A actinomycetemcomitans* in their subgingival biofilm
- Patients with severe chronic periodontitis and generalized deep pocket depths.

There is agreement that patients who fail to respond favorably to SRP, especially those with progressive attachment loss, can benefit from treatment with antibiotics.[24] As previously mentioned, progressive chronic periodontitis is often associated with persistent infections by *Porphyromonas gingivalis*, *A actinomycetemcomitans*, and *Prevotella intermedia*,[10] which invade the soft tissue wall of the periodontal pocket and are difficult to eliminate with SRP. Consistent with this recommendation, patients with chronic periodontitis who have undergone microbiological testing and are positive for *Porphyromonas gingivalis* or *A actinomycetemcomitans* in their subgingival plaque can be expected to benefit from use of antibiotics.[25] Finally, patients with generalized severe chronic periodontitis and multiple deep periodontal pockets may also benefit.[26,27] The common thread in these guidelines is an acknowledgment that SRP has limited ability to eliminate invasive pathogens and remove biofilm from inaccessible sites.

Smokers typically exhibit a less favorable response to periodontal therapy than non-smokers. There is evidence that subgingival pathogens are more difficult to eliminate in smokers.[28,29] Although some studies have suggested that adjunctive systemic antibiotics can improve the responses to periodontal therapy in smokers,[30] a recent systematic review concluded that additional well-designed randomized clinical trials are needed to provide sufficient evidence to support the use of adjunctive antibiotics in the treatment of periodontitis in smokers.[31]

EFFICACY OF SCALING AND ROOT PLANING AS THE SOLE TREATMENT OF PERIODONTITIS

Although SRP is regarded as the gold standard of nonsurgical periodontal treatment, it is a highly demanding therapy. Its effectiveness is limited by anatomic factors (furcation involvement, tooth type, and surface) and the experience of the operator.[32] As previously mentioned, SRP loses some of its ability to eliminate subgingival biofilm as pocket probing depths increase.[33,34] Despite this, the magnitude of probing depth reduction and clinical attachment gain resulting from SRP is greatest at periodontal sites with deep pretreatment probing depths (**Table 3**).[35]

In pockets deeper than 6 mm, SRP provides a mean clinical attachment gain of 1.19 mm and a mean probing depth reduction of 2.19 mm. In pockets of moderate (4–6 mm) depth, the respective values are 0.55 mm and 1.29 mm. SRP also reduces clinical signs of inflammation. As an example, it reduces bleeding on probing to approximately 43% of baseline levels.[35] These outcomes can be consistently achieved with chronic periodontitis patients, independent of the types of instruments used (power-driven or manual).[36,37] Patients with poor oral hygiene, smoking habits, or poor glycemic control exhibit a less favorable response to SRP.

EFFICACY OF SYSTEMIC ANTIBIOTICS AS THE SOLE TREATMENT OF PERIODONTITIS

In patients with advanced chronic periodontitis, diligent treatment with SRP requires a substantial amount of time and effort. It may seem reasonable to consider using systemic antibiotics as a cost-effective alternative to SRP for eliminating subgingival

Table 3			
Summary of clinical outcomes achieved with scaling and root planing when used to treat nonmolar sites			
Pretreatment Status	Number of Clinical Studies Surveyed	Mean Clinical Attachment Level Gain	Mean Probing Depth Reduction
Shallow pockets (1–3 mm)	9	−0.34 mm	0.03 mm
Moderate pockets (4–6 mm)	27	0.55 mm	1.29 mm
Deep pockets (>6 mm)	18	1.19 mm	2.19 mm

Data from Cobb CM. Non-surgical pocket therapy: mechanical. Ann Periodontol 1996;1:443–90.

bacteria. Although this question has been examined in several reviews,[27,38,39] relatively few studies have been specifically designed to address it. As a monotherapy for chronic periodontitis, metronidazole can reduce probing depths, induce modest attachment gains, reduce bleeding on probing, and suppress spirochetes in subgingival biofilm.[38] Comparisons of the efficacy of metronidazole alone with SRP have demonstrated that metronidazole is inferior or, at best, equivalent in improving periodontal status.[40–42] Moreover, a meta-analysis of 4 clinical trials that compared attachment level changes in subjects with untreated periodontitis with that of subjects treated with metronidazole alone or metronidazole in combination with amoxicillin failed to show a statistically significant difference between groups. Thus, there is not sufficient evidence that systemic antibiotics, when used as a monotherapy, are beneficial in the treatment of periodontitis.[27]

In contradistinction to these studies, a more recent study concluded that a combination of metronidazole and amoxicillin as the sole therapy for periodontitis produces changes in clinical and microbiological parameters that are similar to those obtained from conventional SRP.[43] However, every subject in this study received supragingival scaling to facilitate periodontal probing. Thus, the group treated with antibiotics did not actually receive a monotherapy because removal of supragingival biofilm has been shown to alter the number and composition of subgingival bacteria.[44]

Consistent with most clinical studies, microbiological studies have shown that bacteria living in biofilms are more resistant to antimicrobial agents than single, dispersed (planktonic) bacteria.[45–47] This may be related to impairment of antibiotic diffusion into biofilms or to the slower bacterial growth rate secondary to deprivation of nutrients within the biofilm[44]; however, there are other contributing factors. The close association of bacteria living in biofilms facilitates horizontal transfer of genetic information that confers resistance to antibiotics.[48,49] In vitro studies have shown that the antibiotic concentrations found in gingival crevicular fluid (GCF) have limited impact on periodontal pathogens living in biofilms.[50,51] For these reasons, there is a consensus that antibiotics should only be prescribed after biofilm is mechanically disrupted.

EFFICACY OF SCALING AND ROOT PLANING COMBINED WITH SYSTEMIC ANTIBIOTICS

Several comprehensive reviews have evaluated the efficacy of a combination of SRP and systemic antibiotics in treatment of chronic periodontitis.[26,27,39,52–55] Their general conclusions are summarized below:

- Combining systemic antibiotics with SRP can provide a greater therapeutic benefit than SRP alone.
- The combination of antibiotics and SRP provides a greater benefit to patients with aggressive periodontitis than to those with chronic periodontitis.
- The combination of SRP and antibiotics yields its greatest benefit at sites with deep initial probing depths.
- Several different antibiotic regimens are capable of enhancing the treatment response to SRP. Meta-analyses support the use of metronidazole (alone or in combination with amoxicillin) or azithromycin.
- Indirect evidence suggests that antibiotics should be started on the day SRP is completed and that SRP should be completed within a short period (ideally, less than a week).

Meta-analysis is a useful statistical technique for combining results from different studies to achieve higher statistical power. This approach has been used to analyze the benefits of combining antibiotics with SRP. **Table 4** summarizes data from several meta-analyses of the overall effect of combined treatment of chronic periodontitis with SRP and adjunctive antibiotics in comparison with treatment with SRP alone. These studies examined treatment effects throughout the mouth, including sites with only minor attachment loss and shallow probing depths. Based on 2 meta-analyses that considered the effects of a broad range of different antibiotic regimens on treatment of chronic periodontitis, combined therapy can enhance clinical attachment gain by 0.20 to 0.24 mm and decrease probing depth by a mean of 0.28 mm in comparison with SRP alone.[27,54] Neither of these analyses could identify an antimicrobial regimen that was clearly superior to the others. Adjunctive antibiotics seem to consistently enhance the clinical response to SRP for both aggressive and chronic periodontitis patients but patients with aggressive periodontitis seem to derive greater benefit. The mean clinical attachment gain observed in studies of subjects with aggressive periodontitis patients is nearly 3 times greater than that observed in studies of chronic periodontitis.[27]

Regarding the effects of specific antibiotic regimens, treatment with SRP combined with amoxicillin and metronidazole can enhance overall clinical attachment gain by 0.16 to 0.21 mm, and overall probing depth reduction by 0.29 to 0.43 mm, in comparison with SRP alone (see **Table 4**).[52,54] Similarly, the adjunctive benefits of combining metronidazole with SRP correspond to an additional 0.1 mm of attachment gain and 0.15 to 0.18 mm of probing depth reduction.[54,55] The combination of SRP and azithromycin yields a mean attachment gain of 0.11 mm (not statistically significant) and a mean probing depth reduction of 0.39 mm in comparison with SRP alone.[54] Meta-analysis of studies using an adjunctive doxycycline regimen failed to demonstrate a significant overall enhancement of attachment gain or probing depth.[54]

Evidence suggests that the benefits of combining antibiotics with SRP are more substantial at sites with initial probing depths of greater than 6 mm (**Table 5**). At deeper sites, treatment with SRP combined with amoxicillin and metronidazole can enhance clinical attachment gain by 0.45 to 0.67 mm and reduce mean probing depth by 0.92 mm in comparison with treatment with SRP alone.[26,54] Combining metronidazole with SRP results in an additional attachment gain of 0.55 to 0.66 mm and an additional probing depth reduction of 0.83 mm in comparison with SRP alone.[26,54] Use of azithromycin as an adjunct to SRP enhances mean attachment gain and probing depth reduction by 0.43 mm and 0.52 mm, respectively, over SRP alone.[54]

Because many different protocols have been used in studies that evaluated the benefits of combining antibiotics with SRP, there is a lack of evidence pointing to a specific protocol. However, there is indirect evidence that antibiotic therapy should immediately follow the completion of SRP and that SRP should be completed within a reasonably short time (ideally, within 1 week).[39]

TREATMENT COMPLICATIONS AND RESISTANCE

Systemic antibiotics have the potential to produce adverse reactions that must be considered in balance with their expected benefits (see **Table 2**). Direct toxic effects of amoxicillin, metronidazole, doxycycline, or azithromycin are rare. However, all have the potential to induce nausea, vomiting, diarrhea, and abdominal pain in a small percentage of patients.[56] The most common adverse effects associated with amoxicillin and other penicillins are allergic reactions, including skin rashes; serum sickness; and, rarely, anaphylaxis.[57] Patients taking metronidazole often report altered taste sensations and can experience Antabuse effects in response to alcohol ingestion.[38] Photosensitivity can occur in individuals taking doxycycline.[56] In rare instances,

Table 4
Meta-analyses of clinical outcomes associated with combining systemic antibiotics with scaling and root planing to treat chronic periodontitis (overall effects at all sites)

Reference	Dates and Number of Included Studies	Antibiotics Studied	Observation Time (mo)	Mean Clinical Attachment Level Gain (P Value)	Mean Probing Depth Reduction (P Value)
Haffajee et al,[27] 2003[a]	1983–2001 n = 17	MET, SPIR, AMX + MET, AMX + CA, TET, DOX	>1, most ~6	0.24 mm (0.001)	Not analyzed
Keestra et al,[54] 2015[b] (main analysis)	1994–2012 n = 35	AMX, AMX + CA, AMX + MET, MET, AZM, CLR, DOX, SDD, ORN, SPIR, TET, MOX	3	0.20 mm (0.0004)	0.28 mm (<0.00001)
Sgolastra et al,[52] 2012	2001–2011 n = 4	AMX + MET	≥3	0.21 mm (0.03)	0.43 mm (<0.0001)
Keestra et al,[54] 2015 (subanalysis)	1998–2012 n = 7	AMX + MET	3	0.16 mm (0.05)	0.29 mm (0.003)
Sgolastra et al,[55] 2015	1998–2012 n = 6	MET	≥3	0.10 mm (<0.00001)	0.18 mm (0.0001)
Keestra et al,[54] 2015 (subanalysis)	2004–2012 n = 5	MET	3	0.10 mm (0.12)	0.15 mm (0.004)
Keestra et al,[54] 2015 (subanalysis)	2005–2012 n = 6	AZM	3	0.11 mm (0.32)	0.39 mm (0.004)
Keestra et al,[54] 2015 (subanalysis)	1999–2008 n = 4	DOX	3	0.09 mm (0.34)	0.11 mm (0.15)

Abbreviations: AMX, amoxicillin; AZM, azithromycin; CA, clavulanic acid; CLR, clarithromycin; DOX, doxycycline; MET, metronidazole; MOX, moxifloxacin; ORN, ornidazole; SDD, subantimicrobial-dose doxycycline; SPIR, spiramycin; TET, tetracycline.
[a] Main meta-analysis included 3 studies that examined the effect of the antibiotic as a sole treatment.
[b] Main meta-analysis included 9 studies that examined the effect of adjunctive subantimicrobial-dose doxycycline.
Data from Refs.[26,52,54,55]

Table 5
Meta-analyses of clinical outcomes associated with combining systemic antibiotics with scaling and root planing to treat chronic periodontitis (effects at sites with initial probing depths >6 mm)

Reference	Dates and Number of Included Studies	Antibiotics Studied	Observation Time (mo)	Mean Clinical Attachment Level Gain (P Value)	Mean Probing Depth Reduction (P Value)
Herrera et al,[26] 2002 (subanalysis)	1998 n = 2	AMX + MET	12–24	0.45 mm (0.001)	Not analyzed
Keestra et al,[54] 2015 (subanalysis)	2008–2012 n = 4	AMX + MET	3	0.67 mm (0.02)	0.92 mm (0.0003)
Herrera et al,[26] 2002 (subanalysis)	1983–1984 n = 2	MET	2–12	0.55 mm (0.057)	Not analyzed
Keestra et al,[54] 2015 (subanalysis)	2004–2012 n = 5	MET	3	0.66 mm (<0.00001)	0.83 mm (<0.00001)
Keestra et al,[54] 2015 (subanalysis)	2002–2012 n = 5	AZM	3	0.43 mm (0.03)	0.52 mm (0.0003)

Abbreviations: AMX, amoxicillin; AZM, azithromycin; MET, metronidazole.

Data from Herrera D, Sanz M, Jepsen S, et al. A systematic review on the effect of systemic antimicrobials as an adjunct to scaling and root planing in periodontitis patients. J Clin Periodontol 2002;29(Suppl 3):136–59; and Keestra JA, Grosjean I, Coucke W, et al. Non-surgical periodontal therapy with systemic antibiotics in patients with untreated chronic periodontitis: a systematic review and meta-analysis. J Periodont Res 2015;50(3):294–314.

azithromycin may induce angioedema or cholestatic jaundice. In addition, azithromycin can contribute to cardiac arrhythmias and slightly increase the risk of cardiovascular death in individuals with a high baseline risk of cardiovascular disease.[58] Patients should be informed of the potential for adverse reactions; however, these effects typically present as gastrointestinal upsets and most are not serious.[27,39]

Several fundamental issues can, individually or in combination, undermine the therapeutic benefits associated with use of adjunctive antibiotics in periodontal therapy. Lack of patient compliance (adherence) with the prescribed dosage regimen is a major concern. If the antibiotic does not reach optimal concentrations at the infection site or the duration of treatment is too short because the patient does not follow directions, its therapeutic benefit will be compromised. Studies have shown that compliance can be poor with complex regimens that require patients to take multiple doses per day.[59] Thus, it is reasonable to expect that compliance with a combined regimen of amoxicillin and metronidazole will be lower than with a once-a-day azithromycin regimen.

Prescribing an antibiotic will not predictably enhance treatment outcomes if the subgingival biofilm is not thoroughly disrupted before antibiotic treatment or if patients fail to inhibit biofilm reformation by maintaining good oral hygiene.[39,60] An antibiotic's minimal inhibitory concentration (MIC) for bacteria living in a biofilm can be 10 to 1000-fold higher than for bacteria growing in a planktonic state,[61,62] and typically exceeds the concentration that the antibiotic can attain in GCF. In effect, disruption of subgingival biofilm decreases the MIC values and renders the bacteria more susceptible to antibiotics at concentrations found in GCF.[63] There is evidence to suggest that the red complex of subgingival bacteria associated with chronic periodontitis is relatively susceptible to antibiotics.[27] However, other subgingival pathogens found in chronic periodontitis patients, including *Prevotella intermedia*, *Prevotella nigrescens*, and *A actinomycetemcomitans*, are often resistant to doxycycline, amoxicillin, or metronidazole.[64] Failure to eliminate these pathogens could limit the success of SRP combined with an adjunctive antibiotic regimen.

If examination reveals that inflammation has not resolved or attachment loss has not been arrested by treatment with a combined regimen of SRP and antibiotics within 2 to 3 months, 2 different approaches can be used to address resistance to treatment. Microbiological testing could help explain why the original treatment failed and guide additional nonsurgical therapy. Subgingival plaque samples should be collected from progressive disease sites with sterile paper points and shipped to a laboratory that has the specialized expertise needed to identify pathogens that have not been eliminated. Based on this information, an alternative regimen that is appropriate for targeting the remaining pathogens can be selected. Because the subgingival environment progressively recolonizes with bacteria after SRP, subgingival biofilm must be disrupted and dispersed again before administering the alternative antibiotic. At the time the clinical response is reexamined 2 to 3 months later, it may be prudent to conduct another microbiological test to confirm that pathogens have been eliminated. As a second option, periodontal surgery may be used to address persistent pocketing and attachment loss.

There is general agreement that selective, rather than routine use of antibiotics is the best practice. Commensal bacteria living in the intestinal tract contribute to the development, maintenance, and function of the immune system. By disrupting commensal microbiota, antibiotics can perturb host defenses in a detrimental manner.[65] Moreover, antibiotic resistance has become a serious public health issue in recent years. Its economic and social costs are significant. A recent study suggests that subgingival biofilm can serve as a reservoir of β-lactam resistance genes.[66] Dentists can help prevent these issues by prescribing antibiotics only when they are indicated, by prescribing an appropriate antibiotic regimen, and by using antibiotics only after sub-gingival biofilm has been debrided. Patients can help reduce the risk of inducing resis-tance by complying with the recommended dosage and duration of the prescribed regimen.

EVALUATION OF OUTCOME AND LONG-TERM RECOMMENDATIONS

Increased tooth survival is one of the most relevant outcomes for reporting the effec-tiveness of periodontal therapy, and one that patients readily understand. It is rarely used, however, because exceptionally long study periods are required to obtain meaningful data.[26] As a practical matter, increases in clinical attachment level and reduction of probing depths are reasonable proxies for increased tooth survival. In ab-solute terms, a full-mouth attachment gain of only 0.10 to 0.24 mm (see **Table 4**) could be viewed as a modest benefit for using antibiotics in combination with SRP. Consid-ering that patients who are highly susceptible to periodontitis experience a mean full-mouth attachment loss of 0.067 mm per year during supportive therapy after active periodontal treatment,[67] an attachment gain of 0.10 to 0.24 mm effectively off-sets 1.5 to 3.5 years of disease progression.

At periodontal sites with deep (>6 mm) probing depths, combining an antibiotic with SRP can enhance attachment gain by 0.43 to 0.67 mm (see **Table 5**). Because SRP yields a mean attachment gain of 1.19 mm at sites with deep initial probing depths (see **Table 3**), the use of antibiotics in combination with SRP enhances attachment gain by 36% to 56% more than that obtained from SRP alone. In patients with many deep pockets, a benefit of this magnitude is cost-effective and clinically relevant because it could potentially decrease the need for periodontal surgical therapy.[68]

As mentioned previously, patients with mild-to-moderate chronic periodontitis usu-ally respond favorably to initial treatment with SRP alone without adjunctive antibi-otics. Patients with severe chronic periodontitis who have multiple deep pockets, progressive attachment loss, or test positive for invasive subgingival pathogens may benefit from an initial therapy that combines systemic antibiotics with SRP. Consistent with the meta-analyses detailed in **Tables 4** and **5**, a combination of amox-icillin and metronidazole is a reasonable choice for adjunctive use in patients who are not allergic to β-lactam antibiotics. This combination of 2 bactericidal agents has the potential to inhibit a broader spectrum of bacteria than a single agent and is less likely to induce resistance. In patients who are allergic to amoxicillin, an adjunctive regimen of metronidazole or azithromycin is a reasonable alternative. The response to initial periodontal treatment should be evaluated within 2 to 3 months and adjusted as necessary. If progression of attachment loss has been arrested and the outcome is generally favorable, it would be appropriate to treat persistent deep pockets with peri-odontal surgery. Most patients treated with surgical therapy do not require a postop-erative antibiotic regimen.[68] Currently, there is not sufficient evidence to support the adjunctive use of systemic antibiotics in conjunction with periodontal surgery.[39]

SUMMARY

- Although chronic periodontitis often responds to mechanical debridement alone, patients who have progressive attachment loss, invasive subgingival pathogens, or deep pockets may benefit from combining systemic antibiotics with mechan-ical therapy.
- Bacteria in subgingival biofilm are resistant to antibiotics. Antibiotics should only be prescribed after biofilm has been mechanically disrupted, not as the sole approach to treatment.

- Meta-analyses suggest that metronidazole (alone or in combination with amoxicillin) or azithromycin produce statistically significant adjunctive benefits in combination with mechanical therapy.
- When used to treat chronic periodontitis, the combination of mechanical therapy and antibiotics yields its greatest benefit at sites with deep initial probing depths.
- Systemic antibiotics have the potential to produce adverse reactions that must be considered in balance with their expected benefits.

REFERENCES

1. Kassebaum NJ, Bernabe E, Dahiya M, et al. Global burden of severe periodontitis in 1990–2010: a systematic review and meta-regression. J Dent Res 2014;93: 1045–53.
2. Eke PI, Dye BA, Wei L, et al. Prevalence of periodontitis in adults in the United States: 2009 and 2010. J Dent Res 2012;91:914–20.
3. Socransky SS, Haffajee AD. Periodontal microbial ecology. Periodontol 2000 2005;38:135–87.
4. Darveau RP. Periodontitis: a polymicrobial disruption of host homeostasis. Nat Rev Microbiol 2010;8:481–90.
5. Hajishengallis G. Immunomicrobial pathogenesis of periodontitis: keystones, pathobionts, and host response. Trends Immunol 2014;35:3–11.
6. Socransky SS, Haffajee AD, Cugini MA, et al. Microbial complexes in subgingival plaque. J Clin Periodontol 1998;25:134–44.
7. Slots J, Ting M. *Actinobacillus actinomycetemcomitans* and *Porphyromonas gingivalis* in human periodontal disease: occurrence and treatment. Periodontol 2000 1999;20:82–121.
8. Andrian E, Grenier D, Rouabhia M. *Porphyromonas gingivalis*-epithelial cell interactions in periodontitis. J Dent Res 2006;85:392–403.
9. Amano A. Host-parasite interactions in periodontitis: microbial pathogenicity and innate immunity. Periodontol 2000 2010;54:9–14.
10. Bragd L, Dahlen G, Wikstrom M, et al. The capability of *Actinobacillus actinomycetemcomitans, Bacteroides gingivalis* and *Bacteroides intermedius* to indicate progressive periodontitis; a retrospective study. J Clin Periodontol 1987;14:95–9.
11. van Winkelhoff AJ, Rams TE, Slots J. Systemic antibiotic therapy in periodontics. Periodontol 2000 1996;10:45–78.
12. Jain N, Lai PC, Walters JD. Effect of gingivitis on azithromycin concentrations in gingival crevicular fluid. J Periodontol 2012;83:1122–8.
13. Agwuh KN, MacGowan A. Pharmacokinetics and pharmacodynamics of tetracyclines including glycylcyclines. J Antimicrob Chemother 2006;58:256–65.
14. Pajukanta R, Asikainen S, Forsblom B, et al. β-lactamase production and in vitro antimicrobial susceptibility of *Porphyromonas gingivalis*. FEMS Immunol Med Microbiol 1993;6:241–4.
15. Pajukanta R, Asikainen S, Saarela M, et al. In vitro antimicrobial susceptibility of different serotypes of *Actinobacillus actinomycetemcomitans*. Scand J Dent Res 1993;101:299–303.
16. Goldstein EJ, Citron DM, Hunt Gerardo S, et al. Activities of HMR 3004 (RU 64004) and HMR 3647 (RU 66647) compared to those of erythromycin, azithromycin, clarithromycin, roxithromycin and eight other antimicrobial agents against unusual aerobic and anaerobic human and animal bite pathogens isolated from skin and soft tissue infections in humans. Antimicrob Agents Chemother 1998;42: 1127–32.

17. Veloo AC, Seme K, Raangs E, et al. Antibiotic susceptibility profiles of oral pathogens. Int J Antimicrob Agents 2012;40:450–4.
18. Takahashi N, Ishihara K, Kimizuka R, et al. The effects of tetracycline, minocycline, doxycycline and ofloxacin on *Prevotella intermedia* biofilm. Oral Microbiol Immunol 2006;21:366–71.
19. Takemoto T, Kurihara H, Dahlen G. Characterization of *Bacteroides forsythus* isolates. J Clin Microbiol 1997;35:1378–81.
20. Brayton JJ, Yang Q, Nakkula RJ, et al. An in vitro model of ciprofloxacin and minocycline transport by oral epithelial cells. J Periodontol 2002;73:1267–72.
21. Lai PC, Walters JD. Azithromycin kills invasive *Aggregatibacter actinomycetemcomitans* in gingival epithelial cells. Antimicrob Agents Chemother 2013;57:1347–51.
22. Hand WL, King-Thompson NL. The entry of antibiotics into human monocytes. J Antimicrob Chemother 1989;23:681–9.
23. Hand WL, King-Thompson NL. Uptake of antibiotics by human polymorphonuclear leukocyte cytoplasts. Antimicrob Agents Chemother 1990;34:1189–93.
24. Slots J, Research, Science and Therapy Committee. Systemic antibiotics in periodontics. J Periodontol 2004;75:1553–65.
25. Flemmig TF, Milian E, Karch H, et al. Differential clinical treatment outcome after systemic metronidazole and amoxicillin in patients harboring *Aggregatibacter actinomycetemcomitans* and/or *Porphyromonas gingivalis*. J Clin Periodontol 1998;25:380–7.
26. Herrera D, Sanz M, Jepsen S, et al. A systematic review on the effect of systemic antimicrobials as an adjunct to scaling and root planing in periodontitis patients. J Clin Periodontol 2002;29(Suppl 3):136–59.
27. Haffajee AD, Socransky SS, Gunsolley JC. Systemic anti-infective periodontal therapy: a systematic review. Ann Periodontol 2003;8:115–81.
28. Van der Velden U, Varoufaki A, Hutter JW, et al. Effect of smoking and periodontal treatment on the subgingival microflora. J Clin Periodontol 2003;30:603–10.
29. Darby IB, Hodge PJ, Riggio MP, et al. Clinical and microbiological effects of scaling and root planing in smoker and non-smoker chronic and aggressive periodontitis patients. J Clin Periodontol 2005;32:200–6.
30. Mascarenhas P, Gapski R, Al-Shammari K, et al. Clinical response of azithromycin as an adjunct to non-surgical periodontal therapy in smokers. J Periodontol 2005;76:426–36.
31. Angaji M, Gelskey S, Nogueira-Filho G, et al. A systematic review of clinical efficacy of adjunctive antibiotics in the treatment of smokers with periodontitis. J Periodontol 2010;81:1518–28.
32. Brayer WK, Mellonig JT, Dunlap RM, et al. Scaling and root planing effectiveness: the effect of root surface access and operator experience. J Periodontol 1989;60:67–72.
33. Rabbani GM, Ash MM, Caffesse RG. The effectiveness of subgingival scaling and root planing in calculus removal. J Periodontol 1981;52:119–23.
34. Sherman PR, Hutchens LH, Jewson LG, et al. The effectiveness of subgingival scaling and root planing. I. Clinical detection of residual calculus. J Periodontol 1990;61:3–8.
35. Cobb CM. Non-surgical pocket therapy: mechanical. Ann Periodontol 1996;1:443–90.
36. Tunkel J, Heinecke A, Flemmig TF. A systematic review of efficacy of machine-driven and manual subgingival debridement in the treatment of chronic periodontitis. J Clin Periodontol 2002;29(Suppl 3):72–81.

37. Heitz-Mayfield LJ, Lang NP. Surgical and nonsurgical periodontal therapy. Learned and unlearned concepts. Periodontol 2000 2013;62:218–31.
38. Greenstein G. The role of metronidazole in the treatment of periodontal diseases. J Periodontol 1993;64:1–15.
39. Herrera D, Alonso B, Leon R, et al. Antimicrobial therapy in periodontitis: the use of systemic antimicrobials against the subgingival biofilm. J Clin Periodontol 2008;35(Suppl 8):45–66.
40. Lekovic V, Kenney EB, Carranza FA, et al. The effect of metronidazole on human periodontal disease. A clinical and bacteriological study. J Periodontol 1983;54:476–80.
41. Lindhe J, Liljenberg B, Adielson B, et al. Use of metronidazole as a probe in the study of human periodontal disease. J Clin Periodontol 1983;10:100–12.
42. Walsh MM, Buchanan SA, Hoover CI, et al. Clinical and microbiologic effects of single-dose metronidazole or scaling and root planing in treatment of adult periodontitis. J Clin Periodontol 1986;13:151–7.
43. Lopez NJ, Socransky SS, Da Silva I, et al. Effects of metronidazole plus amoxicillin as the only therapy on the microbiological and clinical parameters of untreated chronic periodontitis. J Clin Periodontol 2006;33:648–60.
44. Socransky SS, Haffajee AD. Dental biofilms: difficult therapeutic targets. Periodontol 2000 2002;28:12–55.
45. Anwar H, Dasgupta MK, Costerton JW. Testing the susceptibility of bacteria in biofilms to antibacterial agents. Antimicrob Agents Chemother 1990;34:2043–6.
46. Anwar H, Strap JL, Costerton JW. Establishment of aging biofilms: possible mechanism of bacterial resistance to antibiotic therapy. Antimicrob Agents Chemother 1992;36:1347–51.
47. Marsh PD. Dental plaque: biological significance of a biofilm and community lifestyle. J Clin Periodontol 2005;32(Suppl 6):7–15.
48. Roberts AP, Mullany P. Genetic basis of horizontal gene transfer among oral bacteria. Periodontol 2000 2006;42:36–46.
49. Roberts AP, Kreth J. The impact of horizontal gene transfer on the adaptive ability of the human oral microbiome. Front Cell Infect Microbiol 2014;4:214.
50. Eick S, Seltmann T, Pfister W. Efficacy of antibiotics to strains of periodontopathic bacteria within a single species biofilm - an in vitro study. J Clin Periodontol 2004;31:376–83.
51. Belibasakis GN, Thurnheer T. Validation of antibiotic efficacy on in vitro subgingival biofilms. J Periodontol 2014;85:343–8.
52. Sgolastra F, Gatto R, Petrucci A, et al. Effectiveness of systemic amoxicillin/metronidazole as adjunctive therapy to scaling and root planing in the treatment of chronic periodontitis: a systematic review and meta-analysis. J Periodontol 2012;83:1257–69.
53. Zandbergen D, Slot DE, Cobb CM, et al. The clinical effect of scaling and root planing and the concomitant administration of systemic amoxicillin and metronidazole: a systematic review. J Periodontol 2013;84:332–51.
54. Keestra JA, Grosjean I, Coucke W, et al. Non-surgical periodontal therapy with systemic antibiotics in patients with untreated chronic periodontitis: a systematic review and meta-analysis. J Periodont Res 2015;50(3):294–314.
55. Sgolastra F, Severino M, Petrucci A, et al. Effectiveness of metronidazole as an adjunct to scaling and root planing in the treatment of chronic periodontitis: a systematic review and meta-analysis. J Periodont Res 2014;49:10–9.
56. Walker CB. Selected antimicrobial agents: mechanisms of action, side effects and drug interactions. Periodontol 2000 1996;10:12–28.

57. Idsoe O, Guthe T, Willcox RR, et al. Nature and extent of penicillin side reactions, with particular reference to fatalities from anaphylactic shock. Bull WHO 1968;38: 159–88.
58. Ray WA, Murray KT, Hall K, et al. Azithromycin and the risk of cardiovascular death. N Engl J Med 2012;366:1881–90.
59. Llor C, Sierra N, Hernandez S, et al. The higher the number of daily doses of antibiotic treatment in lower respiratory tract infection, the worse the compliance. J Antimicrob Chemother 2009;63:396–9.
60. Heitz-Mayfield LJ. Systemic antibiotics in periodontal therapy. Aust Dent J 2009; 54:S96–101.
61. Ceri H, Olson ME, Stremick C, et al. The Calgary biofilm device: new technology for rapid determination of antibiotic susceptibilities of bacterial biofilms. J Clin Microbiol 1999;37:1771–6.
62. Costerton JW, Lewandowski Z, Caldwell DE, et al. Microbial biofilms. Annu Rev Microbiol 1995;49:711–45.
63. Pitt WG, McBride MO, Lunceford JK, et al. Ultrasonic enhancement of antibiotic action on Gram-negative bacteria. Antimicrob Agents Chemother 1994;38: 2577–82.
64. Rams TE, Degener JE, van Winkelhoff AJ. Antibiotic resistance in human chronic periodontitis microbiota. J Periodontol 2014;85:160–9.
65. Ubeda C, Pamer EG. Antibiotics, microbiota, and immune defense. Trends Immunol 2012;33:459–66.
66. Dupin C, Tamanai-Shacoori Z, Ehrmann E, et al. Oral gram-negative anaerobic bacilli as a reservoir of β-lactam resistance genes facilitating infections with multi-resistant bacteria. Int J Antimicrob Agents 2015;45:99–105.
67. Rosling B, Serino G, Hellstrom MK, et al. Longitudinal periodontal tissue alterations during supportive therapy. Findings from subjects with normal and high susceptibility to periodontal disease. J Clin Periodontol 2001;28:241–9.
68. Mombelli A, Cionca N, Almaghlouth A. Does adjunctive antimicrobial therapy reduce the perceived need for periodontal surgery? Periodontol 2000 2011;55: 205–16.

Unanswered Questions

Can Bone Lost from Furcations Be Regenerated?

Joseph J. Zambon, DDS, PhD

KEYWORDS

- Furcation defects • Alveolar bone • Animal models • Histology
- Human clinical trials

KEY POINTS

- Histologic demonstration of new bone growth in furcations is the gold standard.
- There is histologic evidence of new bone growth in experimental furcation defects in animal models and in a few reports of furcation defects in humans.
- There are several reported human clinical trials that include surgical reentry and open measurement of furcation defects, but the nature of the hard tissue in the furcation needs to be determined by histology.
- There is a need for more histologic analysis in human clinical studies to confirm the presence and to determine the extent of new bone growth in human furcation defects.

INTRODUCTION

Furcation involvements pose one of the most difficult challenges in periodontal therapy and explain the greater likelihood of molar teeth being lost during the course of chronic periodontitis compared with single-rooted teeth.[1] The architecture of furcation defects plays a major role in disease progression and resistance to therapy.

The architecture of periodontal osseous defects is, by contrast, much simpler than furcation defects. The number of bony walls—1, 2, 3, or a combination—defines periodontal osseous defects. When considering the inferior osseous border is always present, periodontal osseous defects are actually 2-, 3-, or 4-walled defects. Regenerative periodontal therapy typically involves surgical débridement and placement of an autograft, allograft, xenograft, or alloplast into the defects followed by a barrier membrane to obstruct the migration of epithelial cells from the mucoperiosteal flap into the healing site. Over the next several weeks, fibroblasts migrate from the periodontal ligament (PDL) and osteoblasts migrate from the defect osseous walls to

Department of Periodontics and Endodontics, School of Dental Medicine, University at Buffalo, The State University of New York, 3435 Main Street, Buffalo, NY 14214, USA
E-mail address: jjzambon@buffalo.edu

Dent Clin N Am 59 (2015) 935–950
http://dx.doi.org/10.1016/j.cden.2015.06.001
0011-8532/15/$ – see front matter © 2015 Elsevier Inc. All rights reserved.

dental.theclinics.com

colonize the graft scaffold. The migration of host cells into the healing site is sometimes stimulated by biologic agents, such as bone morphogenic or enamel matrix proteins. Over time, osteoblasts may replace the graft material with new bone contiguous with the existing alveolar bone.[2]

Furcation defects present unique challenges. Furcation defects, like osseous defects, are bordered by alveolar bone. In addition, furcation defects are bordered by root surfaces usually covered by cementum but sometimes covered with dentin or even enamel in cases of cervical enamel projections. As periodontal disease progresses, the roots become exposed to the oral environment. They are colonized by oral bacteria and contaminated by bacterial toxins. The furcation fornix may be so narrow that patient oral hygiene is impossible and even professional débridement is difficult. Similar to periodontal osseous defects, cortical bone lines periodontal furcation defects. The procedure for osseous grafts frequently includes cortical (intramarrow) penetration. This causes bleeding from subcortical cancellous bone, clot formation, and migration of osteoblasts into the defect. Intramarrow penetration has been shown to increase clinical bone gain in infrabony defects treated by open flap débridement.[3]

There is a great deal of data on periodontal regeneration in furcation defects. These data are summarized in several excellent reviews (discussed later). This article does not address the entire area of periodontal regeneration. Rather, it focuses on a single but unique and important aspect of periodontal regeneration, that of new bone growth in furcation defects. This article addresses the unanswered question, Can bone lost from furcations be regenerated?

DIAGNOSIS AND CLASSIFICATION OF FURCATION DEFECTS

The diagnosis of furcation defects in dental practice is based primarily on periodontal probing and dental radiographs. Furcation probes (pigtailed explorer and Nabers probe) are used both to detect furcation defects and quantitate the extent of the defect.

Three types of furcation defects were described by Hamp and colleagues[4] based on clinical probing measurements: degree I = horizontal loss of periodontal tissue in the furcation less than 3 mm; degree II = horizontal loss of support in the furcation exceeding 3 mm but not encompassing the total width of the furcation area; and, degree III = horizontal through-and-through loss of the tissue in the furcation. There are several other classification systems (Ramfjord,[5] Tarnow and Fletcher,[6] and Hou and colleagues[7]), some of which provide subcategories to the Hamp classification based on the severity of the furcation defect measured in a vertical direction from the fornix, or roof, of the furcation to the base, or floor, of the defect. The system described by Hamp and colleagues,[4] however, remains widely used in both clinical practice and clinical research.

Standard periapical, bitewing, and panoramic radiographs are used to diagnose furcation defects in dental practice. Like the detection of alveolar bone loss in chronic periodontitis, a significant amount of alveolar bone loss must occur before a furcation defect can be seen on a radiograph. Initial class I furcation defects are only detectable by probing. More severe class II and class III defects maybe evident on radiographs but even then the defects may be hidden by superimposition of roots. Furcation defects might be evident as slight alterations in trabecular radiodensity or they might demonstrate gross radiolucencies. Consequently, the sensitivity of standard radiographs in detecting furcation defects is low but the specificity is high.[8,9]

Besides periodontal probing and radiographs, additional measurements are used to characterize the size of the furcation defects, particularly in clinical studies. These parameters include closed measurements, such as vertical probing depth and horizontal probing depth; vertical attachment level and horizontal attachment level; gingival recession; and open measurements made at the time of surgery or surgical reentry. These vertical and horizontal defect measurements are used to calculate initial defect volume, post-treatment vertical defect fill, and horizontal defect fill as well as overall change in defect volume.

TREATMENT OF FURCATION DEFECTS

Prior to the advent of periodontal regeneration, furcations defects were usually treated by resective surgery, such as tunneling, root resection/amputation, and bicuspidization. These treatments have supplemented by therapies directed toward the regeneration of periodontal tissues. The origin of periodontal regeneration can be traced to studies of new attachment using filters and Teflon membranes.[10,11] This was followed by guided tissue regeneration using nonresorbable and then resorbable barrier membranes followed by combinations of osseous grafts and barrier membranes and, more recently, the use of biologic agents, such as bone morphogenetic proteins and enamel matrix proteins. The field of periodontal regeneration is, therefore, a translational science applying the results of basic laboratory research to clinical practice. For example, peptide-enhanced anorganic bone matrix particulate grafts contain the synthetic biomimetic of the 15 amino acid cell–binding domain of type I collagen bound to bovine hydroxyl apatite. This product is the result of laboratory research that determined the amino acid sequence of type I collagen, pinpointed the cell binding part of the collagen molecule, synthesized the terminal peptide, and linked it to bovine hydroxyl apatite.

THE PROBLEM WITH PROBING

Periodontal probing is the standard method of detecting periodontal furcation defects. With class I defects, there may only be a slight depression indicating the divergence of the roots, whereas the probe may enter the defect to greater depths with class II and III defects. Entry of the probe depends, however, on the absence of obstructing soft tissues, and the depth of penetration depends on the width of the osseous defects and the divergence of the roots. Recent studies using cone-beam CT (CBCT) call into question the accuracy of periodontal probing in the detection of furcation defects.

CBCT enables visualization of slices of the maxilla and mandible in sagittal and horizontal planes. Consequently, furcations that might not be probeable because the defects are too narrow or tortuous are visible on CBCT. Furcations that might be categorized into one class of defect by probing might be categorized into another class of defect by CBCT.

Two recent studies have examined the relationship between clinical probing and CBCT for the detection and classification of furcation defects. Both studies indicate that the clinical diagnosis of furcation defects by periodontal probing can result in significant underestimates and overestimates of the extent of a furcation defect. In one study by Walter and colleagues,[12] CBCT was used to assess 22 maxillary molars in 12 generalized chronic periodontitis patients with clinical furcation defects. There was agreement between clinical probing and CBCT in 27% of the sites, but the clinical diagnoses were overestimated compared with CBCT in 29% of the sites and the clinical diagnoses were underestimated compared with CBCT in of the 44% sites. All the clinically detectable class III furcations were also detected by CBCT but clinical class II and class II to III furcation defects were underestimated by as much as 75%. In a study by Laky and colleagues,[13] 582 molars were clinically examined for class II and class III furcation defects and compared with CT scans. There was agreement between clinical diagnosis and CT in 57% of the sites but the clinical diagnosis was overestimated in 20% of the sites and the clinical diagnosis was underestimated in 23% of the sites. The best correlation between clinical diagnosis and CT was in sites that were the easiest to probe—mandibular and maxillary buccal furcations (correlation coefficients = 0.52 and 0.38, respectively). The worst correlation between clinical diagnosis and diagnosis by CT was in sites that were the hardest to probe—maxillary distal furcations.

The data from these and other studies indicate that furcation defects may be misclassified using standard methods. Zappa and colleagues[14] compared probing with surgical exposure of furcation defects and found that 7% of degree 1 and 24% of degree 2 (Hamp index) were overestimations whereas 27% of degree 3 involvements were not recognized. Pistorius and colleagues[15] compared clinical probing with CT and found a correlation in 69% of defects and an underestimate in 31% of the defects. Accordingly, studies that rely on clinical criteria to classify furcations may have an inherent methodologic error. Misclassification of furcation defects may affect the clinical outcome of treatment studies. For example, a cohort of patients with class II maxillary furcation defects selected on the basis of probing also likely includes some teeth with class III furcation defects. There is known to be significant variability in treatment outcomes for furcation defects. Some of this variability is attributable to patient compliance and some is attributable to unknown factors.[16] Misclassification of periodontal furcation defects may be an as-yet underappreciated source of variability in studies of furcation defects.

POUCHES WITHIN FURCATIONS

In addition to the factors normally associated with the progressing periodontitis—pathogenic plaque bacteria; inadequate oral hygiene; systemic factors, such as diabetes mellitus; habits, such as smoking; local factors, such as open contacts; and overhanging restorations—furcation defects have their own unique factors. These include root morphology, root trunk length, accessory canals, enamel pearls, cemental caries, and pulpal disease manifesting as periodontal-endodontic lesions. The anatomy of the furcation often hinders oral hygiene because it may be too narrow for access by toothbrush bristles or even scalers or curettes during professional treatment. Bower,[17] for example, reported that the width of the furcation entrance in molars is narrower than the width of most curettes.

Another important factor in the etiology of furcation defects is cervical enamel projections—the triangular-shaped extension of enamel from the cementoenamel junction into the furcation. The presence of enamel projections—reported in 15% to 24% of mandibular molars and 9% to 25% of maxillary molars[18]—provides an area devoid of connective tissue attachment and predisposes to the development of furcation defects. Correlations between cervical enamel projections and the presence and severity of furcation defects have been reported by several investigators.[19–21]

Recent electron microscopic studies show that there is even greater complexity to cervical enamel projections than previously thought.[22] Pouchlike openings (**Fig. 1**) have recently been described in association with cervical enamel projections. These anomalies can hide oral biofilms resistant to even the most stringent oral hygiene efforts, thus contributing to the progression of furcation defects.

TYPES OF EVIDENCE FOR NEW BONE GROWTH IN FURCATION DEFECTS

What constitutes evidence for new bone growth in furcation defects? The gold standard for ascertaining the presence and amount of new bone in a furcation defect is

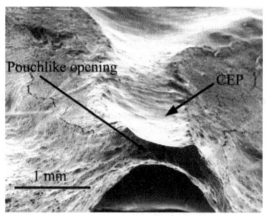

Fig. 1. Electron microscopic view of a furcation. This shows a pouchlike opening apical to the cervical enamel projection that can harbor oral biofilms and lead to progression of furcation defects. CEP, cervical enamel projection. (*From* Blanchard SB, Derderian GM, Averitt TR, et al. Cervical enamel projections and associated pouch-like opening in mandibular furcations. J Periodontol 2012;83(2):198–203; with permission.)

histology—the microscopic identification of bone matrix, osteocytes, osteoblasts, osteoclasts, and haversian canals. The exact nature of the tissue present in a furcation can only be determined by histology. As described by Garrett,[16] "Histological evaluation remains the only reliable method of determining the nature of the attachment apparatus resulting from therapeutic attempts to regenerate the periodontium." Similarly, Eickholz and Hausmann[23] wrote, "the type of tissue recolonizing a periodontal defect after surgical therapy can only be precisely evaluated by histology." Several investigators have recently reaffirmed this view. Nevins and colleagues[24] wrote, "Without histology it would not be possible to evaluate the biological potential of the surgical procedure." Avila-Ortiz and colleagues[25] summarized a systematic review of periodontal regeneration in furcation defects: "These future studies should also have long-term follow-ups, ideally greater than 5 years after baseline, and should place more emphasis on histologic and patient-reported outcomes."

The reason for the dearth of human histologic data on treated furcation defects is self-evident. Material appropriate for histologic examination necessitates surgical exposure and block extraction to preserve tissues relationships. Not many patients or human subject review committees approve block extractions or even extraction of individual teeth that might otherwise be maintained. Hopeless teeth are the exception. Hopeless teeth can be treated with the understanding that they will be subsequently extracted and processed for histologic examination.

The vast majority of histologic and histomorphometric data available in the literature is derived from animal studies. Furcation defects in animal models can be histologically examined to assess periodontal regeneration, including new bone growth, but there are differences between animal and human furcation defects. First, animal teeth have different anatomy. Second, furcation defects in animal models are created surgically rather than the result of chronic periodontitis. There are differences between furcation defects in animal models and humans in types of microorganisms infecting the sites and bacterial toxins on the root surfaces. Also, surgically created furcation defects in animal models are lined by cancellous bone rather than by cortical bone in human furcation defects resulting from chronic periodontitis.

As a consequence of the ethical issues associated with the procurement of human tissue samples for histologic examination, surrogate measures are frequently used to study human furcation defects. These surrogate measures include closed measurements, open measurements made at the time of surgery, and radiographic assessments, including subtraction radiography and micro-CT. The acceptability of surrogate measures in assessing periodontal regeneration in furcation defects can be traced back to the 1996 World Workshop in Periodontics. It was recommended that acceptable proof of periodontal regeneration could include histologic analysis of tissue samples from animal models together with human controlled clinical trials.[26]

Although open measurements made during surgery or surgical reentry provide more evidence for new bone formation in a furcation defect than do closed measurements, it can be difficult to differentiate new bone in a surgically exposed furcation from other tissues, such as cartilage or fibrous connective tissue that may be present in a treated furcation. Consequently, open measurements at surgical reentry may overestimate the amount of bone in a defect. Also, as opposed to histologic analysis in which new bone is measured from a notch placed in the root marking the apical extent of the defect, surgical reentry evaluates changes in probing measurements without actually being able to see the starting point of the furcation defect.

Difficulties in clinically differentiating the type of tissue present in a healing furcation have been reported in several studies. Becker and colleagues[27] reported 3 cases of guided tissue regeneration with surgical reentry at 3 or 6 months. They reported that there were gains in defect fill that they termed, *open probing new attachment*, but that the material "did not have the consistency of bone." Lekovic and colleagues[28] performed intraoperative and reentry measurements of mandibular class II furcation defects. They reported that changes in probing measurements were not due to the growth of new bone in the furcation defect but to new connective tissue attachment. They concluded, "Histologic evaluation of successfully treated Class II furcations in humans will be necessary in the future to verify the possibilities of complete periodontal regeneration with the various techniques."

In their study, Houser and colleagues[29] reported that the "...6-month reentry reveals a bonelike substance that is resistant to probing in the furcation." Clinical reports often refer to hard tissue measurements or hard tissues seen at the time of surgical reentry. These terms are, however, often used interchangeably with *bone*, although there is no histologic basis for this categorization.[30,31]

HISTOLOGIC EVIDENCE FOR NEW BONE GROWTH IN FURCATION DEFECTS IN ANIMAL MODELS

Histologic examination of block sections from animal models provides definitive evidence of bone growth in furcation defects. **Table 1** lists studies of class II and class III furcation defects in animal models—mainly dogs but also baboons and minipigs—treated with a variety of periodontal regenerative agents. The treatments include recombinant human transforming growth factor β3,[32] platelet pellet,[33] polylactide-co-glycolide acid/calcium phosphate bilayered biomaterial,[34] human osteogenic protein-1 and human transforming growth factor-β3,[35] cultured PDL cells,[36] collagen hydrogel/sponge scaffold,[37] enamel matrix derivative with a biphasic calcium phosphate,[38] and bioactive glass/platelet rich plasma.[39]

All these animal studies with histology reported new bone growth in furcation defects. The amount of new bone growth varied. Keles and colleagues[33] reported "limited coronal new bone growth." Suiad and colleagues[39] reported 5.45 mm of new bone in test sites compared with 1.89 mm in control sites. Kosen and

Table 1
Histologic evidence for new bone growth in furcation defects in animal models

Study	Animal Model	Furcation Classification	Treatment	Results
Teare et al,[32] 2008	Baboon	Class II	Surgically created class II furcation defects in maxillary and mandibular molars of 4 adult baboons were treated with heterotopic ossicles and recombinant human transforming growth factor-β3.	After 60 d, recombinant human transforming growth factor-β3, delivered by Matrigel as carrier, was found to induce alveolar bone.
Keles et al,[33] 2009	Dogs	Class II	Surgically created mandibular class II lesions were treated with platelet pellet or platelet pellet and GTR or scaling and root planning.	12 wk postsurgery, there was limited coronal new bone growth in all groups not significantly different from each other.
Carlo Reis et al,[34] 2011	Dogs	Class II	Treated experimental class II furcation defects were treated with semirigid polylactide-co-glycolide acid/calcium phosphate bilayered biomaterial.	Control defects were filled mainly with dense connective tissue. New alveolar bone was evident from the apical limit to the most coronal part of the defect and from lingual to buccal.
Teare et al,[35] 2012	Baboon	Class II	Surgically created class II furcation defects of the first and second mandibular molars of 3 adult baboons	Application of human osteogenic protein-1 and human transforming growth factor-β3 resulted in new bone against the root surfaces.
Suiad et al,[36] 2012	Dogs	Class III	Surgically created class III furcation defects were treated with cultured PDL cells.	After 3 mo, larger area of new bone compared with controls 5.45 ± 1.58 mm^2 vs 1.89 ± 0.95 mm^2 untreated control
Kosen et al,[37] 2012	Dogs	Class II	Surgically created mandibular class II lesions in beagle dogs were treated with collagen hydrogel/sponge scaffold vs untreated control group and evaluated 2 and 4 wk.	Volume of new bone was significantly greater in the test group vs control group—% new bone 51.4 ± 6.4 vs 36.4 ± 5.3.
Mardas et al,[38] 2012	Dogs	Class III	Surgically created 17 mandibular class III lesions in 9 dogs were treated with either enamel matrix derivative with a biphasic calcium phosphate or untreated control.	After 5 mo, new bone formation was observed in both groups—mean new bone height was 4.4 ± 1.3 mm and 4.3 ± 1.6 mm in the control and test groups. There was no significant difference between groups.
Suiad et al,[39] 2012	Dogs	Class II	Surgically created class II lesions were treated with GTR + BG + PRP or with just GTR + BG and B.	There was greater mineralized bone area observed for the GTR + BG + PRP treated defects compared with GTR + BG—10.73 mm^2 vs 7.63 mm^2 after 90 d.

Abbreviations: BG, bioactive glass; GTR, guided tissue regeneration; PRP, platelet-rich plasma.
Data from Refs.[32–39]

colleagues[37] reported that test sites had 51.4% bone fill by volume compared with 36.4% in control sites (**Fig. 2**). Clearly there are numerous literature reports providing histologic evidence of new bone growth in both treated and control furcation defects in animal models.

HISTOLOGIC EVIDENCE FOR NEW BONE GROWTH IN HUMAN FURCATION DEFECTS

In contrast to animal studies, there are few histologic data demonstrating new bone growth in human furcation defects (**Table 2**). Stoller and colleagues[40] (**Fig. 3**) presented histologic data on a furcation in a patient treated 25 months previously during a study of guided tissue regeneration using bioabsorbable polylactic acid–based barrier membranes. The study patients all had class II furcation defects with vertical

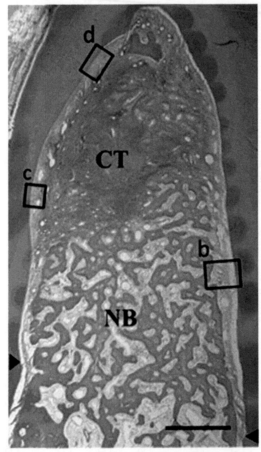

Fig. 2. New bone formation in an experimental dog model 4 weeks after placement of a collagen hydrogel/sponge scaffold. Apical notches marking the apical extent of the original furcation defect are indicated by the arrow heads. New bone fills most of the dimension from the apical notches to the fornix. CT, connective tissue; NB, new bone. (*From* Kosen Y, Miyaji H, Kato A, et al. Application of collagen hydrogel/sponge scaffold facilitates periodontal wound healing in class II furcation defects in beagle dogs. J Periodontal Res 2012;47(5):626–34; with permission.)

Table 2
Histologic evidence for new bone growth in human furcation defects

Study	Type of Study	Furcation Classification	Treatment	Findings
Stoller et al,[40] 2001	Case report	Class II	GTR with bioabsorbable membrane	Bone growth shown in the buccal class II furcation #18, 25 mo after GTR
Mellonig et al,[41] 2009	Four cases	Class III	PDGF and β–tricalcium phosphate	Class III furcations treated in 4 patients with hopeless periodontal prognosis. Some new bone was noted in 3 of 4 teeth ranging from 0 to 2.04 mm.
Nevins et al,[24] 2013	Single-center prospective clinical study	Class III	LANAP in 12 defects in 8 subjects with advanced periodontitis, including 3 teeth with class III furcations	There was some regeneration, including some new bone.

Abbreviations: GTR, guided tissue regeneration; LANAP, laser-assisted new attachment procedure; PGDF, platelet derived growth factor.
 Data from Refs.[24,40,41]

probing depths of at least 5 mm and horizontal probing depths of at least 3 mm. The patient had cracked the treated tooth, a mandibular left second molar, and did not want additional treatment. The tooth was extracted and examined histologically (see **Fig. 3**). PDL and bone were apparent in the furcation. New bone growth could

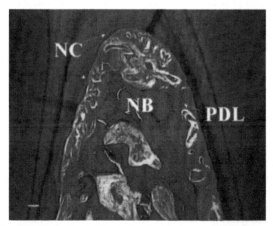

Fig. 3. A histologic section of a buccal furcation in a human mandibular second molar furcation previously by periodontal regenerative surgery. At the time of treatment, the tooth exhibited vertical probing depths of at least 5 mm and horizontal probing depths of at least 3 mm. Twenty-five months after treatment, the tooth cracked. The patient declined treatment. The tooth was extracted and examined histologically. Alveolar bone extends almost to the furcation fornix. NB, new bone; NC, new cementum. (*From* Stoller NH, Johnson LR, Garrett S. Periodontal regeneration of a class II furcation defect utilizing a bioabsorbable barrier in a human. A case study with histology. J Periodontol 2001;72:238–42; with permission.)

be seen coronal to a notch placed in the root at the time of treatment demarcating the apical extent of the furcation defect. The investigators suggest that this particular furcation defect might have been especially favorable to new bone growth because the roots were narrow mesiodistally and there was a 3-wall infrabony defect at the buccal entrance to the furcation.

Mellonig and colleagues[41] examined 4 mandibular first molars with class III furcations and hopeless periodontal and prosthetic prognosis in patients with advanced chronic periodontitis. The furcation defects were treated with a combination of recombinant human platelet-derived growth factor and β–tricalcium phosphate and covered on both facial and lingual surfaces by a collagen membrane. The teeth were extracted after 6 months and evaluated histologically. The investigators found histologic evidence of new bone growth in the furcation: "Foci of new bone were seen almost to the fornix of the furcation."

Nevins and colleagues[24] examined laser-assisted new attachment procedures in 12 hopeless teeth in 8 patients, including 3 teeth with class III furcations. Nine months after treatment, the teeth were extracted and examined histologically. They found new bone growth coronal to the root notch, which was confirmed by micro-CT. Overall, these 3 histologic studies suggest that bone growth is possible in human furcation defects.

EVIDENCE FOR NEW BONE GROWTH IN HUMAN FURCATION DEFECTS OBTAINED BY SURGICAL REENTRY

After histology, the next best evidence for bone growth in furcation defects is surgical reentry. **Table 3** lists studies assessing bone growth in human periodontal furcation defects by surgical reentry, after 6 or 12 months. Most reentry studies examine class II furcations because these are considered especially amenable to periodontal regeneration. As discussed previously, surgical reentry evaluated tissues that feel hard by probing and that may be bone or cartilage or dense connective tissue.

As shown in **Table 3**, surgical reentry studies demonstrated gain of hard tissue in both test and control groups with more gain of hard tissue in the test groups. Although the magnitude of gain in the test sites compared with the control sites was often statistically significant, it was often minimal in terms of real tissue and raises questions as to clinical significance. For example, Houser and colleagues[29] compared the treatment of mandibular class II furcations with either bovine bone xenograft and collagen membranes or open-flap débridement. Surgical reentry after 6 months showed that the test group had decreased vertical probing of 1.5 mm and decreased horizontal probing of 2.1 mm, indicative of new bone growth. This calculated to an 82.7% reduction in the furcation defect in the test group compared with a 42.5% reduction in the furcation defect in the control group. Taheri and colleagues[42] compared anorganic bovine bone xenograft plus bioabsorbable collagen membrane (test) with anorganic bovine bone xenograft alone (control) in human mandibular class II furcations defects. Surgical reentry after 6 months showed decreased probing measurements in both the test and the control groups. The difference between the test and the control groups, however, in both horizontal and vertical measurements was less than 1 mm, suggesting that the amount of new hard tissue may not be clinically significant. Palioto and colleagues[43] (**Fig. 4**) treated class III furcations using a nonresorbable membrane with or without bovine inorganic bone matrix. Surgical reentry at 6 months showed significant gain in terms of reduced vertical probing depths in the test group. There were mean changes of 0.86 and 1.1 mm in horizontal and vertical open probing measurements in the test group compared with −0.03 and 0.84 mm in the control group.

Table 3
Surgical reentry evidence for new bone growth in human furcation defects

Study	Furcation Classification	Treatment	Findings
Houser et al,[29] 2001	Class II	Compared anorganic bovine bone xenograft with a bioabsorbable collagen barrier to open-flap débridement in human mandibular class II furcation; surgical reentry at 6 mo	The test group showed 2.0 mm of vertical and 3.0 mm of horizontal furcation bone fill and an 82.7% defect resolution compared with 0.5 and 0.9 mm and 42.5% in test group.
Lamb et al,[44] 2001	Class II	Compared porous and nonporous Teflon barrier membranes plus demineralized freeze-dried bone allografts in class II buccal/lingual furcation defects; surgical reentry after 9 mo	There was gain of hard tissue (open horizontal probing depth) of 2.33 ± 0.78 mm and 49 ± 12% fill in the nonporous membrane group and 2.75 ± 0.75 mm and 56 ± 12% fill in the porous membrane group.
Pruthi et al,[45] 2002	Class II	Compared ePTFE and collagen membranes in treating class II furcations in human mandibular molars; surgical reentry at 12 mo	There was loss of vertical fill—1.00 ± 2.03 mm in the ePTFE group and gain of 0.81 ± 1.80 mm in the collagen group—and gain of 0.41 ± 0.62, 0.41 ± 0.71 in horizontal fill in the ePTFE and collagen groups, respectively.
Lekovic et al,[46] 2003	Class II	Evaluated platelet-rich plasma, bovine porous bone mineral and guided tissue regeneration in class II molar furcation defects; surgical reentry at 6 mo	There was mean vertical bone level gain of 2.56 ± 0.36 mm in the test vs 0.19 ± 0.02 mm in the control and mean horizontal bone level gain of 2.28 ± 0.33 mm vs 0.08 ± 0.02 mm.
Palioto et al,[43] 2003	Class III	Compared nonresorbable membrane with or without bovine inorganic bone matrix in human class III furcations; surgical reentry at 6 mo	There was a mean change of 0.86 and 1.1 mm in horizontal and vertical open probing measurements in the test group compared with −0.03 and 0.84 mm in the control group. There was significant gain over time for vertical probing depths in the test group.
Taheri et al,[42] 2009	Class II	Compared anorganic bovine bone xenograft plus bioabsorbable collagen membrane (test) to anorganic bovine bone xenograft alone (control) in human mandibular class II furcations defects; surgical reentry after 6 mo	Both groups showed reductions in furcation probing depths at reentry—mean vertical and horizontal reduction of 1.9 ± 1.3 mm, 2.1 ± 0.7 for test and 2.1 ± 1.0, 2.4 ± 1.3 for control, respectively.
Jenabian et al,[47] 2013	Class II	Compared horse bone grafts with either autogenous connective tissue (case) or resorbable membranes (control); surgical reentry procedure after 6 mo	Both groups showed reductions in furcation probing at reentry—mean vertical and horizontal reduction of 0.38 mm and 1 mm for case and 0.51 mm and 0.34 mm for control.

Abbreviation: ePTFE, expanded polytetrafluoroethylene.
Data from Refs.[29,42–47]

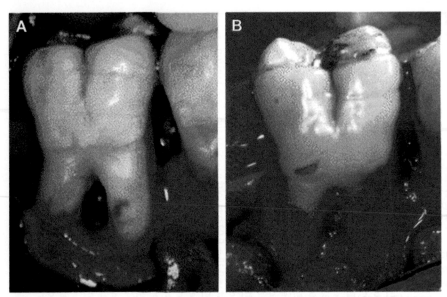

Fig. 4. Periodontal regeneration treatment of a class III mandibular molar furcation. Before (*A*) and after (*B*) treatment of a class III furcation using bovine inorganic bone matrix and nonresorbable membrane. (*From* Palioto DB, Joly JC, deLima AF, et al. Clinical and radiographic treatment evaluation of class III furcation defects using GTR with and without inorganic bone matrix. J Clin Periodontol 2003;30:1–8; with permission.)

PERIODONTAL REGENERATION

There are several recent reviews of periodontal regeneration in furcation defects. Again, periodontal regeneration is defined in histologic terms—new cementum and a functionally oriented periodontal ligament as well as new bone—but the determination of periodontal regeneration is made not by histology but by closed or open clinical measurements and sometimes radiography.

Kinaia and colleagues[48] reviewed randomized controlled human trials for the treatment of class II furcations with surgical reentry at 6 to 12 months. Guided tissue regeneration surgery with resorbable or nonresorbable membranes (13 studies) was better than open flap débridement in reducing vertical probing depth, increasing vertical attachment, and increasing vertical and horizontal bone levels (hard tissues). Horizontal bone increased by 1.85 mm and 1.54 mm whereas vertical bone increased by 1.49 mm and 0.75 mm for resorbable and nonresorbable membranes, respectively. Two studies reported guided tissue regeneration surgery using both graft materials and either resorbable or nonresorbable membranes. Horizontal bone increased by 2.58 and 2.55 mm and vertical bone increased by 2.25 and 1.15 mm for the resorbable and nonresorbable membranes with graft material, respectively.

Chen and colleagues[49] examined randomized controlled clinical trials comparing open flap débridement, guided tissue regeneration, and guided tissue regeneration with osseous grafting in the treatment of class II furcation defects. Meta-analysis of studies with at least 6 months' follow-up showed that guided tissue regeneration and guided tissue regeneration with osseous grafting were both better than open flap débridement in the treatment of mandibular molars in terms of furcation closure rate, vertical and horizontal bone fill, and vertical and horizontal attachment level

Table 4
Efficacy of periodontal regeneration in the treatment of furcation defects

Category	Conclusions
Class I defects Maxillary and mandibular molars	Most defects successfully treated with periodontal nonregenerative surgical therapy; regenerative therapy beneficial in certain cases
Class II defects Maxillary and mandibular molars	Regenerative treatment predictable; periodontal regeneration demonstrated histologically and clinically
Class III defects Mandibular molars	One case report demonstrates periodontal regeneration histologically
Class III defects Maxillary molars	Regenerative therapy not predictable; shown only in clinical case reports

From Avila-Ortiz G, De Buitrago JG, Reddy MS. Periodontal regeneration - furcation defects: a systematic review from the AAP regeneration workshop. J Periodontol 2015;86(2 Suppl):S108–30.

gain. Guided tissue regeneration with osseous grafting was better than guided tissue regeneration without osseous grafting. In maxillary molars, guided tissue regeneration resulted in greater vertical/horizontal bone fill and vertical attachment level gain than the open flap débridement.

In a recent systematic review, Avila-Ortiz and colleagues[25] examined 150 articles with clinical, radiographic, histologic, microbiologic, and patient-reported outcomes in regenerative therapy for different severities of furcation defects in different teeth. As summarized in **Table 4**, the investigators found that most class I mandibular and maxillary molar defects can be treated using standard nonsurgical periodontal therapy. Periodontal regeneration may be useful in specific class I defects. Mandibular and maxillary molar class II defects can be successfully treated by periodontal regeneration. Mandibular and maxillary molar class III furcation defects or maxillary premolar class II and III furcation defects are not predictably treated by periodontal regeneration.

SUMMARY

There is histologic evidence of new bone growth in experimental furcation defects in animal models. There are few reports demonstrating histologic evidence of new bone growth in furcation defects in human. There are also several reports of controlled human clinical trials of hard tissue fill, possibly bone, in furcation defects as determined by surgical reentry. Together the existing data point to the clear need for more histologic analysis for both the presence and the extent of new bone growth in human furcation defects.

REFERENCES

1. Hirschfeld L, Wasserman B. A long-term survey of tooth loss in 600 treated periodontal patients. J Periodontol 1978;49(5):225–37.
2. Melcher AH. Repair potential of periodontal tissues. J Periodontol 1976;47: 256–60.
3. Crea A, Deli G, Littarru C, et al. Intrabony defects, open-flap debridement, and decortication: a randomized clinical trial. J Periodontol 2014;85(1):34–42.
4. Hamp SE, Nyman S, Lindhe J. Periodontal treatment of multirooted teeth. Results after 5 years. J Clin Periodontol 1975;2:126–35.

5. Ramfjord S. Periodontology and periodontics. Philadelphia: W.B. Saunders; 1979.
6. Tarnow D, Fletcher P. Classification of the vertical component of furcation involvement. J Periodontol 1984;55:283–4.
7. Hou GL, Chen YM, Tsai CC, et al. A new classification of molar furcation involvement based on the root trunk and horizontal and vertical bone loss. Int J Periodontics Restorative Dent 1998;18:257–65.
8. Hishikawa T, Izumi M, Naitoh M, et al. The effect of horizontal X-ray beam angulation on the detection of furcation defects of mandibular first molars in intraoral radiography. Dentomaxillofac Radiol 2010;39:85–90.
9. Hishikawa T, Izumi M, Naitoh M, et al. Effects of the vertical projection angle in intraoral radiography on the detection of furcation involvement of the mandibular first molar. Oral Radiol 2011;27(2):102–7.
10. Gottlow J, Nyman S, Karring T, et al. New attachment formation as the result of controlled tissue regeneration. J Clin Periodontol 1984;11(8):494–503.
11. Gottlow J, Nyman S, Lindhe J, et al. New attachment formation in the human periodontium by guided tissue regeneration. Case reports. J Clin Periodontol 1986; 13(6):604–16.
12. Walter C, Kaner D, Berndt DC, et al. Three-dimensional imaging as a pre-operative tool in decision making for furcation surgery. J Clin Periodontol 2009;36:250–7.
13. Laky M, Majdalani S, Kapferer I, et al. Periodontal probing of dental furcations compared with diagnosis by low-dose computed tomography: a case series. J Periodontol 2013;84(12):1740–6.
14. Zappa U, Grosso L, Simona C, et al. Clinical furcation diagnoses and interradicular bone defects. J Periodontol 1993;64(3):219–27.
15. Pistorius A, Patrosio C, Willershausen B, et al. Periodontal probing in comparison to diagnosis by CT-scan. Int Dent J 2001;51:339–47.
16. Garrett S. Periodontal regeneration around natural teeth. Ann Periodontol 1996;1: 621–66.
17. Bower RC. Furcation morphology relative to periodontal treatment. Furcation entrance architecture. J Periodontol 1979;50:23–7.
18. Masters D, Hoskin S. Projection of cervical enamel into molar furcations. J Periodontol 1964;35:49–53.
19. Bissada NF, Abdelmalek RG. Incidence of cervical enamel projections and its relationship to furcation involvement in Egyptian skulls. J Periodontol 1973;44(9):583–5.
20. Grewe JM, Meskin LH, Miller T. Cervical enamel projections: prevalence, location, and extent; with associated periodontal implications. J Periodontol 1965;36(6): 460–5.
21. Swan RH, Hurt WC. Cervical enamel projections as an etiologic factor in furcation involvement. J Am Dent Assoc 1976;93(2):342–5.
22. Blanchard SB, Derderian GM, Averitt TR, et al. Cervical enamel projections and associated pouch-like opening in mandibular furcations. J Periodontol 2012; 83(2):198–203.
23. Eickholz P, Hausmann E. Evidence for healing of Class II and Class III furcations 24 months after guided tissue regeneration therapy: digital subtraction and clinical measurements. J Periodontol 1999;70(12):1490–500.
24. Nevins ML, Camelo M, Schupbach P, et al. Human clinical and histologic evaluation of laser-assisted new attachment procedure. Int J Periodontics Restorative Dent 2012;32(5):497–507.
25. Avila-Ortiz G, De Buitrago JG, Reddy MS. Periodontal regeneration - furcation defects: a systematic review from the AAP regeneration workshop. J Periodontol 2015;86(2 Suppl):S108–30.

26. Consensus report. Periodontal regeneration around natural teeth. Ann Periodontol 1996;1(1):667–70.

27. Becker W, Becker BE, Prichard JF, et al. Root isolation for new attachment procedures. A surgical and suturing method: three case reports. J Periodontol 1987;58: 819–26.

28. Lekovic V, Kenney EB, Kovacevic K, et al. Evaluation of guided tissue regeneration in Class II furcation defects. A clinical re-entry study. J Periodontol 1989;60: 694–8.

29. Houser BE, Mellonig JT, Brunsvold MA, et al. Clinical evaluation of anorganic bovine bone xenograft with a bioabsorbable collagen barrier in the treatment of molar furcation defects. Int J Periodontics Restorative Dent 2001;21(2): 161–9.

30. Anderegg CR, Martin SJ, Gray JL, et al. Clinical evaluation of the use of decalcified freeze-dried bone allograft with guided tissue regeneration in the treatment of molar furcation invasions. J Periodontol 1991;62(4):264–8.

31. Gantes B, Martin M, Garrett S, et al. Treatment of periodontal furcation defects. (II). Bone regeneration in mandibular class II defects. J Clin Periodontol 1988; 15(4):232–9.

32. Teare JA, Ramoshebi LN, Ripamonti U. Periodontal tissue regeneration by recombinant human transforming growth factor-beta 3 in *Papio ursinus*. J Periodontal Res 2008;43(1):1–8.

33. Keles GC, Cetinkaya BO, Baris S, et al. Comparison of platelet pellet with or without guided tissue regeneration in the treatment of class II furcation defects in dogs. Clin Oral Investig 2009;13(4):393–400.

34. Carlo Reis EC, Borges AP, Araújo MV, et al. Periodontal regeneration using a bilayered PLGA/calcium phosphate construct. Biomaterials 2011;32:9244–53.

35. Teare JA, Petit JC, Ripamonti U. Synergistic induction of periodontal tissue regeneration by binary application of human osteogenic protein-1 and human transforming growth factor-β3 in Class II furcation defects of *Papio ursinus*. J Periodontal Res 2012;47:336–44.

36. Suaid FF, Ribeiro FV, Gomes TR, et al. Autologous periodontal ligament cells in the treatment of Class III furcation defects: a study in dogs. J Clin Periodontol 2012;39(4):377–84.

37. Kosen Y, Miyaji H, Kato A, et al. Application of collagen hydrogel/sponge scaffold facilitates periodontal wound healing in class II furcation defects in beagle dogs. J Periodontal Res 2012;47(5):626–34.

38. Mardas N, Kraehenmann M, Dard M. Regenerative wound healing in acute degree III mandibular defects in dogs. Quintessence Int 2012;43(5):e48–59.

39. Suaid FF, Carvalho MD, Ambrosano GM, et al. Platelet-rich plasma in the treatment of Class II furcation defects: a histometrical study in dogs. J Appl Oral Sci 2012;20(2):162–9.

40. Stoller NH, Johnson LR, Garrett S. Periodontal regeneration of a class II furcation defect utilizing a bioabsorbable barrier in a human. A case study with histology. J Periodontol 2001;72:238–42.

41. Mellonig JT, Valderrama Mdel P, Cochran DL. Histological and clinical evaluation of recombinant human platelet-derived growth factor combined with beta tricalcium phosphate for the treatment of human Class III furcation defects. Int J Periodontics Restorative Dent 2009;29:169–77.

42. Taheri M, Molla R, Radvar M, et al. An evaluation of bovine derived xenograft with and without a bioabsorbable collagen membrane in the treatment of mandibular Class II furcation defects. Aust Dent J 2009;54:220–7.

43. Palioto DB, Joly JC, deLima AF, et al. Clinical and radiographic treatment evaluation of class III furcation defects using GTR with and without inorganic bone matrix. J Clin Periodontol 2003;30:1–8.
44. Lamb JW 3rd, Greenwell H, Drisko C, et al. A comparison of porous and nonporous Teflon membranes plus demineralized freeze-dried bone allograft in the treatment of Class II buccal/lingual furcation defects: A clinical reentry study. J Periodontol 2001;72:1580–7.
45. Pruthi VK, Gelskey SC, Mirbod SM. Furcation therapy with bioabsorbable collagen membrane: a clinical trial. J Can Dent Assoc 2002;68:610–5.
46. Lekovic V, Camargo PM, Weinlaender M, et al. Effectiveness of a combination of platelet-rich plasma, bovine porous bone mineral and guided tissue regeneration in the treatment of mandibular grade II molar furcations in humans. J Clin Periodontol 2003;30:746–51.
47. Jenabian N, Haghanifar S, Maboudi A, et al. Clinical and radiographic evaluation of Bio-Gen with biocollagen compared with Bio-Gen with connective tissue in the treatment of class II furcation defects: a randomized clinical trial. Appl Oral Sci 2013;21(5):422–9.
48. Kinaia BM, Steiger J, Neely AL, et al. Treatment of Class II molar furcation involvement: meta-analyses of reentry results. J Periodontol 2011;82(3):413–28.
49. Chen TS, Tu YK, Yen CC, et al. A systematic review and meta-analysis of guided tissue regeneration/osseous grafting for the treatment of Class II furcation defects. J Dent Sci 2013;8:209–24.

Can Periimplantitis Be Treated?

Jia-Hui Fu, BDS, MS[a], Hom-Lay Wang, DDS, MSD, PhD[b],*

KEYWORDS

- Periimplantitis • Peri-implant bone loss • Infection • Guided bone regeneration
- Surgery

KEY POINTS

- Periimplantitis can be treated, but the treatment outcome is not always successful or predictable.
- The combination of resective and regenerative surgical techniques seemed to have favorable treatment outcomes in the management of periimplantitis.
- It is best to prevent peri-mucositis, which is the precursor of periimplantitis. This prevention can be achieved by eliminating bacterial plaque through meticulous oral hygiene practices and professional mechanical debridement. In addition, other contributing factors, such as wrong implant position, poor patient selection, and the presence of residual cement or deep probing depths, should be corrected.

INTRODUCTION

Over the past few decades, dental implants have been found to have high predictability and survival rates because of improvements in knowledge and clinical expertise, together with technological advances in implant designs.[1] They are thus integrated into the clinical management of fully or partially edentulous patients. However, having a high implant survival rate is not equivalent to long-term implant success, which is defined as having a functional and esthetic implant restoration with no pain, mobility, and suppuration and no more than 2 mm of radiographic peri-implant bone loss.[2] Also, despite the high early survival rates, dental implants do have their fair share of long-term esthetic, biological, and mechanical complications. The incidence of esthetic complications might have reduced because of the recent introduction of zirconia,

Disclaimer: The authors do not have any financial interests, either directly or indirectly, in the products or information listed in the paper.

[a] Discipline of Periodontics, Faculty of Dentistry, National University of Singapore, 11 Lower Kent Ridge Road, Singapore 119083, Singapore; [b] Department of Periodontics and Oral Medicine, University of Michigan, School of Dentistry, 1011 North University Avenue, Ann Arbor, MI 48109-1078, USA
* Corresponding author.
E-mail address: homlay@umich.edu

but the incidence of biological and mechanical complications remained high.[1] Therefore, this paper aims to review the current evidence on the management of peri-implant diseases in an attempt to answer the following question: Can periimplantitis be treated?

Definition

Peri-implant diseases, which are infectious inflammatory diseases of the peri-implant tissues,[3] can be broadly categorized into peri-implant mucositis and periimplantitis. In sites with peri-implant mucositis, the inflammatory lesion is found to be limited to the peri-implant soft tissues with no evidence of progressive peri-implant bone loss beyond the initial physiologic bone remodeling that occurred following implant placement (**Fig. 1**).[4] Sites with periimplantitis, on the other hand, exhibit progressive peri-implant bone loss following the initial physiologic bone remodeling that occurred after implant placement as the inflammatory lesion progresses in both the mucosa and bone (**Fig. 2**).[4] As the discriminating feature is progressive bone loss beyond physiologic bone remodeling, it is, thus, important to establish baseline peri-implant bone levels, which is recommended to best occur at the time of prosthesis installation.[5] Changes in bone levels from the time of implant placement to prosthesis installation are considered the result of physiologic bone remodeling or early implant failure.[6] Therefore, it is challenging to determine the baseline peri-implant bone levels for immediately loaded implants, as time is not allowed for physiologic bone remodeling.

Diagnosis

Based on the abovementioned definitions, peri-implant mucositis is diagnosed by the presence of bleeding on probing, which is a key clinical parameter that indicates gingival inflammation. In addition, the presence of suppuration and/or increase in probing pocket depth (eg, ≥ 4 mm) are also used to detect peri-implant mucositis.[4] Periimplantitis often presents with similar clinical signs as peri-implant mucositis but with progressive bone loss as the main feature that distinguishes periimplantitis from peri-implant mucositis. Baseline and follow-up radiographs are needed to detect changes in peri-implant bone levels over time, however, these are only useful for assessing the interproximal regions. Changes in buccal or lingual bone levels can be determined by probing depths or recession of the peri-implant mucosa resulting in exposure of the implant threads. When the baseline peri-implant bone levels cannot be accurately determined, for example, in immediately loaded implants or when baseline radiographs are not taken, it is recommended to consider 2-mm vertical bone loss from the expected bone level as a threshold for the diagnosis of periimplantitis.[7] In

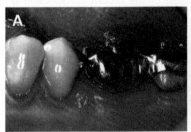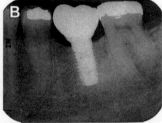

Fig. 1. (*A*) Clinical presentation of peri-implant mucositis at mandibular left first molar. Probing depth of 3 mm with bleeding on probing detected. (*B*) Radiographic presentation of peri-implant mucositis at mandibular left first molar with no evidence of progressive bone loss.

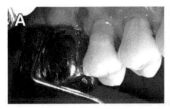
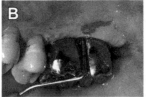
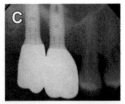

Fig. 2. Clinical presentation of periimplantitis at maxillary right first and second molars. Probing depth of 9 mm with bleeding on probing detected. (*A*) Buccal view. (*B*) Palatal view. (*C*) Radiographic presentation of periimplantitis at maxillary right first and second molars with progressive radiographic bone loss.

addition, marginal peri-implant bone loss of more than 0.44 mm per year has been suggested to be an indication of progressive bone loss.[8] Clinical detection of mobility of the implant fixture signifies failure of the implant restoration, which is the end point of peri-implant diseases.

Classification

A newly proposed classification schema for periimplantitis has attempted to categorize periimplantitis into early, moderate, and advanced based on the percentage of bone loss, which is differentiated as less than 25%, 25% to 50%, and greater than 50% of the implant length[9] (**Fig. 3**) and the probing depth of 4 mm or greater, 6 mm or greater, and 8 mm or greater with the presence of bleeding or suppuration on probing, respectively.[10] This classification hopes to provide a standardized method for clinicians and researchers to better share information relevant to the management of periimplantitis.[9] Considering different defect configurations, several investigators have endeavored to categorize the pattern of peri-implant bone loss. In a human and dog comparative model, peri-implant bone defects were divided into well-defined intrabony defects (class Ia–e) and horizontal bone loss (class II). Circumferential bone loss with buccal and lingual dehiscences was the most common defect configuration.[11] Another classification system described the radiographic presentation of peri-implant bone loss as 5 main types, namely, saucer-shaped, wedge-shaped, flat, undercut, and slitlike defects. It was found that the saucer-shaped

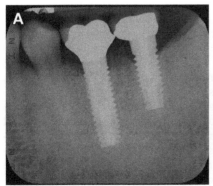
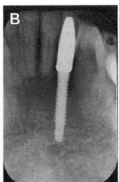
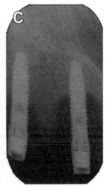

Fig. 3. Radiographic presentation of varying degrees of periimplantitis. (*A*) Early (<25% bone loss). (*B*) Moderate (25%–50% bone loss). (*C*) Advanced (>50% bone loss).

defects were the most common.[12] This finding is important because the defect config-uration may impact the chosen treatment approach.

Epidemiology

Epidemiologic studies on peri-implant diseases often report varying prevalence rates because of the distinct differences in the disease case definitions, sample size, sample population, and follow-up periods.[4,13] In particular, the different case definitions resulted only in an average agreement (52%) among examiners.[14] **Table 1** clearly demonstrates the wide variation in the prevalence of peri-implant mucositis and peri-implantitis from epidemiologic studies published from 2011 to 2015. In attempt to reduce the effects of confounders, the 11th European Workshop on Periodontology recently published a meta-analysis of the current epidemiology of peri-implant diseases.[13] An estimated weighted mean prevalence of 43% (range: 19%–65%) for peri-implant mucositis was reported in a European, South American, and North American sample population consisting of 4209 implants in 1196 patients.[15] For periimplantitis, it was 22% (range: 1%–47%) in a similar ethnic sample population of 8893 implants in 2131 patients.[15] These values seemed to concur with those reported by the American Academy of Periodontology.[4]

Goals of Treatment

The progression of peri-implant diseases is assumed to be similar to that of periodontal diseases, whereby healthy peri-implant mucosa under persistent inflammatory challenge can transform into peri-implant mucositis and eventually periimplantitis.[13] Therefore, the primary goal of the management of peri-implant disease is clearly to eradicate the inflammatory lesions so that healthy and stable peri-implant tissues can be achieved in the long-term.[16] The secondary goals are the elimination of potential contributing factors to prevent recurrence of disease and the reestablishment of function and esthetics, so that long-term clinical success can be acheived.[6]

CONTROL OF CONTRIBUTING FACTORS

Several contributing factors that were thought to facilitate the initiation and progression of peri-implant disease have been identified, and they can be broadly categorized into patient- and implant-related factors (**Table 2**).[4,6]

Patient-Related Factors

Smoking
Numerous studies have demonstrated that smoking is associated with increased implant failure rates and periimplantitis,[5,17–20] with an odds ratio of 3.6 to 4.6.[21] This finding may be attributed to the increased levels of inflammatory cytokines in the peri-implant crevicular fluids in smokers compared with nonsmokers,[22] thus leading to an increased rate of peri-implant bone loss of 0.164 mm per year[23] and compromised midfacial and interproximal soft tissue remodeling[22,24] adversely affecting the long-term functional and esthetic stability of the implant restoration. Some recent studies showed that smoking did not exert a significant effect on the risk of periimplantitis.[25–27] A recent patient-based meta-analysis reported that smoking had no significant effect on the risk of periimplantitis (risk ratio of 1.7). However, an implant-based analysis showed that smoking significantly increased the risk of periimplantitis (risk ratio of 2.1).[28] The conflicting results might be caused by heterogeneous case definitions for smoking and periimplantitis, small study sample sizes, and inferior patient

compliance to regular periodontal maintenance.[19,27,28] Future studies in this area are required.

Periodontal status

Longitudinal studies,[29,30] systematic reviews,[5,31–33] and meta-analyses[34–36] have stressed that the history of treated periodontitis is a major risk factor in the development of periimplantitis leading to implant loss. Patients with compromised periodontal status were more susceptible to peri-implant diseases compared with periodontally healthy patients with an odds ratio of 3.1 to 4.7[21] and a risk ratio of 2.17.[37] A recent systematic review reported that plaque accumulation around the implant restoration initiates the development of peri-implant mucositis,[38] presaging periimplantitis.[39] Patients with poor plaque control were associated with an increased risk of periimplantitis (odds ratio of 14.1).[40] Those with a full-mouth plaque score of less than 25% had only 5% of their implants with periimplantitis compared with 23% in patients with a full-mouth plaque score of 25% or greater.[27] Patients with residual probing depths and noncompliance to a strict periodontal maintenance program are at risk of developing peri-implant diseases, with a lower 10-year implant survival rate of 92.1%[41] and approximately 3-times greater marginal peri-implant bone loss over time.[41,42] In contrast, patients who adhered to a periodontal maintenance program had a 2.5-times lower risk of periimplantitis.[39] Therefore, the value of good periodontal health before implant placement and after prosthetic installation is paramount to long-term implant success; this can be achieved by stringent periodontal maintenance.[30,43,44]

Implant-Related Factors

Implant position

In order to achieve a stable functional and esthetic restoration for the long-term, the dental implant has to be placed in a prosthetically driven position. This position will ensure that the restoration has an appropriate emergence profile and occlusal loading so that maintenance of healthy peri-implant tissues is feasible. In addition, implant placement is governed by rules so that adjacent anatomic tissues are not violated.[45,46] Mesiodistally, there should be at least 1.5 mm of space between implant and adjacent teeth. This dimension may be increased to 3 mm in the posterior region in order to accommodate the emergence profile of the restoration. It is recommended that at least 3 mm of space be kept between 2 implants. These dimensions allow for proper bone remodeling and osseointegration with minimal risk of damage to adjacent teeth or implant. Buccolingually, the implant shoulder should be about 1.5 to 2.0 mm palatal to the buccal plate to compensate for buccal bone remodeling[47] and to provide support for the overlying soft tissue. Implants that are buccally placed have a 3-times greater risk of esthetic complications, such as midfacial mucosal recession.[48] In general, the implant platform should be placed 2 mm below the expected cementoenamel junction or the midfacial gingival margin.[45] However, in the esthetic zone, it may be prudent to place the implant shoulder 0.5 to 1.0 mm subcrestal[47] so that a proper emergence profile can be achieved. Recent literature also found that subcrestal placement of the microgap[49,50] and the presence of a platform switch[51,52] aid in the preservation of the marginal bone level and, therefore, can be a useful feature in the anterior region where the implant can be placed slightly subcrestal. If the implant is placed too shallow, esthetic complications, such as poor contours of the restoration and visible metal margins, may ensue. Also, any physiologic bone and soft tissue remodeling may result in exposure of the implant threads to the oral environment,[53] leading to increased plaque accumulation and subsequent peri-implant bone and soft tissue loss. If the implant is placed too deep, the peri-implant sulcular depth will increase,

Table 1
Prevalence of peri-implant mucositis and periimplantitis from epidemiologic studies published from 2011 to 2015

Authors/Year	Study Population	Implant System	Number of Subjects/Implants	Mean Follow-up Period (y)	Case Definition		Percentage of Peri-Implant Mucositis (Subjects/Implants [%])	Percentage of Periimplantitis (Subjects/Implants [%])
					Peri-Implant Mucositis	Periimplantitis		
Rinke et al,[119] 2011	German	Ankylos	89/Estimated 347	5.7 Range: 2–11.3	BOP and PPD ≥4 mm	BOP and PPD ≥4 mm with BL ≥3.5 mm	44.9/—	11.2/—
Cho-Yan Lee et al,[42] 2012	Australian	Straumann	60/117	8 Range: 5–14	—	BOP and PPD ≥5 mm with BL >2–3 mm	—	16.7/13.1
Mir-Mari et al,[120] 2012	Spanish	Brånemark TiUnite Osseotite	245/964	6.3 Range: 1–18	BL <2 threads with BOP	BL ≥2 threads with BOP or suppuration	38.8/21.6	16.3/9.1
Casado et al,[121] 2013	Brazilian	—	103/392	Range: 1–5	BOP and/or gingival inflammation with no BL	BOP and gingival inflammation, implant mobility, suppuration with BL	19.4/24.7	30.1/43.6

Marrone et al,[122] 2013	Belgian	Steri-Oss Nobel Replace Straumann Frialit 2 Ankylos IMZ Zimmer TSV	103/266	8.5 Range: 5–18	BOP with no PPD >5 mm and no BL or BL ≤2 mm	31/38	BL >2 mm with BOP and PPD >5 mm	37/23
Daubert et al,[123] 2014	North American	Brånemark Straumann Nobel Biocare Steri-Oss Centerpulse Astra Tech Sulzer	96/225	10.9	BOP and/or gingival inflammation with no BL	48/33	BOP and/or suppuration with 2 mm of BL and PPD ≥4 mm	26/13
Aguirre-Zorzano et al,[27] 2014	Spanish	Astra Tech Nobel Replace	239/786	5.3	BOP with no BL	24.7/12.8	BOP and/or suppuration and BL >1.5 mm	15.1/9.8

Abbreviations: BL, bone loss; BOP, bleeding on probing; PPD, probing pocket depth; TSV, tapered screw vent.
Data from Refs.[27,42,119–123]

Table 2	
Risk factors of peri-implant diseases	
Patient-Related Factors	**Implant-Related Factors**
• Smoking	• Implant position
• History of periodontitis	• Residual cement
• Lack of regular periodontal maintenance	• Implant surface
• Poor plaque control	• Poor emergence profile
	• Occlusal overloading

Data from Rosen P, Clem D, Cochran D, et al. Peri-implant mucositis and peri-implantitis: a current understanding of their diagnoses and clinical implications. J Periodontol 2013;84(4):436–43; and Padial-Molina M, Suarez F, Rios HF, et al. Guidelines for the diagnosis and treatment of peri-implant diseases. Int J Periodontics Restorative Dent 2014;34(6):e102–11.

thus favoring the growth of anaerobic microbiota,[54] which will facilitate peri-implant tissue breakdown.[53]

Prosthetic considerations

Although peri-implant tissue response around screw-retained restorations seems to be more favorable compared with that around cement-retained restorations,[55] a recent systematic review and meta-analysis[56] found no difference in peri-implant marginal bone loss around cement- and screw-retained implant restorations. Studies have shown that, in the presence of excess cement at the crown-abutment interface, peri-implant mucosal inflammation or bone loss occurs 80% to 85% of the time.[57–59] The use of certain cement, for example, methacrylate-based cement, is associated with increased residual cement and consequently a higher prevalence for peri-implant diseases[57,60] because they are less viscous[60] and also more susceptible to bacterial invasion.[61] In contrast, zinc oxide eugenol–containing cements are more viscous, thus, easier to remove and can inhibit biofilm growth at the crown-abutment interface.[62] Customized abutments that bring the restorative margins coronally or screw-retained restorations may be considered[57] if the restorative margins are located more subgingivally,[63] as it is technically more challenging to remove excess cement around such restorations.

The ability to clean around the implant restoration plays a role in the development of peri-implant diseases. A poor emergence profile impedes proper plaque control and, thus, expedites the progression of peri-implant diseases. A clinical trial demonstrated a 12-times reduction in prevalence of peri-implants in patients who were able to effectively clean their implant restorations (4%) as compared with those who could not maintain good plaque control (48%).[64]

Bone formation can result from mild occlusal overloading of 1500 to 3000 microstrain. When the strain in bone exceeds 3000 microstrain, bone resorption occurs.[65,66] However, most studies have not measured or defined the amount of occlusal overload on implant restorations. It is thought that bacterial plaque is the main causative factor of peri-implant bone loss. However, a recent case report demonstrated that occlusal overloading in the absence of peri-implant mucosal inflammation resulted in bone loss along the implant surface without affecting marginal bone levels. In addition, reosseointegration occurred after removal of the heavy occlusal forces.[67] Therefore, it might be possible to have peri-implant bone loss along the implant surface and not on the crestal region in the absence of mucosal inflammation. On the other hand, if there is peri-implant mucosal inflammation, marginal bone loss will ensue.[68,69] More clinical trials are needed to investigate the effect of occlusal overloading on dental implants as current systematic reviews showed limited and conflicting results.[68,70,71]

THERAPEUTIC OPTIONS AND THEIR CLINICAL OUTCOMES

Similar to the treatment of periodontal diseases, the management of periimplantitis can be categorized into nonsurgical and surgical interventions (**Table 3**). Frequently, the nonsurgical interventions, also known as antiinfective measures, are also used in combination with surgical interventions to eliminate biofilm on the implant and restore peri-implant tissue health. An ideal treatment outcome will include a shallow probing sulcular depth of less than 5 mm with no bleeding on probing and stable peri-implant bone and soft tissue levels. Alternative treatment outcomes that are reported in the literature include implant loss, persistent or recurrent periimplantitis, changes in bleeding on probing, and diminished peri-implant mucosal level and marginal bone level.[72] Various therapeutic options used in the management of peri-implant diseases are discussed next.

Nonsurgical Interventions

Antiinfective measures
Mechanical debridement Bacterial challenge within the peri-implant tissues is the main cause of peri-implant diseases. Therefore, the main aim of mechanical debridement is the restitution of peri-implant tissue health with the removal of peri-implant biofilm from the implant and/or abutment surface.[73] This procedure can be achieved by using specific instruments that are softer than titanium to avoid damage to the implant and abutment surfaces, which would otherwise promote bacterial colonization. These instruments can be coated with titanium, carbon fiber, polytetrafluoroethylene, plastic, polyetheretherketone, or silicon. Ultrasonic tips or polishing cups coated with carbon fiber or plastic ultrasonic and/or air abrasive systems that use low abrasive amino acid glycine powder are also useful.[74] In general, instruments that are softer than the implant fixture are recommended for mechanical debridement to minimize damage to the implant surface.[75] However, as these instruments have often been found to be ineffective,[76] the use of stainless steel curettes and an air-powder abrasive system are advocated for the debridement of rough implant surfaces, as any resultant implant surface modification will not increase the susceptibility of the surfaces to bacterial adhesion.[77] The effectiveness of mechanical debridement in recent randomized clinical trials is summarized in **Table 4**.

Chemotherapeutics Chemotherapeutics can be used adjunctively to mechanical debridement. They can be categorized into antiseptics, which are germicides used on skin or living tissues to inhibit or destroy microorganisms, and antibiotics, which can inhibit or kill selective bacteria by affecting their metabolic processes.[78] In both cases, the aim is to eliminate invasive pathogens and prevent recolonization of these pathogens in the peri-implant tissues so that long-term peri-implant health is sustained.[74,79] The main types of antiseptics used are topically applied essential oils,

Table 3 Therapeutic approaches	
Nonsurgical	**Surgical**
Disinfective Interventions	• Access flap
• Mechanical debridement	• Resective
• Chemotherapeutics	• Regenerative
• Lasers	

Table 4
Evaluation of the effectiveness of mechanical debridement on the management of peri-implant diseases based on randomized clinical trials in the past 5 years (2011–2015)

Authors/Year	Sample Size	Case Definition	Intervention	Follow-up (mo)	Results	Conclusion
Sahm et al,[124] 2011	30 Patients with 41 implants	PPD ≥4 mm with BOP and suppuration and radiographic BL ≤30%	Nonsurgical therapy Amino acid glycine powder vs carbon curettes with 0.1% chlorhexidine irrigation	6	NSSD between the 2 groups • Mean plaque index: 0.1 (air polishing) vs 0.2 (curette) • PPD reduction: 0.6 mm (air polishing) vs 0.5 mm (curette) • Mucosal recession: −0.2 mm (air polishing) vs 0.0 mm (curette) • CAL: 0.4 mm (air polishing) vs 0.5 mm (curette) SSD between the 2 groups: • BOP reduction: 43.5% (air polishing) vs 11.0% (curette)	Between air polishing and debridement with curettes, SSD for BOP only
John et al,[125] 2015	25 Patients with 36 implants	PPD ≥4 mm with BOP and suppuration and radiographic BL ≤30%	Nonsurgical therapy Air-powder mixture polishing vs carbon curettes with 0.1% chlorhexidine irrigation	12	NSSD between the 2 groups • Mean plaque index: −0.6 (air polishing) vs 0.3 (curette) • PPD reduction: 0.5 mm (air polishing) vs 0.4 mm (curette) • Mucosal recession: 0.1 mm (air polishing) vs 0.1 mm (curette) • CAL: 0.6 mm (air polishing) vs 0.5 mm (curette) SSD between the 2 groups: • BOP reduction: 41.2% (air polishing) vs 16.6% (curette)	

Abbreviations: BL, bone loss; BOP, bleeding on probing; CAL, clinical attachment loss; NSSD, no statistical significant difference; PPD, probing pocket depth; SSD, statistical significant difference.

Data from Sahm N, Becker J, Santel T, et al. Non-surgical treatment of peri-implantitis using an air-abrasive device or mechanical debridement and local application of chlorhexidine: a prospective, randomized, controlled clinical study. J Clin Periodontol 2011;38(9):872–8; and John G, Sahm N, Becker J, et al. Nonsurgical treatment of peri-implantitis using an air-abrasive device or mechanical debridement and local application of chlorhexidine. Twelve-month follow-up of a prospective, randomized, controlled clinical study. Clin Oral Investig 2015. [Epub ahead of print].

triclosan, and chlorhexidine. Antibiotics can be delivered either locally or systemically. Locally delivered antibiotics are typically minocycline microspheres or doxycycline hyclate gel. Systemic antibiotics are typically from the penicillin, erythromycin, or tetracycline classes. Other agents that have been used in implant surface decontamination are saline, citric acid, and hydrogen peroxide.[80] The effectiveness of these agents in recent randomized clinical trials is summarized in **Table 5**.

Lasers The use of lasers in dentistry has gained popularity in recent years. The commonly used lasers for the decontamination of the implant surface are Nd:YAG (2940 nm), erbium:yttrium-aluminium-garnet (Er:YAG) (2940 nm), diode (660 nm), and carbon dioxide (10600 nm) lasers. Both the Nd:YAG and Er:YAG lasers have high bactericidal potential on implant surfaces at low-energy density,[81,82] but there may be some titanium surface alterations if the power settings for the Er:YAG laser are greater than 300 mJ/10 Hz.[83] Thus, it is recommended to use 100 mJ/10 Hz for not more than 2 minutes to decontaminate the implant surface safely.[84] It was reported that ablation of the titanium surface occurs easily regardless of the power settings for the Nd:YAG laser.[85] In addition, the Nd:YAG, diode, and carbon dioxide lasers are less effective in removing calculus compared with the Er:YAG laser.[86–88] A recent case report demonstrated that the Er:YAG laser could remove the bacterial-contaminated titanium oxide layer, thus promoting reosseointegration and healthy soft tissue adaptation around a failing implant.[89] Consequently, the Er:YAG laser seems to be the laser of choice in the management of peri-implant disease.

The laser-assisted periimplantitis protocol is a variation of the laser-assisted new attachment protocol. In this technique, the Nd:YAG laser is used to remove inflamed peri-implant tissues and decontaminate the implant surface during mechanical debridement.[10] However, this application is still in its infancy as no clinical trial has been reported.

Photodynamic therapy involves the use of a specific wavelength of light (630–700 nm) to activate photosensitive dyes that are placed at the site of interest, for example, periodontal pockets. The activation of these dyes, such as toluidine blue O, causes the release of oxygen radicals that will decimate periodontal pathogens.[90] The effectiveness of lasers and photodynamic therapy in recent randomized clinical trials is summarized in **Table 6**.

Summary Nonsurgical interventions, such as mechanical debridement with good oral hygiene practices, are effective in reducing bleeding on probing and mucosal inflammation in peri-implant mucositis.[73,91] The use of a powered toothbrush and adjunctive use of chemotherapeutics or lasers required further validation.[91] Also, as there is no one superior reagent or methodology,[80] additional well-designed randomized clinical trials are needed to validate the effectiveness of various methodologies used in the surface decontamination of dental implants.[80]

Surgical Interventions

Nonsurgical treatment of periimplantitis shows limited improvement in clinical parameters with no particular treatment having superior performance than mechanical debridement alone.[92] It is, thus, ineffective in arresting disease progression, achieving disease resolution, and preventing disease recurrence.[74] Therefore, similar to the treatment of chronic periodontitis, surgical interventions are needed to gain access to the peri-implant defect in an attempt to debride the implant surface and promote reosseointegration or soft tissue reattachment.[74]

Table 5
Evaluation of the effectiveness of chemotherapeutics on the management of peri-implant diseases based on randomized clinical trials in the past 5 years (2011–2015)

Authors/Year	Sample Size	Case Definition	Intervention	Follow-up (mo)	Results	Conclusion
Heitz-Mayfield et al,[73] 2011	29 Patients with 29 implants	BOP with no BL	Nonsurgical therapy with curettes 0.5% Chlorhexidine gel vs placebo gel for brushing	3	NSSD between the 2 groups • BOP reduction • PPD reduction • Total DNA count	It seemed that the use of chlorhexidine had no significant influence on clinical and radiographic outcomes, but there was reported better suppression of anaerobic bacteria.
Machtei et al,[126] 2012	60 Patients with 77 implants	PPD 6–10 mm with BOP and radiographic BL	Nonsurgical therapy Chlorhexidine chip vs cross-linked gelatin matrix chip	6	NSSD between the 2 groups • BOP reduction: 57.5% (chlorhexidine) vs 45.5% (matrix) • PPD reduction: 2.13 mm (chlorhexidine) vs 1.73 mm (matrix) • Change in CAL: 2.18 mm (chlorhexidine) vs 1.69 mm (matrix)	
Hallström et al,[133] 2012	43 Patients with 43 implants	PPD ≥5 mm with BOP and/or suppuration	Nonsurgical therapy with titanium curettes and rubber cups with polishing paste With or without systemic azithromycin	6	NSSD between the 2 groups • PPD reduction • BOP reduction • Bacterial count	
de Waal et al,[127] 2013	30 Patients with 79 implants	PPD ≥5 mm with BOP and/or suppuration and radiographic BL ≥2 mm	Surgical therapy with bone recontouring, debridement with curettes, and decontamination with saline-soaked gauze 0.12% Chlorhexidine with 0.05% cetylpyridinium chloride irrigation vs a placebo solution irrigation	12	NSSD between the 2 groups: • Bacteria cultured on implant surface • Plaque: 38.7 (chlorhexidine) vs 50 (placebo) • BOP: 96.8% (chlorhexidine) vs 94.7% (placebo) • Suppuration on probing: 29% (chlorhexidine) vs 15.8% (placebo)	

| de Waal et al,[134] 2014 | 44 Patients with 108 implants | PPD ≥5 mm with BOP and/or suppuration and radiographic BL ≥2 mm | Surgical therapy with bone recontouring, debridement with curettes, and decontamination with saline-soaked gauze 0.12% Chlorhexidine with 0.05% cetylpyridinium chloride irrigation vs 2% chlorhexidine irrigation | 12 | NSSD between the 2 groups:
• Bacteria cultured on implant surface
• Plaque: 37.0 (0.12% chlorhexidine) vs 31.2 (2% chlorhexidine)
• BOP: 68.5% (0.12% chlorhexidine) vs 77.1% (2% chlorhexidine)
• Suppuration on probing: 1.9% (0.12% chlorhexidine) vs 10.4% (2% chlorhexidine)
• PPD: 2.9 mm (0.12% chlorhexidine) vs 3.0 mm (2% chlorhexidine)
• BL: 4.1 mm (0.12% chlorhexidine) vs 4.3 mm (2% chlorhexidine)
SSD between the 2 groups
• For mean reduction of bacterial load on implant surface: 3.37 (0.12% chlorhexidine) vs 3.65 (2% chlorhexidine) |

(partial row, top):
• PPD: 4.3 mm (chlorhexidine) vs 3.7 mm (placebo)
• BL: 5.0 mm (chlorhexidine) vs 3.9 mm (placebo)
SSD between the 2 groups
• For mean reduction of bacterial load on implant surface: 4.21 (chlorhexidine) vs 2.77 (placebo)

Abbreviations: BL, bone loss; BOP, bleeding on probing; CAL, clinical attachment loss; NSSD, no statistical significant difference; PPD, probing pocket depth; SSD, statistical significant difference.
Data from Refs.[73,126,127]

Table 6
Evaluation of the effectiveness of lasers on the management of peri-implant diseases based on randomized clinical trials in the past 5 years (2011–2015)

Authors/Year	Sample Size	Case Definition	Intervention	Follow-up (mo)	Results	Conclusion
Persson et al,[128] 2011	42 Patients with 100 implants	PPD ≥5 mm with BOP at ≥1 peri-implant site with radiographic BL of ≥2 mm	Nonsurgical therapy Glycine-based powder air polishing vs Er:YAG laser	6	NSSD between the 2 groups • PPD reduction: 0.9 mm (Er:YAG) vs 0.8 mm (air polishing) • For bone level • For bacterial counts	The use of lasers did not seem to have any additional benefits on clinical or radiographic outcomes.
Renvert et al,[135] 2011	42 Patients with 100 implants	PPD ≥5 mm with BOP with radiographic BL of >3 mm	Nonsurgical therapy Hydrophobic powder air polishing vs Er:YAG laser	6	NSSD between the 2 groups • BOP reduction • Visible plaque • Presence of suppuration • PPD reduction: 0.8 mm (Er:YAG) vs 0.9 mm (air polishing) • BL: 0.3 mm (Er:YAG) vs 0.1 mm (air polishing)	
Schwarz et al,[129] 2011	32 Patients with 35 implants	PPD >6 mm with intrabony bone defect of >3 mm and supracrestal defect of >1 mm	Surgical therapy Access flap with implantoplasty and guided bone regeneration and decontamination with plastic curettes Cotton pellets and sterile saline vs Er:YAG laser	6	NSSD between the 2 groups • BOP reduction: 47.8% (Er:YAG) vs 55.0% (CPS) • CAL: 1.5 mm (Er:YAG) vs 2.2 mm (CPS)	
Schwarz et al,[102] 2012	24 Patients with 24 implants	PPD >6 mm with intrabony bone defect of >3 mm and supracrestal defect of >1 mm	Surgical therapy Access flap with implantoplasty and guided bone regeneration and decontamination with plastic curettes Cotton pellets and sterile saline vs Er:YAG laser	24	NSSD between the 2 groups • BOP reduction: 75.0% (Er:YAG) vs 54.9% (CPS) • CAL: 1.0 mm (Er:YAG) vs 1.2 mm (CPS)	

Study	Patients/implants	Inclusion criteria	Treatment	Duration (mo)	Results
Schwarz et al,[130] 2013	21 Patients with 21 implants	PPD >6 mm with intrabony bone defect of >3 mm and supracrestal defect of >1 mm	Surgical therapy Access flap with implantoplasty and guided bone regeneration and decontamination with plastic curettes Cotton pellets and sterile saline vs Er:YAG laser	48	NSSD between the 2 groups • BOP reduction: 47.8% (Er:YAG) vs 55.0% (CPS) • CAL: 1.5 mm (Er:YAG) vs 2.2 mm (CPS)
Schär et al,[131] 2013	40 Patients with 40 implants	PPD 4–6 mm with BOP at ≥1 peri-implant site with radiographic BL of 0.5–2.0 mm	Nonsurgical therapy Mechanical debridement with titanium curettes and glycine-based powder air polishing and Adjunctive PDT vs adjunctive minocycline hydrochloride microspheres	6	NSSD between the 2 groups • BOP reduction: 50% (MD) vs 40% (PDT) • PPD reduction: 0.49 mm (MD) vs 0.36 mm (PDT) • CAL: 2.53 mm (MD) vs 2.50 mm (PDT) • Mucosal recession: 1.38 mm (MD) vs 1.33 mm (PDT) SSD: no bacterial plaque found in the PDT group • Complete resolution of mucosal inflammation: 15% (MD) vs 30% (PDT)
Bassetti et al,[132] 2014	40 Patients with 40 implants	PPD 4–6 mm with BOP at ≥1 peri-implant site and radiographic BL of 0.5–2.0 mm	Nonsurgical therapy Mechanical debridement with titanium curettes and glycine-based powder air polishing and Adjunctive PDT vs adjunctive minocycline hydrochloride microspheres	12	NSSD between the 2 groups • BOP reduction: 65% (MD) vs 57% (PDT) • PPD reduction: 0.56 mm (MD) vs 0.11 mm (PDT) • CAL: 2.41 mm (MD) vs 2.58 mm (PDT) • Mucosal recession: 1.41 mm (MD) vs 1.50 mm (PDT) • Modified plaque index: 0.00 (MD) vs 0.01 (PDT) • For bacterial counts • For IL-1b, MMP-1, and MMP-8 • Complete resolution of mucosal inflammation: 35.0% (MD) vs 36.1% (PDT)

(continued on next page)

Table 6
(continued)

Authors/Year	Sample Size	Case Definition	Intervention	Follow-up (mo)	Results	Conclusion
Papadopoulos et al,[136] 2015	16 Patients with 16 implants	PPD ≥6 mm with BOP or suppuration and radiographic BL of ≥2 mm	Surgical therapy with mechanical debridement using plastic curettes and decontamination with saline-soaked sterile gauze With vs without diode laser	6	NSSD between the 2 groups • CAL: 4.77 mm (no laser) vs 4.46 mm (laser) • BOP: 31.3% (no laser) vs 23.8% (laser) • PPD reduction: 4.31 mm (no laser) vs 4.44 mm (laser) • Plaque index: 20.8 (no laser) vs 7.1 (laser)	

Abbreviations: BL, bone loss; BOP, bleeding on probing; IL, interleukin; MD, mechanical debridement with air polishing; NSSD, no statistical significant difference; PDT, photodynamic therapy; PPD, probing pocket depth; SSD, statistical significant difference.
Data from Refs.[102,128–132]

Access flap

The objective of the access flap is to gain contact to the supracrestal but submucosal implant surface for debridement and decontamination (**Fig. 4**). Debridement can be achieved with the use of curettes, ultrasonic tips, and air abrasive systems. A recent multicentered clinical trial evaluated the effectiveness of an antiinfective protocol in the management of periimplantitis defects. The protocol involved elevation of full-thickness mucoperiosteal flaps at the implants with periimplantitis, debridement of the implant surface with titanium coated or carbon fiber curettes, and decontamination using copious sterile saline irrigation and rubbing the implant surface with saline-soaked sterile gauze before replacing and suturing the flap. Patients were also given postoperative antimicrobial and antiseptic mouth rinses. The results of this trial demonstrated reduction in probing depths, bleeding on probing, and suppuration on probing from baseline to 1 year after surgery. Bone levels were stable, but there was significant facial mucosal recession of 1 mm. Therefore, the investigators concluded that periimplantitis could be successfully managed with this specific anti-infective protocol.[93] The advantage of this protocol is that it is straightforward, safe, and economical and yet delivered sustainable clinical outcomes.

Resective and regenerative

Treatment of teeth with horizontal bone loss and deep probing depths involves an access flap or apically positioned flap with osseous bone recontouring to achieve a biologically compatible and maintainable periodontal architecture.[94] Likewise for the management of periimplantitis defects with horizontal bone loss and deep probing depths, which are categorized as class II defects,[11] an apically positioned flap with osseous recontouring is a treatment option. However, in order to facilitate optimal plaque control around the exposed roughened implant surface, implantoplasty is recommended. Implantoplasty is a resective procedure that involves the smoothening of the roughened implant surface or threads with a high-speed diamond or tungsten carbide bur to create a polished implant surface that is not plaque retentive (**Fig. 5**).[95] A 3-year

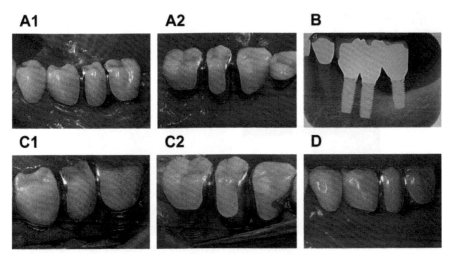

Fig. 4. Clinical case illustrating access flap surgery at mandibular left second premolar, first molar, and second molar. (*A*) Clinical presentation with 5- to 10-mm probing depths around the implants: (1) buccal view and (2) lingual view. (*B*) Radiographic presentation. (*C*) Access flap surgery: (1) buccal view and (2) lingual view. (*D*) Clinical presentation at 9 months after surgery with 3 to 4 mm probing depths around the implants.

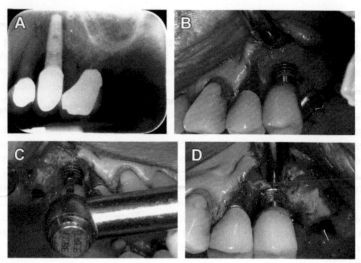

Fig. 5. Clinical case illustrating implantoplasty on implant at maxillary left second premolar. (*A*) Radiographic presentation showing horizontal bone loss around the implant. (*B*) Clinical presentation of the peri-implant defect. (*C*) Smoothening of the exposed implant threads. (*D*) Smoothened implant surface.

clinical trial reported that implants treated with implantoplasty had a higher implant survival rate compared with those that were treated with an apically positioned flap only.[95]

Regenerative surgical techniques have been proposed for the management of the intrabony component of peri-implant defects (**Fig. 6**). Its aim is to regenerate lost

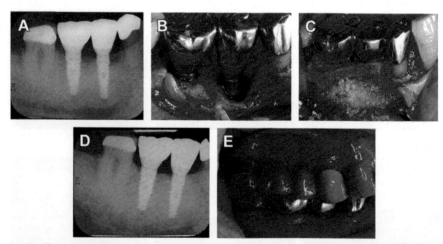

Fig. 6. Clinical case illustrating guided bone regeneration around implants replacing the mandibular right second premolar and first molar. (*A*) Radiographic presentation showing cratering bone loss around the implants. (*B*) Clinical presentation of the peri-implant defects. (*C*) Guided bone regeneration performed around the implants using allogenic cancellous bone and a collagen membrane. (*D*) Radiographic bone fill seen at the 4-year follow-up. (*E*) Clinical presentation at the 4-year follow-up.

peri-implant bone and increase the chance of reosseointegration. Diverse antiinfective methods have been proposed, but no one superior method has been described.[80] Likewise, different grafting materials and barrier membranes have been used.[96–98] A recent clinical trial found that the additional use of a barrier membrane did not improve the clinical outcomes as both groups demonstrated similar bone fill and reductions in probing depth and bleeding on probing.[97] This finding concurred with the reported results from a review on surgical therapy for the management of periimplantitis.[99] Also, the defect configuration may influence the regenerative potential of the site. Defects that were noncontained, such as class Ib, Ie, and II,[11] tend to have lesser probing depth reduction and clinical attachment gain.[100]

Recently, a combination treatment approach comprising implantoplasty (resective) and guided bone regeneration (regenerative) demonstrated favorable clinical outcomes in terms of probing depth reduction, resolution of inflammation, and defect fill.[101–103] Therefore, this approach was suggested in the management of periimplantitis defects with suprabony and intrabony components. Unfortunately there is paucity of current literature comparing the effectiveness of various surgical techniques and grafting materials to treat periimplantitis. In addition, a recent systematic review found that there was only partial bone regeneration in most studies[104]; thus, it is uncertain if guided bone regeneration is superior to other nonsurgical or surgical methods for treating periimplantitis.[105]

Summary Surgical interventions are more effective in the management of periimplantitis compared with nonsurgical interventions.[106] Periimplantitis defects can be managed conservatively with an access flap and an antiinfective protocol.[93,107] Alternatively, regenerative procedures are recommended for periimplantitis defects that have an intrabony component. Through a network meta-analysis, it was found that guided bone regeneration with nonresorbable membranes or resorbable membranes had 3.52 mm and 2.40 mm greater probing depth reduction compared with nonsurgical therapy, respectively.[106] Recent systematic reviews and meta-analyses showed a weighted mean probing depth reduction of 2.97 mm (2.04 mm [33.4%] for surgical resection and 3.16 mm [48.2%] for guided bone regeneration), clinical attachment level gain of 1.65 mm, bleeding on probing reduction of 45.8%, and a weighted mean radiographic bone fill of 2.1 to 2.17 mm for guided bone regeneration.[108,109] It is important to realize that there are several limitations associated with the analyses, such as inclusion of case series and cohort studies, a limited number of high-quality studies available, and vast heterogeneity in the study designs and treatment modalities. Therefore, further validation of the various surgical techniques is necessary.

PROPOSED WORKFLOW

Based on the available evidence and consensus statement,[110] the authors proposed the following workflow for the management of peri-implant diseases (**Fig. 7**) as a guide to clinicians. Similar to conventional periodontal therapy, the management of peri-implant diseases should start with the initial therapy, which involves the identification of disease and elimination or reduction of etiologic and contributing factors. This step is crucial in achieving predictable and stable long-term clinical outcomes. Therefore, in the management of peri-implant diseases, the first step is to determine the nature of the disease and identify, remove, or correct the causative and contributing factors, such as bacterial plaque, smoking, and undesirable prosthetic designs. Subsequently, patients should go through mechanical debridement with or without the adjunctive use of chemotherapeutics or lasers. Evaluation of disease resolution, that is, elimination or

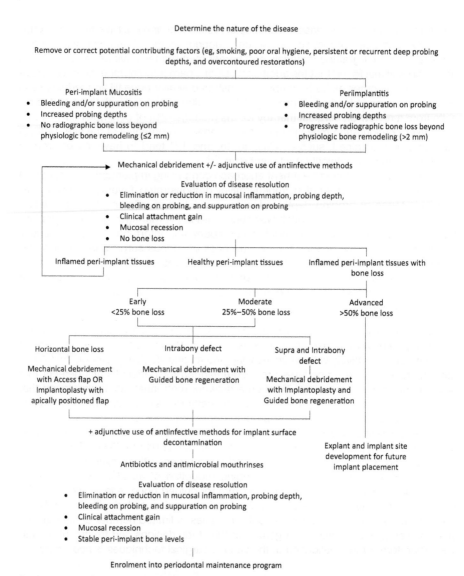

Fig. 7. Proposed treatment workflow for the management of peri-implant diseases. (*From* Heitz-Mayfield LJ, Needleman I, Salvi GE, et al. Consensus statements and clinical recommendations for prevention and management of biologic and technical implant complications. Int J Oral Maxillofac Implants 2014;29(Suppl):346–50; with permission.)

reduction in mucosal inflammation, probing depths, suppuration on probing and bleeding on probing, presence of clinical attachment gain, and/or mucosal recession and no bone loss, should be performed 2 to 4 weeks after therapy.

At sites with periimplantitis, mechanical debridement alone is generally unable to eradicate the disease progression; further surgical interventions are commonly necessary. Clinicians can decide on the surgical intervention based on the degree of peri-implant bone loss. In advanced cases, whereby there is greater than 50%

bone loss or if the implant is mobile, explantation and implant site development with guided bone regeneration for future implant placement is recommended. The rationale is to remove the existing inflammation early and prevent further bone loss, especially in the vertical dimension, so that future prosthetic rehabilitation is possible. At sites with early (<25% bone loss) or moderate (25%–50% bone loss), the defect configuration will aid in the selection of the surgical intervention. When there is horizontal peri-implant bone loss, an access flap or implantoplasty with an apically positioned flap can be performed to debride the exposed implant surfaces and promote soft tissue readhesion. Sites with an intrabony defect can be managed with guided bone regeneration to promote reosseointegration and soft tissue readhesion. Combination defects that have both suprabony and intrabony components can be treated with implantoplasty on the supracrestal exposed implant surface and guided bone regeneration in the intrabony component. This combined approach will facilitate good plaque control and reosseointegration. Surgical interventions are accompanied by postoperative antiinfective approaches that may include antibiotics and/or antimicrobial mouth rinses. Patients are subsequently reviewed for disease resolution, which, in cases of periimplantitis, includes radiographic examination to ensure that there is no further peri-implant bone loss. Consequently, patients who have regained healthy peri-implant tissues will, thus, be enrolled into a strict periodontal maintenance program.

SUMMARY

Systematic reviews and meta-analyses concluded that

- Mechanical plaque control, either professionally or home care, should be the goal in the management of peri-implant mucositis and the prevention of the development of periimplantitis. Therefore, strict adherence to periodontal maintenance is of paramount importance.[91]
- The evidence to support the use of systemic or locally delivered antibiotics in the management of peri-implant diseases is inconclusive.[111]
- The use of locally delivered antibiotics (minocycline or doxycycline hyclate), Er:YAG laser treatment, or submucosal air polishing with glycine powder together with mechanical debridement using curettes show greater reductions in probing depth and bleeding on probing compared with adjunctive submucosal chlorhexidine irrigation.[112]
- The use of lasers for nonsurgical debridement in the management of periimplantitis offered no additional benefits over conventional mechanical debridement with curettes.[113–115]
- There is no single superior antiinfective method available.[80]
- Surgical interventions achieved greater probing depth reduction and clinical attachment gain compared with nonsurgical interventions.[106]
- Access flap surgery shows resolution in only 58% of the lesions.[107]
- The combination of resective and regenerative surgical techniques seemed to have favorable treatment outcomes in the management of periimplantitis.[109]
- Reosseointegration of a previously contaminated implant surface is possible but highly variable and unpredictable.[116]

The question posed for the paper was as follows: Can periimplantitis be treated? Based on the available evidence, the authors have found that periimplantitis could be treated to a certain extent; but the treatment outcome is not always successful or predictable,[116] as indicated by favorable short-term treatment outcomes and further progression or recurrence of the disease.[72] A mean patient-based success rate of 69% was reported, with periodontal access flap surgery being the most frequently performed procedure (47%) compared with regenerative therapy (20%). Also, the success rate was significantly reduced in patients with severe periodontitis, severe marginal bone loss, poor oral hygiene, and low compliance.[117] Therefore, it is best to prevent peri-mucositis, which is the precursor of periimplantitis. This prevention can be achieved by eliminating bacterial plaque through meticulous oral hygiene practices and professional mechanical debridement.[91] In addition, other contributing factors, such as unfavorable implant position, poor patient selection, and presence of residual cement or probing depths, should be eradicated.[13,118] Patients who maintained excellent oral hygiene standards and are enrolled in a strict periodontal maintenance program exhibited stable peri-implant tissues over time.[118]

REFERENCES

1. Pjetursson BE, Asgeirsson AG, Zwahlen M, et al. Improvements in implant dentistry over the last decade: comparison of survival and complication rates in older and newer publications. Int J Oral Maxillofac Implants 2014; 29(Suppl):308–24.
2. Misch CE, Perel ML, Wang HL, et al. Implant success, survival, and failure: the International Congress of Oral Implantologists (ICOI) Pisa Consensus Conference. Implant Dent 2008;17(1):5–15.
3. Lindhe J, Meyle J, Group D of European Workshop on Periodontology. Peri-implant diseases: consensus report of the sixth European Workshop on Periodontology. J Clin Periodontol 2008;35(8 Suppl):282–5.
4. Rosen P, Clem D, Cochran D, et al. Peri-implant mucositis and peri-implantitis: a current understanding of their diagnoses and clinical implications. J Periodontol 2013;84(4):436–43.
5. Heitz-Mayfield LJ. Peri-implant diseases: diagnosis and risk indicators. J Clin Periodontol 2008;35(8 Suppl):292–304.
6. Padial-Molina M, Suarez F, Rios HF, et al. Guidelines for the diagnosis and treatment of peri-implant diseases. Int J Periodontics Restorative Dent 2014;34(6): e102–11.
7. Sanz M, Chapple IL, Working Group 4 of the VIII European Workshop on Periodontology. Clinical research on peri-implant diseases: consensus report of Working Group 4. J Clin Periodontol 2012;39(Suppl 12):202–6.
8. Galindo-Moreno P, Leon-Cano A, Ortega-Oller I, et al. Marginal bone loss as success criterion in implant dentistry: beyond 2 mm. Clin Oral Implants Res 2015;26(4):e28–34.
9. Froum SJ, Rosen PS. A proposed classification for peri-implantitis. Int J Periodontics Restorative Dent 2012;32(5):533–40.
10. Romanos GE, Javed F, Delgado-Ruiz RA, et al. Peri-implant diseases: a review of treatment interventions. Dent Clin North Am 2015;59(1):157–78.
11. Schwarz F, Herten M, Sager M, et al. Comparison of naturally occurring and ligature-induced peri-implantitis bone defects in humans and dogs. Clin Oral Implants Res 2007;18(2):161–70.
12. Zhang L, Geraets W, Zhou Y, et al. A new classification of peri-implant bone morphology: a radiographic study of patients with lower implant-supported mandibular overdentures. Clin Oral Implants Res 2014;25(8):905–9.

13. Jepsen S, Berglundh T, Zitzmann NU, Group 3 of the 11th European Workshop on P. Primary prevention of peri-implantitis: managing peri-implant mucositis. J Clin Periodontol 2015;42(Suppl 16):S152-7.
14. Merli M, Bernardelli F, Giulianelli E, et al. Inter-rater agreement in the diagnosis of mucositis and peri-implantitis. J Clin Periodontol 2014;41(9):927-33.
15. Derks J, Tomasi C. Peri-implant health and disease. A systematic review of current epidemiology. J Clin Periodontol 2015;42(Suppl 16):S158-71.
16. Heitz-Mayfield LJ. Diagnosis and management of peri-implant diseases. Aust Dent J 2008;53(Suppl 1):S43-8.
17. Levin L, Hertzberg R, Har-Nes S, et al. Long-term marginal bone loss around single dental implants affected by current and past smoking habits. Implant Dent 2008;17(4):422-9.
18. Saaby M, Karring E, Schou S, et al. Factors influencing severity of peri-implantitis. Clin Oral Implants Res 2014. [Epub ahead of print].
19. Klokkevold PR, Han TJ. How do smoking, diabetes, and periodontitis affect outcomes of implant treatment? Int J Oral Maxillofac Implants 2007;22(Suppl): 173-202.
20. French D, Larjava H, Ofec R. Retrospective cohort study of 4591 Straumann implants in private practice setting, with up to 10-year follow-up. Part 1: multivariate survival analysis. Clin Oral Implants Res 2014. [Epub ahead of print].
21. Heitz-Mayfield LJ, Huynh-Ba G. History of treated periodontitis and smoking as risks for implant therapy. Int J Oral Maxillofac Implants 2009;24(Suppl): 39-68.
22. Tatli U, Damlar I, Erdogan O, et al. Effects of smoking on periimplant health status and IL-1beta, TNF-alpha, and PGE2 levels in periimplant crevicular fluid: a cross-sectional study on well-maintained implant recall patients. Implant Dent 2013;22(5):519-24.
23. Clementini M, Rossetti PH, Penarrocha D, et al. Systemic risk factors for peri-implant bone loss: a systematic review and meta-analysis. Int J Oral Maxillofac Surg 2014;43(3):323-34.
24. Raes S, Rocci A, Raes F, et al. A prospective cohort study on the impact of smoking on soft tissue alterations around single implants. Clin Oral Implants Res 2014. [Epub ahead of print].
25. Renvert S, Aghazadeh A, Hallstrom H, et al. Factors related to peri-implantitis - a retrospective study. Clin Oral Implants Res 2014;25(4):522-9.
26. Koldsland OC, Scheie AA, Aass AM. The association between selected risk indicators and severity of peri-implantitis using mixed model analyses. J Clin Periodontol 2011;38(3):285-92.
27. Aguirre-Zorzano LA, Estefania-Fresco R, Telletxea O, et al. Prevalence of peri-implant inflammatory disease in patients with a history of periodontal disease who receive supportive periodontal therapy. Clin Oral Implants Res 2014. [Epub ahead of print].
28. Sgolastra F, Petrucci A, Severino M, et al. Smoking and the risk of peri-implantitis. A systematic review and meta-analysis. Clin Oral Implants Res 2015;26(4):e62-7.
29. Carcuac O, Jansson L. Peri-implantitis in a specialist clinic of periodontology. Clinical features and risk indicators. Swed Dent J 2010;34(2):53-61.
30. Roccuzzo M, De Angelis N, Bonino L, et al. Ten-year results of a three-arm prospective cohort study on implants in periodontally compromised patients. Part 1: implant loss and radiographic bone loss. Clin Oral Implants Res 2010; 21(5):490-6.

31. Karoussis IK, Kotsovilis S, Fourmousis I. A comprehensive and critical review of dental implant prognosis in periodontally compromised partially edentulous patients. Clin Oral Implants Res 2007;18(6):669–79.

32. Schou S, Holmstrup P, Worthington HV, et al. Outcome of implant therapy in patients with previous tooth loss due to periodontitis. Clin Oral Implants Res 2006; 17(Suppl 2):104–23.

33. Ong CT, Ivanovski S, Needleman IG, et al. Systematic review of implant outcomes in treated periodontitis subjects. J Clin Periodontol 2008;35(5): 438–62.

34. Chrcanovic BR, Albrektsson T, Wennerberg A. Periodontally compromised vs. periodontally healthy patients and dental implants: a systematic review and meta-analysis. J Dent 2014;42(12):1509–27.

35. Ramanauskaite A, Baseviciene N, Wang HL, et al. Effect of history of periodontitis on implant success: meta-analysis and systematic review. Implant Dent 2014;23(6):687–96.

36. Wen X, Liu R, Li G, et al. History of periodontitis as a risk factor for long-term survival of dental implants: a meta-analysis. Int J Oral Maxillofac Implants 2014;29(6):1271–80.

37. Sgolastra F, Petrucci A, Severino M, et al. Periodontitis, implant loss and peri-implantitis. A meta-analysis. Clin Oral Implants Res 2015;26(4):e8–16.

38. Renvert S, Polyzois I. Risk indicators for peri-implant mucositis: a systematic literature review. J Clin Periodontol 2015;42(Suppl 16):S172–86.

39. Costa FO, Takenaka-Martinez S, Cota LO, et al. Peri-implant disease in subjects with and without preventive maintenance: a 5-year follow-up. J Clin Periodontol 2012;39(2):173–81.

40. Ferreira SD, Silva GL, Cortelli JR, et al. Prevalence and risk variables for peri-implant disease in Brazilian subjects. J Clin Periodontol 2006;33(12): 929–35.

41. Zangrando MS, Damante CA, Sant'Ana AC, et al. Long-term evaluation of periodontal parameters and implant outcomes in periodontally compromised patients: a systematic review. J Periodontol 2015;86(2):201–21.

42. Cho-Yan Lee J, Mattheos N, Nixon KC, et al. Residual periodontal pockets are a risk indicator for peri-implantitis in patients treated for periodontitis. Clin Oral Implants Res 2012;23(3):325–33.

43. Roccuzzo M, Bonino L, Dalmasso P, et al. Long-term results of a three arms prospective cohort study on implants in periodontally compromised patients: 10-year data around sandblasted and acid-etched (SLA) surface. Clin Oral Implants Res 2014;25(10):1105–12.

44. Roccuzzo M, Bonino F, Aglietta M, et al. Ten-year results of a three arms prospective cohort study on implants in periodontally compromised patients. Part 2: clinical results. Clin Oral Implants Res 2012;23(4):389–95.

45. Buser D, Martin W, Belser UC. Optimizing esthetics for implant restorations in the anterior maxilla: anatomic and surgical considerations. Int J Oral Maxillofac Implants 2004;19(Suppl):43–61.

46. Bashutski JD, Wang HL. Common implant esthetic complications. Implant Dent 2007;16(4):340–8.

47. Ishikawa T, Salama M, Funato A, et al. Three-dimensional bone and soft tissue requirements for optimizing esthetic results in compromised cases with multiple implants. Int J Periodontics Restorative Dent 2010;30(5):503–11.

48. Evans CD, Chen ST. Esthetic outcomes of immediate implant placements. Clin Oral Implants Res 2008;19(1):73–80.

49. Schwarz F, Alcoforado G, Nelson K, et al. Impact of implant-abutment connection, positioning of the machined collar/microgap, and platform switching on crestal bone level changes. Camlog Foundation Consensus Report. Clin Oral Implants Res 2014;25(11):1301–3.
50. Schwarz F, Hegewald A, Becker J. Impact of implant-abutment connection and positioning of the machined collar/microgap on crestal bone level changes: a systematic review. Clin Oral Implants Res 2014;25(4):417–25.
51. Palaska I, Tsaousoglou P, Vouros I, et al. Influence of placement depth and abutment connection pattern on bone remodeling around 1-stage implants: a prospective randomized controlled clinical trial. Clin Oral Implants Res 2014. [Epub ahead of print].
52. Pozzi A, Agliardi E, Tallarico M, et al. Clinical and radiological outcomes of two implants with different prosthetic interfaces and neck configurations: randomized, controlled, split-mouth clinical trial. Clin Implant Dent Relat Res 2014; 16(1):96–106.
53. Grunder U. Stability of the mucosal topography around single-tooth implants and adjacent teeth: 1-year results. Int J Periodontics Restorative Dent 2000; 20(1):11–7.
54. Rismanchian M, Shahabouei MH, Yaghinei J, et al. Comparative microflora assessment of natural sulci vs. deep and shallow implant sulci in partial edentulousness. J Oral Implantol 2013. [Epub ahead of print].
55. Weber HP, Kim DM, Ng MW, et al. Peri-implant soft-tissue health surrounding cement- and screw-retained implant restorations: a multi-center, 3-year prospective study. Clin Oral Implants Res 2006;17(4):375–9.
56. de Brandao ML, Vettore MV, Vidigal Junior GM. Peri-implant bone loss in cement- and screw-retained prostheses: systematic review and meta-analysis. J Clin Periodontol 2013;40(3):287–95.
57. Korsch M, Obst U, Walther W. Cement-associated peri-implantitis: a retrospective clinical observational study of fixed implant-supported restorations using a methacrylate cement. Clin Oral Implants Res 2014;25(7):797–802.
58. Wilson TG Jr. The positive relationship between excess cement and peri-implant disease: a prospective clinical endoscopic study. J Periodontol 2009;80(9): 1388–92.
59. Linkevicius T, Puisys A, Vindasiute E, et al. Does residual cement around implant-supported restorations cause peri-implant disease? A retrospective case analysis. Clin Oral Implants Res 2013;24(11):1179–84.
60. Korsch M, Walther W. Peri-implantitis associated with type of cement: a retrospective analysis of different types of cement and their clinical correlation to the peri-implant tissue. Clin Implant Dent Relat Res 2014. [Epub ahead of print].
61. Korsch M, Walther W, Marten SM, et al. Microbial analysis of biofilms on cement surfaces: an investigation in cement-associated peri-implantitis. J Appl Biomater Funct Mater 2014;12(2):70–80.
62. Raval NC, Wadhwani CP, Jain S, et al. The interaction of implant luting cements and oral bacteria linked to peri-implant disease: an in vitro analysis of planktonic and biofilm growth - a preliminary study. Clin Implant Dent Relat Res 2014. [Epub ahead of print].
63. Linkevicius T, Vindasiute E, Puisys A, et al. The influence of margin location on the amount of undetected cement excess after delivery of cement-retained implant restorations. Clin Oral Implants Res 2011;22(12):1379–84.
64. Serino G, Strom C. Peri-implantitis in partially edentulous patients: association with inadequate plaque control. Clin Oral Implants Res 2009;20(2):169–74.

65. Frost HM. From Wolff's law to the mechanostat: a new "face" of physiology. J Orthop Sci 1998;3(5):282–6.

66. Frost HM. A 2003 update of bone physiology and Wolff's law for clinicians. Angle Orthod 2004;74(1):3–15.

67. Mattheos N, Schittek Janda M, Zampelis A, et al. Reversible, non-plaque-induced loss of osseointegration of successfully loaded dental implants. Clin Oral Implants Res 2013;24(3):347–54.

68. Naert I, Duyck J, Vandamme K. Occlusal overload and bone/implant loss. Clin Oral Implants Res 2012;23(Suppl 6):95–107.

69. Klinge B, Meyle J, Working G. Peri-implant tissue destruction. The Third EAO Consensus Conference 2012. Clin Oral Implants Res 2012;23(Suppl 6):108–10.

70. Fu JH, Hsu YT, Wang HL. Identifying occlusal overload and how to deal with it to avoid marginal bone loss around implants. Eur J Oral Implantol 2012;5(Suppl): S91–103.

71. Chambrone L, Chambrone LA, Lima LA. Effects of occlusal overload on peri-implant tissue health: a systematic review of animal-model studies. J Periodontol 2010;81(10):1367–78.

72. Heitz-Mayfield LJ, Mombelli A. The therapy of peri-implantitis: a systematic review. Int J Oral Maxillofac Implants 2014;29(Suppl):325–45.

73. Heitz-Mayfield LJ, Salvi GE, Botticelli D, et al. Anti-infective treatment of peri-implant mucositis: a randomised controlled clinical trial. Clin Oral Implants Res 2011;22(3):237–41.

74. Figuero E, Graziani F, Sanz I, et al. Management of peri-implant mucositis and peri-implantitis. Periodontol 2000 2014;66(1):255–73.

75. Louropoulou A, Slot DE, Van der Weijden FA. Titanium surface alterations following the use of different mechanical instruments: a systematic review. Clin Oral Implants Res 2012;23(6):643–58.

76. Louropoulou A, Slot DE, Van der Weijden F. The effects of mechanical instruments on contaminated titanium dental implant surfaces: a systematic review. Clin Oral Implants Res 2014;25(10):1149–60.

77. Duarte PM, Reis AF, de Freitas PM, et al. Bacterial adhesion on smooth and rough titanium surfaces after treatment with different instruments. J Periodontol 2009;80(11):1824–32.

78. Slots J, Research S, Therapy C. Systemic antibiotics in periodontics. J Periodontol 2004;75(11):1553–65.

79. Socransky SS, Haffajee AD. Dental biofilms: difficult therapeutic targets. Periodontol 2000 2002;28:12–55.

80. Suarez F, Monje A, Galindo-Moreno P, et al. Implant surface detoxification: a comprehensive review. Implant Dent 2013;22(5):465–73.

81. Kreisler M, Kohnen W, Marinello C, et al. Bactericidal effect of the Er:YAG laser on dental implant surfaces: an in vitro study. J Periodontol 2002;73(11): 1292–8.

82. Giannelli M, Bani D, Tani A, et al. In vitro evaluation of the effects of low-intensity Nd:YAG laser irradiation on the inflammatory reaction elicited by bacterial lipopolysaccharide adherent to titanium dental implants. J Periodontol 2009;80(6): 977–84.

83. Stubinger S, Etter C, Miskiewicz M, et al. Surface alterations of polished and sandblasted and acid-etched titanium implants after Er:YAG, carbon dioxide, and diode laser irradiation. Int J Oral Maxillofac Implants 2010;25(1):104–11.

84. Kim JH, Herr Y, Chung JH, et al. The effect of erbium-doped: yttrium, aluminium and garnet laser irradiation on the surface microstructure and

roughness of double acid-etched implants. J Periodontal Implant Sci 2011; 41(5):234–41.

85. Kreisler M, Gotz H, Duschner H. Effect of Nd:YAG, Ho:YAG, Er:YAG, CO2, and GaAlAs laser irradiation on surface properties of endosseous dental implants. Int J Oral Maxillofac Implants 2002;17(2):202–11.

86. Moritz A, Schoop U, Goharkhay K, et al. Treatment of periodontal pockets with a diode laser. Lasers Surg Med 1998;22(5):302–11.

87. Liu CM, Hou LT, Wong MY, et al. Comparison of Nd:YAG laser versus scaling and root planing in periodontal therapy. J Periodontol 1999;70(11):1276–82.

88. Tucker D, Cobb CM, Rapley JW, et al. Morphologic changes following in vitro CO2 laser treatment of calculus-ladened root surfaces. Lasers Surg Med 1996;18(2):150–6.

89. Nevins M, Nevins ML, Yamamoto A, et al. Use of Er:YAG laser to decontaminate infected dental implant surface in preparation for reestablishment of bone-to-implant contact. Int J Periodontics Restorative Dent 2014;34(4):461–6.

90. Konopka K, Goslinski T. Photodynamic therapy in dentistry. J Dent Res 2007; 86(8):694–707.

91. Salvi GE, Ramseier CA. Efficacy of patient-administered mechanical and/or chemical plaque control protocols in the management of peri-implant mucositis. A systematic review. J Clin Periodontol 2015;42(Suppl 16):S187–201.

92. Faggion CM Jr, Listl S, Fruhauf N, et al. A systematic review and Bayesian network meta-analysis of randomized clinical trials on non-surgical treatments for peri-implantitis. J Clin Periodontol 2014;41(10):1015–25.

93. Heitz-Mayfield LJ, Salvi GE, Mombelli A, et al. Anti-infective surgical therapy of peri-implantitis. A 12-month prospective clinical study. Clin Oral Implants Res 2012;23(2):205–10.

94. Ochsenbein C. A primer for osseous surgery. Int J Periodontics Restorative Dent 1986;6(1):8–47.

95. Romeo E, Ghisolfi M, Murgolo N, et al. Therapy of peri-implantitis with resective surgery. A 3-year clinical trial on rough screw-shaped oral implants. Part I: clinical outcome. Clin Oral Implants Res 2005;16(1):9–18.

96. Froum SJ, Froum SH, Rosen PS. Successful management of peri-implantitis with a regenerative approach: a consecutive series of 51 treated implants with 3- to 7.5-year follow-up. Int J Periodontics Restorative Dent 2012;32(1):11–20.

97. Roos-Jansaker AM, Persson GR, Lindahl C, et al. Surgical treatment of peri-implantitis using a bone substitute with or without a resorbable membrane: a 5-year follow-up. J Clin Periodontol 2014;41(11):1108–14.

98. Wiltfang J, Zernial O, Behrens E, et al. Regenerative treatment of peri-implantitis bone defects with a combination of autologous bone and a demineralized xenogenic bone graft: a series of 36 defects. Clin Implant Dent Relat Res 2012;14(3):421–7.

99. Renvert S, Polyzois I, Claffey N. Surgical therapy for the control of peri-implantitis. Clin Oral Implants Res 2012;23(Suppl 6):84–94.

100. Schwarz F, Sahm N, Schwarz K, et al. Impact of defect configuration on the clinical outcome following surgical regenerative therapy of peri-implantitis. J Clin Periodontol 2010;37(5):449–55.

101. Schwarz F, Sahm N, Becker J. Combined surgical therapy of advanced peri-implantitis lesions with concomitant soft tissue volume augmentation. A case series. Clin Oral Implants Res 2014;25(1):132–6.

102. Schwarz F, John G, Mainusch S, et al. Combined surgical therapy of peri-implantitis evaluating two methods of surface debridement and decontamination. A two-year clinical follow up report. J Clin Periodontol 2012;39(8):789–97.

103. Matarasso S, Iorio Siciliano V, Aglietta M, et al. Clinical and radiographic outcomes of a combined resective and regenerative approach in the treatment of peri-implantitis: a prospective case series. Clin Oral Implants Res 2014; 25(7):761–7.

104. Sahrmann P, Attin T, Schmidlin PR. Regenerative treatment of peri-implantitis using bone substitutes and membrane: a systematic review. Clin Implant Dent Relat Res 2011;13(1):46–57.

105. Elangovan S. Complete regeneration of peri-implantitis-induced bony defects using guided bone regeneration is unpredictable. J Am Dent Assoc 2013; 144(7):823–4.

106. Faggion CM Jr, Chambrone L, Listl S, et al. Network meta-analysis for evaluating interventions in implant dentistry: the case of peri-implantitis treatment. Clin Implant Dent Relat Res 2013;15(4):576–88.

107. Claffey N, Clarke E, Polyzois I, et al. Surgical treatment of peri-implantitis. J Clin Periodontol 2008;35(8 Suppl):316–32.

108. Khoshkam V, Chan HL, Lin GH, et al. Reconstructive procedures for treating peri-implantitis: a systematic review. J Dent Res 2013;92(12 Suppl):131S–8S.

109. Chan HL, Lin GH, Suarez F, et al. Surgical management of peri-implantitis: a systematic review and meta-analysis of treatment outcomes. J Periodontol 2014; 85(8):1027–41.

110. Heitz-Mayfield LJ, Needleman I, Salvi GE, et al. Consensus statements and clinical recommendations for prevention and management of biologic and technical implant complications. Int J Oral Maxillofac Implants 2014;29(Suppl): 346–50.

111. van Winkelhoff AJ. Antibiotics in the treatment of peri-implantitis. Eur J Oral Implantol 2012;5(Suppl):S43–50.

112. Muthukuru M, Zainvi A, Esplugues EO, et al. Non-surgical therapy for the management of peri-implantitis: a systematic review. Clin Oral Implants Res 2012; 23(Suppl 6):77–83.

113. Kotsakis GA, Konstantinidis I, Karoussis IK, et al. Systematic review and meta-analysis of the effect of various laser wavelengths in the treatment of peri-implantitis. J Periodontol 2014;85(9):1203–13.

114. Mailoa J, Lin GH, Chan HL, et al. Clinical outcomes of using lasers for peri-implantitis surface detoxification: a systematic review and meta-analysis. J Periodontol 2014;85(9):1194–202.

115. Yan M, Liu M, Wang M, et al. The effects of Er:YAG on the treatment of peri-implantitis: a meta-analysis of randomized controlled trials. Lasers Med Sci 2014. [Epub ahead of print].

116. Renvert S, Polyzois I, Maguire R. Re-osseointegration on previously contaminated surfaces: a systematic review. Clin Oral Implants Res 2009;20(Suppl 4): 216–27.

117. Lagervall M, Jansson LE. Treatment outcome in patients with peri-implantitis in a periodontal clinic: a retrospective study. J Periodontol 2013;84(10): 1365–73.

118. Serino G, Turri A, Lang NP. Maintenance therapy in patients following the surgical treatment of peri-implantitis: a 5-year follow-up study. Clin Oral Implants Res 2015;26(8):950–6.

119. Rinke S, Ohl S, Ziebolz D, et al. Prevalence of periimplant disease in partially edentulous patients: a practice-based cross-sectional study. Clin Oral Implants Res 2011;22(8):826–33.

120. Mir-Mari J, Mir-Orfila P, Figueiredo R, et al. Prevalence of peri-implant diseases. A cross-sectional study based on a private practice environment. J Clin Periodontol 2012;39(5):490–4.
121. Casado PL, Villas-Boas R, de Mello W, et al. Peri-implant disease and chronic periodontitis: is interleukin-6 gene promoter polymorphism the common risk factor in a Brazilian population? Int J Oral Maxillofac Implants 2013;28(1): 35–43.
122. Marrone A, Lasserre J, Bercy P, et al. Prevalence and risk factors for peri-implant disease in Belgian adults. Clin Oral Implants Res 2013;24(8):934–40.
123. Daubert DM, Weinstein BF, Bordin S, et al. Prevalence and predictive factors for peri-implant disease and implant failure: a cross-sectional analysis. J Periodontol 2015;86:337–47.
124. Sahm N, Becker J, Santel T, et al. Non-surgical treatment of peri-implantitis using an air-abrasive device or mechanical debridement and local application of chlorhexidine: a prospective, randomized, controlled clinical study. J Clin Periodontol 2011;38(9):872–8.
125. John G, Sahm N, Becker J, et al. Nonsurgical treatment of peri-implantitis using an air-abrasive device or mechanical debridement and local application of chlorhexidine. Twelve-month follow-up of a prospective, randomized, controlled clinical study. Clin Oral Investig 2015. [Epub ahead of print].
126. Machtei EE, Frankenthal S, Levi G, et al. Treatment of peri-implantitis using multiple applications of chlorhexidine chips: a double-blind, randomized multicentre clinical trial. J Clin Periodontol 2012;39(12):1198–205.
127. de Waal YC, Raghoebar GM, Huddleston Slater JJ, et al. Implant decontamination during surgical peri-implantitis treatment: a randomized, double-blind, placebo-controlled trial. J Clin Periodontol 2013;40(2):186–95.
128. Persson GR, Roos-Jansaker AM, Lindahl C, et al. Microbiologic results after non-surgical erbium-doped:yttrium, aluminum, and garnet laser or air-abrasive treatment of peri-implantitis: a randomized clinical trial. J Periodontol 2011; 82(9):1267–78.
129. Schwarz F, Sahm N, Iglhaut G, et al. Impact of the method of surface debridement and decontamination on the clinical outcome following combined surgical therapy of peri-implantitis: a randomized controlled clinical study. J Clin Periodontol 2011;38(3):276–84.
130. Schwarz F, Hegewald A, John G, et al. Four-year follow-up of combined surgical therapy of advanced peri-implantitis evaluating two methods of surface decontamination. J Clin Periodontol 2013;40(10):962–7.
131. Schär D, Ramseier CA, Eick S, et al. Anti-infective therapy of peri-implantitis with adjunctive local drug delivery or photodynamic therapy: six-month outcomes of a prospective randomized clinical trial. Clin Oral Implants Res 2013;24(1):104–10.
132. Bassetti M, Schar D, Wicki B, et al. Anti-infective therapy of peri-implantitis with adjunctive local drug delivery or photodynamic therapy: 12-month outcomes of a randomized controlled clinical trial. Clin Oral Implants Res 2014; 25(3):279–87.
133. Hallstrom H, Persson GR, Lindgren S, et al. Systemic antibiotics and debridement of peri-implant mucositis. A randomized clinical trial. J Clin Periodontol 2012;39(6):574–81.
134. de Waal YC, Raghoebar GM, Meijer HJ, et al. Implant decontamination with 2% chlorhexidine during surgical peri-implantitis treatment: a randomized, double-blind, controlled trial. Clin Oral Implants Res 2014. [Epub ahead of print].

135. Renvert S, Lindahl C, Roos Jansaker AM, et al. Treatment of peri-implantitis using an Er:YAG laser or an air-abrasive device: a randomized clinical trial. J Clin Periodontol 2011;38(1):65–73.
136. Papadopoulos CA, Vouros I, Menexes G, et al. The utilization of a diode laser in the surgical treatment of peri-implantitis. A randomized clinical trial. Clin Oral Investig 2015. [Epub ahead of print].

Does Gingival Recession Require Surgical Treatment?

Hsun-Liang Chan, DDS, MS[a],
Yong-Hee Patricia Chun, DDS, MS, PhD[b,c], Mark MacEachern, MLIS[d],
Thomas W. Oates, DMD, PhD[b,*]

KEYWORDS

- Gingival recession • Periodontal attachment loss • Esthetics • Surgical flaps

KEY POINTS

- Gingival recession is defined as when "the location of the gingival margin is apical to the cemento-enamel junction (CEJ)."
- About 23% of adults in the United States have one or more tooth surfaces with 3 mm or more gingival recession.
- The cause of gingival recession is multifactorial, confounded by poorly defined contributions from predisposing and precipitating factors.
- Predisposing factors include bone dehiscence, tooth malposition, thin soft and hard tissues, inadequate keratinized/attached mucosa, and frenum pull.
- Precipitating factors include traumatic forces (eg, excessive brushing), habits (eg, smoking, oral piercing), plaque-induced inflammation, and dental treatment (eg, certain types of orthodontic tooth movement, equal/subgingival restorations).
- Surgical correction of a gingival recession is often considered when (1) a patient raises a concern about esthetics or tooth hypersensitivity, (2) there is active gingival recession, and (3) orthodontic/restorative treatment will be implemented on a tooth with presence of predisposing factors. The benefits of these treatment approaches are not well supported in current literature relative to alternative approaches with control of possible etiologic factors.

Continued

[a] Department of Periodontics and Oral Medicine, University of Michigan School of Dentistry, R3323B 1011 North University Avenue, Ann Arbor, MI 48105, USA; [b] Department of Periodontics, University of Texas Health Science Center at San Antonio, 7703 Floyd Curl Drive, San Antonio, TX 78229, USA; [c] Department of Cellular and Structural Biology, University of Texas Health Science Center at San Antonio, 7703 Floyd Curl Drive, San Antonio, TX 78229, USA; [d] Taubman Health Sciences Library, University of Michigan, 1135 East Catherine Street, Ann Arbor, MI 48109, USA
* Corresponding author.
E-mail address: oates@uthscsa.edu

Dent Clin N Am 59 (2015) 981–996
http://dx.doi.org/10.1016/j.cden.2015.06.010
0011-8532/15/$ – see front matter © 2015 Elsevier Inc. All rights reserved.

dental.theclinics.com

Continued

- Possible surgical modalities for treating a gingival recession include root coverage or keratinized tissue augmentation.
- A root coverage procedure is to augment soft tissues coronal to the gingival margin. Examples include coronally advanced flap with or without a subepithelial connective tissue graft and an allograft.
- A keratinized tissue augmentation procedure is to provide qualitative changes to the soft tissues apical to the gingival margin. Examples include a free gingival graft and subepithelial connective tissue graft.

INTRODUCTION

Gingival recession is defined as when "the location of the gingival margin is apical to the cemento-enamel junction (CEJ)."[1] It is a common dental condition that affects a large number of patients. A survey of adults ranging from 30 to 90 years of age estimated that 23% of adults in the United States have one or more tooth surfaces with 3 mm or more gingival recession.[2] The prevalence, extent, and severity of gingival recession increased with age, with at least 40% of young adults and up to 88% of older adults having at least 1 site with 1 mm or more of recession (**Table 1**).[3–5] Other periodontal (eg, oral hygiene and gingival bleeding) and health parameters (eg, diabetes and alcohol intake) were not associated with the extent of recession.[4]

Therapeutic options for recessions have been well documented with a high degree of success. Soft-tissue grafting procedures represent one of the most common periodontal surgical procedures performed in the United States, with periodontists performing on average more than 100 of these procedures per year (American Dental Association survey 2005–06).[6] What is not so clear is the cause of this condition, the role of possible causative factors, and the need for treatment. With such a prevalent condition, it is critical to discriminate when to treat these lesions and which types of lesions require surgical treatment. This review examines these questions regarding

Table 1			
Study documentation of prevalence of gingival recession			
Study Reference	**Prevalence (%)**	**Adult Population Defined by**	**Comments**
2	23	≥3 mm of recession	• NHANES survey 1988–1994
3	50	>50 y of age with ≥1 site	• Found in patients with both good and poor oral hygiene
	88	>65 y of age with ≥1 site	• Facial surfaces most commonly affected
4	85	Adults with ≥1 site	• French population studied • Risk factors: age, gender, plaque index, smoking, missing teeth, and gingival bleeding
5,7	40	16–25 y of age	• Evaluated facially positioned teeth
	80	36–86 y of age	

Abbreviation: NHANES, National Health and Nutrition Examination Survey.
   Data from Refs.[2–5,7]

this common oral condition as well as provides an overview of what is known about gingival recession defects and their treatment.

ETIOLOGY

The cause of gingival recession is multifactorial; therefore, a single factor alone may not necessarily result in the development of gingival recession. Factors associated with gingival recession are broadly categorized into 2 types, predisposing factors and precipitating factors, as summarized in **Table 2**. Predisposing factors are mainly variations of developmental morphology that may impose a higher risk of recession, whereas precipitating factors are acquired habits or conditions that introduce gingival recession.

Predisposing Factors

As the alveolar bone supports the overlying soft tissue, conditions that may cause bone dehiscence/fenestration defects are thought to increase the risk of developing gingival recession. Malpositioned teeth, especially facially positioned teeth are likewise thought susceptible to recession over time.[5,7]

Although it seems obvious that the lack of facial alveolar bone would lead to increased risk of gingival recession, it is not so simple. The prevalence of recession in these studies is not different from the overall prevalence rates for recession.[3–5,7] Furthermore, as any practitioner of periodontal surgery can attest, patients frequently have no facial alveolar bone without any signs of recession (**Fig. 1**). Therefore, although the lack of alveolar bone may be a predisposing factor, there must be other factors that more directly contribute to this type of loss of gingival tissues.

Gingival recession is thought to be more common in patients with thinner gingival tissues than in those with thicker gingival tissues. Facial gingival thickness has been positively associated with its underlying alveolar plate thickness.[8] It seems likely that thinner tissue would be more susceptible to recession than thicker tissue, after nonsurgical or surgical periodontal treatment.[9,10] Teeth with more prominent roots may have thinner alveolar bone and gingival tissues on the facial aspect creating a predisposing condition for recession, but as with alveolar bone, it is not clear whether lack of tissue thickness alone causes facial recession. Again, with thin gingival tissue as a predisposing factor, recession may develop only in the presence of concurrent precipitating factors, for example, inflammation and trauma. Although unproven, any differences in risk of gingival recession apparent between thin and thick tissue may be due more directly to precipitating factors involved. Without these precipitating factors, the gingival margin with thin tissues or lack of alveolar bone could remain unchanged.

Another factor frequently cited as a predisposing factor leading to gingival recession is a frenum pull. It is thought that when the attachment of the frenum is proximate to the gingival margin, the repeated stretch of the frenum during oral function could exert

Table 2
Common risk factors of gingival recession

Predisposing Factors	Precipitating Factors
1. Bone dehiscence	1. Traumatic forces, eg, excessive brushing
2. Tooth malposition	2. Habits, eg, smoking, oral piercing
3. Thin tissue	3. Plaque-induced inflammation
4. Inadequate keratinized/attached mucosa	4. Dental treatment, eg, certain types of orthodontic tooth movement, subgingival restorations
5. Frenum pull	

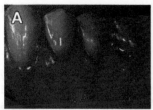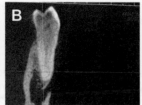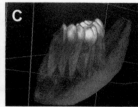

Fig. 1. Differences between bone thickness and soft-tissue recession. Clinical appearance (*A*) of lower left posterior quadrant of a 40-year-old patient showing minimal signs of gingival recession in the absence of buccal bone over the teeth as evident in cone beam computer tomographic images (*B, C*).

forces somehow compromising the mucosal tissue margin or oral hygiene in leading to gingival recession. However, cross-sectional studies failed to demonstrate an association of recessions with high frenum attachment.[11,12]

Inadequate keratinized mucosa (KM), most commonly defined as equal or less than 2 mm, is frequently observed concurrently with gingival recession. Historically, it has been considered a predisposing factor of gingival recession. A cross-sectional study[13] established a correlation between inadequate KM and increased gingival inflammation, which is a precursor of periodontal diseases leading to gingival recession. However, inadequate KM might simply be a consequence of gingival recession, rather than a cause of gingival recession. This point is supported by an interventional, longitudinal study[14] that concluded that the attachment level could be maintained with control of gingival inflammation, even without adequate KM. This study with 32 subjects concluded that sites with insufficient attached mucosa (≤2 mm) due to gingival recession did not lose attachment or have additional recession over a period of 6 years. In the presence of inflammation, patients without adequate KM showed continuous attachment loss and additional recession. Therefore, poor oral hygiene may be considered a precipitating factor for gingival recession. However, another split-mouth design study[15] following up 73 subjects for 10 to 27 years found that teeth with recessions without receiving surgical treatment experienced an increase of the recession by 0.7 to 1.0 mm. Further, new recessions developed in 15 sites during the study period in the absence of inflammation. In contrast, teeth with gingival recession receiving a free gingival graft had a reduction of gingival recession by approximately 1.5 mm through creeping attachment. Therefore, although anatomic variants considered to be predisposing factors leading to recession do not always require treatment, with concurrent precipitating factors, surgical intervention may be indicated.

Precipitating Factors

The role of oral hygiene practices as contributing to the occurrence of gingival recession remains a major consideration in the understanding of the cause, the prognosis, and the treatment. It is important to recognize that gingival recession may be associated with both extremes of oral hygiene, one occurring in patients with extremely good oral hygiene and the other in those with unfavorable oral hygiene as described earlier. In the former type, meticulous brushing is thought to introduce trauma to the gingiva leading to recession.[16,17] This type of recession is commonly seen on the facial side of canines and premolars and associated with overzealous brushing habits. Contrarily, poor oral hygiene is associated with recession due to plaque-induced inflammation and subsequent attachment loss. Although the role of traumatic tooth brushing as a precipitating factor to gingival recession is well accepted, the evidence in support of this concept remains limited. It seems that several factors related to tooth brushing may contribute to recession. These factors include brushing force and brush hardness, frequency and duration of tooth brushing, as well as frequency of changing tooth brushes and the brushing techniques and types of manual or electric brushes used.[18] In cases of both overzealous and insufficient oral hygiene, an underlying inflammatory response is likely to contribute to tissue destruction resulting in gingival recession. Another precipitating factor for recession is alveolar bone and soft-tissue remodeling associated with generalized periodontal disease (**Fig. 2**) or tooth extraction. This condition commonly occurs in the proximal sites of teeth adjacent to the extraction site and often results in circumferential exposure of root surfaces of involved teeth.

Less commonly found, but clinically important, local gingival tissue trauma or irritation as found with tobacco chewing and oral piercing can lead to inflammatory changes in the tissues resulting in gingival recession.[19] When smokeless tobacco is used, the tobacco is kept in the vestibule adjacent to mandibular incisors or premolars for a prolonged time. The gingival tissues can experience mechanical or chemical injury with the consequence of a recession.[20] In the presence of labial or lingual piercings, gingival recession is found in up to 80% of pierced individuals in mandibular and maxillary teeth.[20] In addition, oral piercing poses a 11-fold greater risk for developing gingival recession.[20]

One frequent concern for gingival recession is with orthodontic tooth movement (**Fig. 3**).[21] The risk for gingival recession in the mandibular incisors during or after orthodontic therapy is much studied, yet research in this area remains inconclusive. Most commonly, studies have evaluated orthodontic repositioning of the mandibular incisors as proclination, with the forward tipping or bodily movement more likely to lead to thinner alveolar bone and soft tissues on the facial aspect of the tooth, and retroclination, leading to an increased thickness of facial tissues. Studies evaluating the effects of orthodontic treatment on gingival recession typically suggest an incidence of 10% to 20% when evaluated for as long as 5 years after the completion of orthodontic therapy.[22–26] These rates of occurrence, considered relative to the overall high prevalence found in adults, suggest that orthodontic tooth movement may provide only a minor contribution to the overall prevalence of gingival recession. Two recent studies have taken this discussion a step further in suggesting that the extent

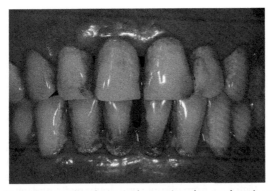

Fig. 2. Demonstration of generalized gingival recession due to chronic periodontitis, especially the mandibular anterior teeth. The chronic and horizontal pattern of the periodontium and the alveolar bone often result in circumferential exposure of root surfaces of several teeth.

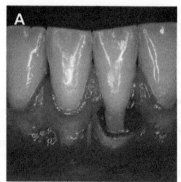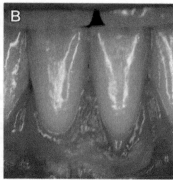

Fig. 3. Illustration of an orthodontics-associated gingival recession and treatment. (*A*) Gingival recession with clinically evident inflammation around tooth #24 developed during orthodontic treatment, leaving minimal amount of attached mucosa (*B*) A free gingival graft was placed with a primary aim of increasing the attached mucosa apical to the gingival margin. The soft tissue can be coronally advanced in the future to cover the root. (*Courtesy of* Dr Jeff Li, DMD, Graduate Periodontics Resident, University of Michigan School of Dentistry, Ann Arbor, MI.)

of gingival recession when it occurs after orthodontics may be small and of limited clinical concern, affecting only 10% of patients, with most cased being readily treatable as Miller class I lesions.[25,27] These findings suggest that preorthodontic periodontal procedures directed at minimizing recession may not be justified in most cases. A systematic review of this literature confirmed that, although soft-tissue augmentation as a preorthodontic procedure may be a clinically viable option, this treatment is not based on solid scientific evidence.[28]

Repeated scaling and root planning or periodontal surgeries on shallow pockets may induce clinical attachment loss, partially manifested by gingival recession.[29] It was concluded that the critically probing depth that determines if a certain procedure will gain or lose clinical attachment is 2.9 and 4.2 mm for scaling and root planning and the modified Widman flap procedure, respectively. It is thought that tissue remodeling in sites with shallow pockets during healing following these periodontal procedures may result in minor clinical attachment loss.

PATHOGENESIS OF GINGIVAL RECESSION

The loss of clinical attachment is apparent either as increased probing depth or as gingival recession.[30] A preclinical study[31] inducing gingival recession by replacing rat incisors with acrylic resin implants suggested that gingival recession is associated with (1) local inflammation characterized by mononuclear cells, (2) breakdown of connective tissue, and (3) proliferation of the oral and junctional epithelia into the site of connective tissue destruction. The 2 epithelial layers eventually fuse together, encroaching on the intervening connective tissue. The common keratinized layer differentiated and separated, forming a narrow cleft, bringing about a reduction in height of the gingival margin, which is manifest clinically as gingival recession. Thin tissue seems to recede more often in response to inflammation as a result of trauma to the tissues. Human histology from chronic and acute clefts and wide recessions confirms the relevance of an inflammatory infiltrate in the pathogenesis of clefts versus wide recessions.[32] In all subtypes of recessions, the epithelium is acanthotic and proliferative and surrounded by an inflammatory infiltrate. In addition, in acute clefts associated with tooth brushing trauma, necrotic cells can be found. In wide recessions, the dentogingival epithelium penetrates into the lamina propria, thereby decreasing the width of the lamina propria and allowing the dentogingival and oral epithelia to coalesce, resulting in loss of attachment to the tooth. The inflammatory infiltrate can span the entire thickness of the width of the gingiva thus promoting a recession. In thicker gingiva, connective tissue free of inflammatory infiltrate may be interposed between oral and junctional epithelia preventing a recession.[33]

FACTORS TO BE CONSIDERED FOR TREATING GINGIVAL RECESSION

Does gingival recession require surgical treatment? To address the question, the authors first conducted targeted searches in PubMed and Embase to capture a narrow set of studies focused on surgical treatment of gingival recession (**Box 1**). Reference lists of key studies from this result set were checked for additional studies relevant to the cause, contributing factors of gingival recession, and indications of surgical interventions. Subsequent searches were run in PubMed on themes identified during the initial literature review. An analysis of the search results identified factors that influence the decisions of whether or not to treat gingival recession, based on which a stratified, evidence-based decision-making process (**Fig. 4**) was formulated. Recessions adjacent to implants were excluded.

The flowchart starts with a consideration of patient's concerns, followed by a consideration of the stability of the lesion, whether other dental needs are required, and, lastly, existing predisposing morphologic factors that may trigger further gingival recession. The factors are described in detail in the following.

Classification of Recession Defects

Clinically, a widely used classification system was proposed in 1985 by Dr P. D. Miller, based on the predictability of achieving root coverage (**Box 2**).[34] Full root coverage is anticipated in class I and II recessions, in which interproximal tissues are still intact; on the other hand, in class III recessions, only partial coverage is expected. Minimal root coverage is expected in class IV recessions.

Patient's Concerns

Although dentists view esthetics as the most important reason for root coverage procedures,[35] patients are often not even aware of recessions on their teeth because most of them are asymptomatic.[36] Only 28% of the clinically identified recession sites were perceived by patients as such, with a fraction being associated with dentin hypersensitivity or unaesthetic appearance. Women were more concerned about esthetics than men. Dentin hypersensitivity associated with gingival recession is more common in younger patients. The large discrepancy in the number of diagnosed recessions and patient-perceived recessions should prompt the dentist to be mindful when suggesting a root coverage procedure.

Box 1
PubMed search designed to capture a narrow set of studies on surgical interventions for gingival recession

("gingival recession/surgery"[mh] OR ("gingival recession"[majr] OR ("gingival"[ti] AND ("recession"[ti] OR "recessions"[ti]))) AND ("oral surgical procedures"[majr] OR surgery[ti] OR surgeries[ti] OR surgic*[ti] OR operati*[ti])) AND english[la] NOT (animals[mh] NOT humans[mh]) NOT (case reports[pt] OR "case report"[ti]).

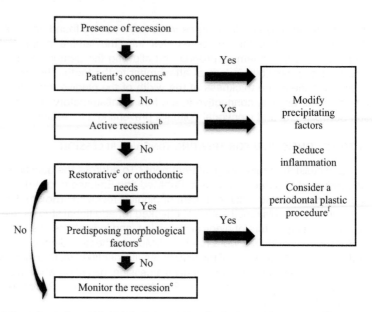

Fig. 4. A flow chart of considerations for treating gingival recession. Generally, a periodontal plastic surgery is rendered only to address patients' concerns or halt an active lesion. As the recession is confounded by multiple factors, there is no effective way to predict the occurrence of gingival recession. A preventive procedure is generally not recommended. Clinicians should make the best judgment by taking considerations of various predisposing and precipitating factors. Control of precipitating factors and reduction of periodontal inflammation should always precede a corrective surgery. [a]Patient concerns may include esthetics or root sensitivity. [b]Active recession may be determined by comparing the size of the current lesion to previous records or judged by patient's impression. [c]Restorative needs with an equal or subgingival margin, abutment for a removable partial denture, especially an RPI-bar denture, and overdenture abutment. [d]Predisposing morphologic factors may include inadequate keratinized mucosa, frenum pull, and thin tissue-type, which might increase the risk of future recession. [e]Periodontal plastic surgery is not likely needed. However, regular prophylaxis/periodontal maintenance and modifying precipitating factors are required. [f]It is performed to augment the soft tissue either apical (eg, a free gingival graft to increase the width of the keratinized mucosa) or coronal (a root coverage procedure) to the free gingival margin. RPI, mesial rest, disto-lingual guide plate, I-bar.

Box 2
Diagnosis/prognosis for gingival recession

Miller classification

- Class 1: recession not beyond MGJ; no interproximal tissue loss; 100% coverage expected

- Class 2: recession extend to or beyond mucogingival junction (MGJ); no interproximal tissue loss; 100% coverage expected

- Class 3: recession extend to or beyond MGJ; presence of loss of interproximal tissue and/or tooth malposition; partial coverage expected

- Class 4: recession extend to or beyond MGJ; presence of loss of interproximal tissue and/or tooth malposition; coverage not expected

From Miller PD Jr. Root coverage using the free soft tissue autograft following citric acid application. III. A successful and predictable procedure in areas of deep-wide recession. Int J Periodontics Restorative Dent 1985;5(2):14–37.

Unsatisfactory esthetics

In the event of gingival recession, the affected tooth looks longer and the free gingival margin may become asymmetric comparing right and left quadrants. Because of this unaesthetic appearance, patients may seek dental treatment with sites having an esthetic concern highly variable between patients.[37] Few patients may seek esthetic treatment of recession on the mandibular teeth (**Fig. 5**).

Root hypersensitivity

Root hypersensitivity (RS) affects from 3% to 57% of population.[38] It is an unpleasant experience that may be initiated by various stimuli, such as cold. It is primarily caused by the exposure of root surfaces to the oral environment as a result of gingival recession.

Surgical root coverage procedures have been used to treat RS. A systematic review[39] evaluated the effect of root coverage procedures for treating RS. Nine studies were included in this review, using various techniques for Miller class 1 and 2 root coverage, including coronally advanced flap (CAF) alone, CAF + enamel matrix derivative (EMD), CAF + subepithelial connective tissue graft (SCTG), semilunar coronally positioned flap, and SCTG with resin-modified glass-ionomer restoration. RS was evaluated as being present or absent, directly from the subjects' opinions in most included articles. The results showed that in 55.55 % to 100 % of the cases, RS decreased after a root coverage procedure. From a clinical point of view, it seems that surgical root coverage procedures may treat RS with more than 50% of success rate. This rate of reduction in symptoms may not be different from that found for topical interventions; however, there are no studies to date directly making this comparison.[40]

A multicenter study[41] with 85 subjects demonstrated the benefit of performing root coverage procedures for reduction of RS. At the baseline, approximately 40% of the

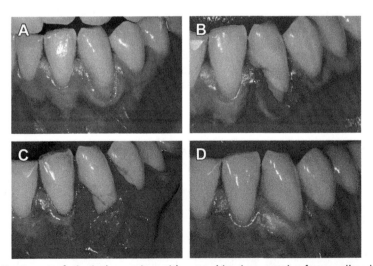

Fig. 5. Treatment of gingival recession with a combined approach of coronally advanced flap and subepithelial connective tissue graft. (A) An unaesthetic gingival recession site on tooth #22 is possibly due to excessive brushing and labial positioning. Note the potential for the frenum attachment to contribute to future complications. (B) A recipient bed was prepared. (C) A connective graft was harvested and transferred to the recipient site. (D) Six months after the surgery, the root was covered.

subjects reported RS as a reason for seeking treatment. At 6 months after randomly treating with CAF or CAF + SCTG, the prevalence of RS reduced to approximately 10%. However, a systematic review[39] found conflicting evidences for surgical root coverage procedures to reduce RS, reflecting the limited evidence confounded by the subjective nature of patients' perceptions of RS along with extent of the defect and treatment variabilities in obtaining the complete coverage needed for resolution.[42,43]

Active Recession (Progression)

A progressive lesion may warrant a surgical intervention to improve periodontal support by increasing the amount of soft-tissue attachment and to halt disease progression (**Fig. 6**).[44] A longitudinal study[45] showed that sites with recession had a higher risk of additional recession. A split-mouth design study[15] following 73 subjects for 10 to 27 years found that teeth with gingival recession receiving a free gingival graft had a reduction of gingival recession by approximately 1.5 mm. The contralateral homogenous sites not receiving surgical treatment experienced an increase in the recession by 0.7 to 1.0 mm during the same time frame. The clinical ramifications on tooth loss or patient-centered outcomes for this difference were not determined.

Restorative or Orthodontic Needs

Teeth with gingival recession may be at a higher risk of developing further recession when receiving a restoration with the potential to compromise the gingival tissues.[46,47] Valderhaug and Birkeland[48] evaluated 329 crowns, most of which (59%) were placed subgingivally at the beginning of the study. After 5 years, only 32% of the crown margins remained below the gingival margin, suggesting that almost half of the teeth developed recession, with more attachment loss associated with subgingival restorations. Similarly, studies[49,50] comparing periodontal conditions between abutment and nonabutment teeth of removable partial dentures concluded that significantly more plaque accumulation and inflammation, deeper probing depths, and more recession were associated with abutment teeth.

It has been discussed in an earlier section that orthodontic treatment may present a risk factor for gingival recession, although it may affect only 10% to 20% of patients. Therefore, patients with orthodontic or restorative needs should be closely monitored for signs of recession and may be suggested of surgical intervention, if indicated, especially for those with presence of other risk factors, for example, thin tissue type.

TREATMENT GOALS

There are generally 2 goals for performing a surgery, and depending on the goals an appropriate procedure is chosen: (1) augment soft tissues coronal to the gingival

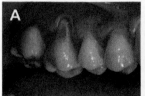 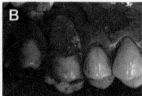 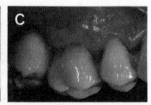

Fig. 6. Treatment of an active or progressing gingival recession site. (*A*) A decision was made to perform a coronally advanced flap and subepithelial connective tissue graft on tooth #3. (*B*) The graft was secured in place. (*C*) Results 2 years after the surgery showed a reversal of the gingival recession.

margin (root coverage) and (2) augment soft tissues apical to the gingival margin, that is, provide a qualitative change to the existing soft tissues. A root coverage procedure is preferred, especially if the patient's main concern is the recession itself. However, there are some limitations with which one may not be able to achieve root coverage or the outcome is not predictable, for example, Miller class 3 and 4 recessions.[34] Although the second goal does not attempt to reduce the amount of recession, it could increase the thickness and width of the attached mucosa, preventing further recession. Many surgical procedures have been developed over the years to reach these goals. Because these procedures are not the focus of this article, only a brief summary of the commonly performed procedures are included in **Table 3**.[51,52]

TREATMENT OUTCOMES OF VARIOUS SURGICAL PROCEDURES

The effectiveness of various surgical procedures for correcting Miller class I or II recessions have been investigated in a few systematic reviews.[43,52–56] The mean percentage of root coverage ranges widely from 50% to 97.3%. The CAF + SCTG is considered the gold standard for root coverage, which achieves approximately 80% root coverage. There is some evidence to suggest that the application of biologics, for example, EMD or PDGF, may promote tissue regeneration and increase the prevalence of complete coverage; however, definitive studies remain to be done.[43,57] For augmenting soft tissues apical to gingival margin, free gingival graft (FGG) is still considered the gold standard for increasing the amount of KM.[44] The second-generation (allografts/xenografts) (**Fig. 7**)

Table 3
Modalities of treating a gingival recession

Modality	Root Coverage	Augment Keratinized Tissue
Goals	Augment soft tissues coronal to the gingival margin	Provide qualitative changes to the soft tissues apical to the gingival margin
Purposes	• Root coverage • Increase tissue thickness • Increase keratinized tissue width	• Increase tissue thickness • Increase keratinized tissue width
Predictability	• Miller class I and II: favorable • Miller class III and IV: less to unfavorable	More predictable than root coverage procedures
Available procedures	• Pedicle flaps (CAF, lateral sliding flap) • CAF + SCTG • CAF + allografts/xenografts • CAF + biologics • Tissue engineering	• FGG • Allografts/xenografts • Tissue engineering

Determining factors	• Systemic factors: smoking
	• Surgeon experience
	• Local factors:
	  ○ Oral hygiene
	  ○ Interproximal soft/hard tissue
	  ○ Flap thickness
	  ○ Flap tension
	  ○ Amount of recession
		• Systemic factors: smoking
		• Surgeon experience
		• Local factors:
		  ○ Oral hygiene
		  ○ Graft thickness
		  ○ Graft stability

Data from Tatakis DN, Chambrone L, Allen EP, et al. Periodontal soft tissue root coverage procedures: a consensus report from the AAP regeneration workshop. J Periodontol 2015;86(2 Suppl):S52–5; and Oates TW, Robinson M, Gunsolley JC. Surgical therapies for the treatment of gingival recession. A systematic review. Ann Periodontol 2003;8(1):303–20.

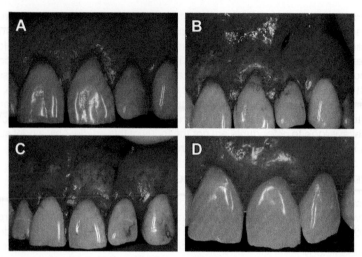

Fig. 7. Demonstration of a root coverage procedure with an allograft. (*A*) Gingival recession was found on teeth #8 and #9. (*B*) A coronally advanced flap was planned. (*C*) An allograft was placed on #9. (*D*) Results after 12 months showed satisfactory root coverage. (*Courtesy of* Prof H-L Wang, DDS, MSD, PhD, Director of Graduate Periodontics Program, University of Michigan, Ann Arbor, MI.)

and third-generation (tissue-engineering) procedures eliminate the need of harvesting autogenous tissues and show promising outcomes.

Regarding patient morbidity, it was reported that more than half of the subjects experienced interference of daily life activities from these surgical procedures.[41] Approximately 25% to 35% of subjects reported some pain after the surgery for about 1 to 2 days, which prompted the use of some pain medications. Therefore, the benefits of receiving a surgery should be weighed carefully with the limited understanding of risks for progression, costs, and possible morbidities.

SUMMARY AND FINAL REMARKS

Given the high prevalence of gingival recession, and the therapeutic potential to successfully manage this condition, it is critical that we continue to improve our understanding of the cause, prognosis, and treatment of this condition to assure that we continue to provide the best, evidence-based care possible. This review of predisposing and precipitating factors discusses common perceptions regarding these factors leading to the development of gingival recession. However, this review also represents how little is truly known in this regard. The most recent and thorough evaluations of the evidence fail to clarify the role of toothbrushing, frenum attachment, and orthodontic movement in the progression of gingival recession. Furthermore, there is little evidence regarding the effectiveness of common treatments to prevent gingival recession relative to patient-centered outcomes.

Although much remains to be known, it is clear that surgical interventions can successfully reduce recession. It is also clear that a small percentage of sites clearly benefit from these interventions. What is less clear is the benefit of the broad application of these interventions in sites with recession. Findings from several studies have suggested limited benefits from surgical interventions. Pini Prato (2000)[58] found only 2 of 8 nontreated buccally erupting premolar sites to show 1 mm of gingival recession after 2 years, suggesting progression, even minor amounts, is not easily predicted in the absence of treatment. The benefits may also be in question relative to the amount of recession that may occur in the absence of treatment. After 10 to 27 years, although 34 of 55 untreated sites showed some recession, the amounts of recession recorded after this extended period averaged 0.7 mm and ranged between 0 and 2 mm.[15]

As one looks toward the continued development of evidence-based care, one needs to look for new information to clarify these many unanswered questions but must always look to offer the best treatment options available to patients based on what is known at that time within the context of the limitations in our knowledge. Understanding the cause, prognosis, and treatment of gingival recession continues to offer many unanswered questions and challenges in periodontics as we strive to provide the best care possible for our patients.

REFERENCES

1. Peridontology AAP. Glossary of periodontal terms. Chicago (IL): The American Academy of Periodontology; 2001.
2. Albandar JM, Kingman A. Gingival recession, gingival bleeding, and dental calculus in adults 30 years of age and older in the United States, 1988-1994. J Periodontol 1999;70(1):30–43.
3. Kassab MM, Cohen RE. The etiology and prevalence of gingival recession. J Am Dent Assoc 2003;134(2):220–5.
4. Sarfati A, Bourgeois D, Katsahian S, et al. Risk assessment for buccal gingival recession defects in an adult population. J Periodontol 2010;81(10):1419–25.
5. Gorman WJ. Prevalence and etiology of gingival recession. J Periodontol 1967; 38(4):316–22.
6. American Dental Association. 2005-06 Survey of Dental Services Rendered. Chicago, IL; 2007.
7. Bernimoulin J, Curilovie Z. Gingival recession and tooth mobility. J Clin Periodontol 1977;4(2):107–14.
8. Fu JH, Yeh CY, Chan HL, et al. Tissue biotype and its relation to the underlying bone morphology. J Periodontol 2010;81(4):569–74.
9. Anderegg CR, Metzler DG, Nicoll BK. Gingiva thickness in guided tissue regeneration and associated recession at facial furcation defects. J Periodontol 1995; 66(5):397–402.
10. Claffey N, Shanley D. Relationship of gingival thickness and bleeding to loss of probing attachment in shallow sites following nonsurgical periodontal therapy. J Clin Periodontol 1986;13(7):654–7.
11. Lafzi A, Abolfazli N, Eskandari A. Assessment of the etiologic factors of gingival recession in a group of patients in northwest Iran. J Dent Res Dent Clin Dent Prospects 2009;3(3):90–3.
12. Nguyen-Hieu T, Ha Thi BD, Do Thu H, et al. Gingival recession associated with predisposing factors in young Vietnamese: a pilot study. Oral Health Dent Manag 2012;11(3):134–44.
13. Lang NP, Loe H. The relationship between the width of keratinized gingiva and gingival health. J Periodontol 1972;43(10):623–7.
14. Kennedy JE, Bird WC, Palcanis KG, et al. A longitudinal evaluation of varying widths of attached gingiva. J Clin Periodontol 1985;12(8):667–75.
15. Agudio G, Nieri M, Rotundo R, et al. Periodontal conditions of sites treated with gingival-augmentation surgery compared to untreated contralateral

homologous sites: a 10- to 27-year long-term study. J Periodontol 2009;80(9): 1399–405.

16. Addy M, Mostafa P, Newcombe RG. Dentine hypersensitivity: the distribution of recession, sensitivity and plaque. J Dent 1987;15(6):242–8.

17. Niemi ML, Sandholm L, Ainamo J. Frequency of gingival lesions after standardized brushing as related to stiffness of toothbrush and abrasiveness of dentifrice. J Clin Periodontol 1984;11(4):254–61.

18. Rajapakse PS, McCracken GI, Gwynnett E, et al. Does tooth brushing influence the development and progression of non-inflammatory gingival recession? A systematic review. J Clin Periodontol 2007;34(12):1046–61.

19. Campbell A, Moore A, Williams E, et al. Tongue piercing: impact of time and barbell stem length on lingual gingival recession and tooth chipping. J Periodontol 2002;73(3):289–97.

20. Robertson PB, Walsh M, Greene J, et al. Periodontal effects associated with the use of smokeless tobacco. J Periodontol 1990;61(7):438–43.

21. Wennstrom JL, Lindhe J, Sinclair F, et al. Some periodontal tissue reactions to orthodontic tooth movement in monkeys. J Clin Periodontol 1987;14(3):121–9.

22. Slutzkey S, Levin L. Gingival recession in young adults: occurrence, severity, and relationship to past orthodontic treatment and oral piercing. Am J Orthod Dentofacial Orthop 2008;134(5):652–6.

23. Renkema AM, Fudalej PS, Renkema A, et al. Gingival recessions and the change of inclination of mandibular incisors during orthodontic treatment. Eur J Orthod 2013;35(2):249–55.

24. Aziz T, Flores-Mir C. A systematic review of the association between appliance-induced labial movement of mandibular incisors and gingival recession. Aust Orthod J 2011;27(1):33–9.

25. Vasconcelos G, Kjellsen K, Preus H, et al. Prevalence and severity of vestibular recession in mandibular incisors after orthodontic treatment. Angle Orthod 2012;82(1):42–7.

26. Renkema AM, Fudalej PS, Renkema AA, et al. Gingival labial recessions in orthodontically treated and untreated individuals: a case-control study. J Clin Periodontol 2013;40(6):631–7.

27. Joss-Vassalli I, Grebenstein C, Topouzelis N, et al. Orthodontic therapy and gingival recession: a systematic review. Orthod Craniofac Res 2010;13(3):127–41.

28. Kloukos D, Eliades T, Sculean A, et al. Indication and timing of soft tissue augmentation at maxillary and mandibular incisors in orthodontic patients. A systematic review. Eur J Orthod 2014;36(4):442–9.

29. Lindhe J, Nyman S, Karring T. Scaling and root planning in shallow pockets. J Clin Periodontol 1982;9(5):415–8.

30. Beck JD, Koch GG. Characteristics of older adults experiencing periodontal attachment loss as gingival recession or probing depth. J Periodontal Res 1994;29(4):290–8.

31. Baker DL, Seymour GJ. The possible pathogenesis of gingival recession. A histological study of induced recession in the rat. J Clin Periodontol 1976;3(4): 208–19.

32. Smukler H, Landsberg J. The toothbrush and gingival traumatic injury. J Periodontol 1984;55(12):713–9.

33. Baker P, Spedding C. The aetiology of gingival recession. Dent Update 2002; 29(2):59–62.

34. Miller PD Jr. A classification of marginal tissue recession. Int J Periodontics Restorative Dent 1985;5(2):8–13.

35. Zaher CA, Hachem J, Puhan MA, et al. Interest in periodontology and preferences for treatment of localized gingival recessions. J Clin Periodontol 2005; 32(4):375–82.
36. Nieri M, Pini Prato GP, Giani M, et al. Patient perceptions of buccal gingival recessions and requests for treatment. J Clin Periodontol 2013;40(7):707–12.
37. Tjan AH, Miller GD, The JG. Some esthetic factors in a smile. J Prosthet Dent 1984;51(1):24–8.
38. West NX. Dentine hypersensitivity: preventive and therapeutic approaches to treatment. Periodontol 2000 2008;48:31–41.
39. Douglas de Oliveira DW, Oliveira-Ferreira F, Flecha OD, et al. Is surgical root coverage effective for the treatment of cervical dentin hypersensitivity? A systematic review. J Periodontol 2013;84(3):295–306.
40. Acharya AB, Surve SM, Thakur SL. A clinical study of the effect of calcium sodium phosphosilicate on dentin hypersensitivity. J Clin Exp Dent 2013;5(1): e18–22.
41. Cortellini P, Tonetti M, Baldi C, et al. Does placement of a connective tissue graft improve the outcomes of coronally advanced flap for coverage of single gingival recessions in upper anterior teeth? A multi-centre, randomized, double-blind, clinical trial. J Clin Periodontol 2009;36(1):68–79.
42. Clauser C, Nieri M, Franceschi D, et al. Evidence-based mucogingival therapy. Part 2: Ordinary and individual patient data meta-analyses of surgical treatment of recession using complete root coverage as the outcome variable. J Periodontol 2003;74(5):741–56.
43. Cairo F, Pagliaro U, Nieri M. Treatment of gingival recession with coronally advanced flap procedures: a systematic review. J Clin Periodontol 2008;35(8 Suppl):136–62.
44. Greenwell H, Fiorellini J, Giannobile W, et al. Oral reconstructive and corrective considerations in periodontal therapy. J Periodontol 2005;76(9):1588–600.
45. Serino G, Wennstrom JL, Lindhe J, et al. The prevalence and distribution of gingival recession in subjects with a high standard of oral hygiene. J Clin Periodontol 1994;21(1):57–63.
46. Waerhaug J. Healing of the dento-epithelial junction following subgingival plaque control. I. As observed in human biopsy material. J Periodontol 1978;49(1):1–8.
47. Silness J. Fixed prosthodontics and periodontal health. Dent Clin North Am 1980; 24(2):317–29.
48. Valderhaug J, Birkeland JM. Periodontal conditions in patients 5 years following insertion of fixed prostheses. Pocket depth and loss of attachment. J Oral Rehabil 1976;3(3):237–43.
49. Zlataric DK, Celebic A, Valentic-Peruzovic M. The effect of removable partial dentures on periodontal health of abutment and non-abutment teeth. J Periodontol 2002;73(2):137–44.
50. Wright PS, Hellyer PH. Gingival recession related to removable partial dentures in older patients. J Prosthet Dent 1995;74(6):602–7.
51. Tatakis DN, Chambrone L, Allen EP, et al. Periodontal soft tissue root coverage procedures: a consensus report from the AAP regeneration workshop. J Periodontol 2015;86(2 Suppl):S52–5.
52. Oates TW, Robinson M, Gunsolley JC. Surgical therapies for the treatment of gingival recession. A systematic review. Ann Periodontol 2003;8(1):303–20.
53. Roccuzzo M, Bunino M, Needleman I, et al. Periodontal plastic surgery for treatment of localized gingival recessions: a systematic review. J Clin Periodontol 2002;29(Suppl 3):178–94 [discussion: 95–6].

54. Chambrone L, Sukekava F, Araujo MG, et al. Root-coverage procedures for the treatment of localized recession-type defects: a Cochrane systematic review. J Periodontol 2010;81(4):452–78.
55. Thoma DS, Benic GI, Zwahlen M, et al. A systematic review assessing soft tissue augmentation techniques. Clin Oral Implants Res 2009;20(Suppl 4):146–65.
56. Chambrone L, Tatakis DN. Periodontal soft tissue root coverage procedures: a systematic review from the AAP Regeneration Workshop. J Periodontol 2015; 86(2 Suppl):S8–51.
57. McGuire MK, Scheyer ET, Schupbach P. Growth factor-mediated treatment of recession defects: a randomized controlled trial and histologic and microcomputed tomography examination. J Periodontol 2009;80(4):550–64.
58. Pini Prato G, Bacetti T, Magnani C, et al. Mucogingival interceptive surgery of buccally-erupted premolars in patients scheduled for orthodontic treatment. I. A 7-year longitudinal study. J Perio 2000;71(2):172–1781.

Index

Note: Page numbers of article titles are in **boldface** type.

Dent Clin N Am 59 (2015) 997–1002
http://dx.doi.org/10.1016/S0011-8532(15)00105-6
0011-8532/15/$ – see front matter © 2015 Elsevier Inc. All rights reserved.

dental.theclinics.com

United States Postal Service

Statement of Ownership, Management, and Circulation
(All Periodicals Publications Except Requestor Publications)

1. Publication Title	2. Publication Number	3. Filing Date
Dental Clinics of North America	5 6 6 - 4 8 0	9/18/15

4. Issue Frequency	5. Number of Issues Published Annually	6. Annual Subscription Price
Jan, Apr, Jul, Oct	4	$280.00

7. Complete Mailing Address of Known Office of Publication (Not printer) (Street, city, county, state, and ZIP+4®)

Elsevier Inc.
360 Park Avenue South
New York, NY 10010-1710

Contact Person
Stephen R. Bushing
Telephone (Include area code)
215-239-3688

8. Complete Mailing Address of Headquarters or General Business Office of Publisher (Not printer)

Elsevier Inc._360 Park Avenue South, New York, NY 10010-1710

9. Full Names and Complete Mailing Addresses of Publisher, Editor, and Managing Editor (Do not leave blank)

Publisher (Name and complete mailing address)

Linda Belfus, Elsevier Inc., 1600 John F. Kennedy Blvd., Suite 1800, Philadelphia, PA 19103

Editor (Name and complete mailing address)

John Vassallo, Elsevier Inc., 1600 John F. Kennedy Blvd., Suite 1800, Philadelphia, PA 19103-2899

Managing Editor (Name and complete mailing address)

Adrianne Brigido, Elsevier Inc., 1600 John F. Kennedy Blvd., Suite 1800, Philadelphia, PA 19103-2899

10. Owner (Do not leave blank. If the publication is owned by a corporation, give the name and address of the corporation immediately followed by the names and addresses of all stockholders owning or holding 1 percent or more of the total amount of stock. If not owned by a corporation, give the names and addresses of the individual owners. If owned by a partnership or other unincorporated firm, give its name and address as well as those of each individual owner. If the publication is published by a nonprofit organization, give its name and address.)

Full Name	Complete Mailing Address
Wholly owned subsidiary of	1600 John F. Kennedy Blvd. Ste. 1800
Reed/Elsevier, US holdings	Philadelphia, PA 19103-2899

11. Known Bondholders, Mortgagees, and Other Security Holders Owning or Holding 1 Percent or More of Total Amount of Bonds, Mortgages, or Other Securities. If none, check box. ☐ None

Full Name	Complete Mailing Address
N/A	

12. Tax Status (For completion by nonprofit organizations authorized to mail at nonprofit rates) (Check one)
The purpose, function, and nonprofit status of this organization and the exempt status for federal income tax purposes:
☐ Has Not Changed During Preceding 12 Months
☐ Has Changed During Preceding 12 Months (Publisher must submit explanation of change with this statement)

PS Form 3526, July 2014 (Page 1 of 3 (Instructions Page 3)) PSN 7530-01-000-9931 PRIVACY NOTICE: See our Privacy policy in www.usps.com

---

13. Publication Title		14. Issue Date for Circulation Data Below
Dental Clinics of North America		July 2015

15. Extent and Nature of Circulation			Average No. Copies Each Issue During Preceding 12 Months	No. Copies of Single Issue Published Nearest to Filing Date
a. Total Number of Copies (Net press run)			900	750
b. Legitimate Paid and/Or Requested Distribution (By Mail and Outside the Mail)	(1)	Mailed Outside-County Paid/Requested Mail Subscriptions stated on PS Form 3541. (Include paid distribution above nominal rate, advertiser's proof copies and exchange copies)	354	260
	(2)	Mailed In-County Paid/Requested Mail Subscriptions stated on PS Form 3541. (Include paid distribution above nominal rate, advertiser's proof copies and exchange copies)		
	(3)	Paid Distribution Outside the Mails Including Sales Through Dealers And Carriers, Street Vendors, Counter Sales, and Other Paid Distribution Outside USPS®	191	243
	(4)	Paid Distribution by Other Classes of Mail Through the USPS (e.g. First-Class Mail®)		
c. Total Paid or Requested Circulation (Sum of 15a (1), (2), (3), and (4))			545	503
d. Free or Nominal Rate Distribution (By Mail and Outside the Mail)	(1)	Free or Nominal Rate Outside-County Copies included on PS Form 3541	58	61
	(2)	Free or Nominal Rate In-County Copies included on PS Form 3541		
	(3)	Free or Nominal Rate Copies mailed at Other classes Through the USPS (e.g. First-Class Mail®)		
	(4)	Free or Nominal Rate Distribution Outside the Mail (Carriers or Other means)		
e. Total Nonrequested Distribution (Sum of 15d (1), (2), (3) and (4)			58	61
f. Total Distribution (Sum of 15c and 15e)			603	564
g. Copies not Distributed (See instructions to publishers #4 (page #3))			297	186
h. Total (Sum of 15f and g)			900	750
i. Percent Paid and/or Requested Circulation (15c divided by 15f times 100)			90.38%	89.18%

* If you are claiming electronic copies go to line 16 on page 3. If you are not claiming Electronic copies, skip to line 17 on page 3

16. Electronic Copy Circulation	Average No. Copies Each Issue During Preceding 12 Months	No. Copies of Single Issue Published Nearest to Filing Date
a. Paid Electronic Copies		
b. Total paid Print Copies (Line 15c) + Paid Electronic copies (Line 16a)		
c. Total Print Distribution (Line 15f) + Paid Electronic Copies (Line 16a)		
d. Percent Paid (Both Print & Electronic copies) (16b divided by 16c X 100)		

I certify that 50% of all my distributed copies (electronic and print) are paid above a nominal price

17. Publication of Statement of Ownership
If the publication is a general publication, publication of this statement is required. Will be printed in the _October 2015_ issue of this publication.

18. Signature and Title of Editor, Publisher, Business Manager, or Owner

Stephen R. Bushing – Inventory Distribution Coordinator

Stephen R. Bushing – Inventory Distribution Coordinator

Date: September 18, 2015

I certify that all information furnished on this form is true and complete. I understand that anyone who furnishes false or misleading information on this form or who omits material or information requested on the form may be subject to criminal sanctions (including fines and imprisonment) and/or civil sanctions (including civil penalties).

PS Form 3526, July 2014 (Page 3 of 3)

Moving?

Make sure your subscription moves with you!

To notify us of your new address, find your **Clinics Account Number** (located on your mailing label above your name), and contact customer service at:

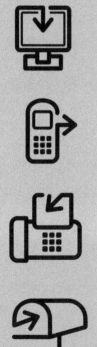

Email: journalscustomerservice-usa@elsevier.com

800-654-2452 (subscribers in the U.S. & Canada)
314-447-8871 (subscribers outside of the U.S. & Canada)

Fax number: 314-447-8029

Elsevier Health Sciences Division
Subscription Customer Service
3251 Riverport Lane
Maryland Heights, MO 63043

*To ensure uninterrupted delivery of your subscription, please notify us at least 4 weeks in advance of move.

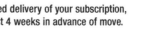

Moving?